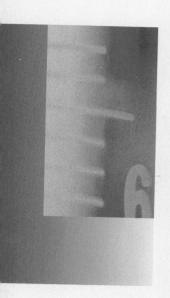

Calculation *of* Medication Dosages

Practical Strategies to Ensure Safety and Accuracy

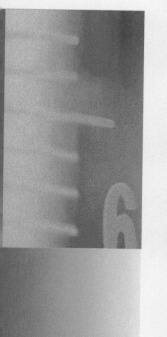

Calculation *of* Medication Dosages

Practical Strategies to Ensure Safety and Accuracy

Janice F. Boundy, PhD, RN
Professor and Associate Dean, Graduate Program
Saint Francis Medical Center College of Nursing
Peoria, Illinois

Patricia A. Stockert, PhD, RN
Professor and Associate Dean, Undergraduate Program
Saint Francis Medical Center College of Nursing
Peoria, Illinois

Wolters Kluwer | Lippincott Williams & Wilkins
Health

Philadelphia · Baltimore · New York · London
Buenos Aires · Hong Kong · Sydney · Tokyo

Senior Acquisitions Editor: Hilarie Surrena
Managing Editor: Betsy Gentzler
Production Project Manager: Cynthia Rudy
Director of Nursing Production: Helen Ewan
Senior Managing Editor/Production: Erika Kors
Art Director: Joan Wendt
Manufacturing Coordinator: Karin Duffield
Production Services/Compositor: TechBooks
Printer: R.R. Donnelley–Willard

9 8 7 6 5 4 3 2 1

Library of Congress Cataloging-in-Publication Data

Boundy, Janice F.
    Calculation of medication dosages : practical strategies to ensure
    safety and accuracy / Janice F. Boundy, Patricia A. Stockert.
        p. ; cm.
    Includes index.
    ISBN-13: 978-0-7817-5854-3
    ISBN-10: 0-7817-5854-8
    1. Pharmaceutical arithmetic. I. Stockert, Patricia A. II. Title.
    [DNLM: 1. Nursing Care--methods--Programmed Instruction.
  2. Pharmaceutical Preparations--administration & dosage—
Programmed Instruction. 3. Algorithms—Programmed Instruction.
  WY 18.2 B765c 2008]
  RS57.B68 2008
  615′.1401513—dc22

                                                                                    2006028270

Reviewers

Celeste Baldwin, PhD, RN, CNS
Director of Nursing
The University of Toledo
Toledo, Ohio

Rita Bergevin, MA, RN, BC
Clinical Assistant Professor
Binghamton University, Decker School of Nursing
Binghamton, New York

Sally Hill Boyster, MS, RNC
Professor of Nursing
Rose State College
Midwest City, Oklahoma

Pat Bradley, MEd, MS, RN
Nursing Faculty
Grossmont College
El Cajon, California

Sandra Cole, BSN, MSN
Nursing Instructor
Delaware Technical & Community College
Georgetown, Delaware

Laura Cralle, MSN, RN, GNP-BC
Associate Professor
Odessa College
Midland, Texas

Gina Doyle
Practical Nursing Coordinator/Instructor
Mid-America Technology Center
Wayne, Oklahoma

Karen Driol, MS, BSN, RN
Faculty
British Columbia Institute of Technology,
    School of Nursing
Burnaby, British Columbia, Canada

Laurie Fontenot, RN-C
Department Head
Louisiana Technical College, T. H. Harris Campus
Opelousas, Louisiana

Irene Henderson, EdD, RN
Chairperson, Department of Nursing
University of Arkansas at Pine Bluff
Pine Bluff, Arkansas

Marie Hess, EdD, RN
Professor of Nursing
Jefferson Community College
Watertown, New York

Susan Holmes, MSN, CNS, TFNP
Instructor
Auburn University, School of Nursing
Auburn, Alabama

Cheryl Karl, MSN, RN, MA
Assistant Professor of Nursing
Anne Arundel Community College
Arnold, Maryland

Richard Keller, MSN, BA, ASN, LNC
Nursing Faculty
Drexel University
Philadelphia, Pennsylvania

Gail Kost, MSN, RN
Clinical Lecturer
Indiana University
Indianapolis, Indiana

Ramona Lazenby, EdD, CRNP
Assistant Professor of Nursing
Auburn University, Montgomery School of Nursing
Montgomery, Alabama

Laura Lenau, MS, RN
Learning Resources Coordinator, Nursing Department
Salish Kootenai College
Pablo, Montana

Linda McIntosh Liptok, MSN, RN, BMus, APRN-BC
Assistant Professor
Kent State University, Tuscarawas
New Philadelphia, Ohio

Dorothy Mathers, MSN, RN
Associate Professor
Pennsylvania College of Technology
Williamsport, Pennsylvania

Kim McCarron, MS, RN
Clinical Assistant Professor
Towson University
Towson, Maryland

Teresa Moore, BS, PharmD
Nursing Pharmacology Instructor
Albany State University
Albany, Georgia

Bonnie Nelson, MSN, RN
Director, Instructional Services
Medical College of Ohio
Toledo, Ohio

Eva Ann Pihlgren, BSN, MN
Professor of Nursing
Antelope Valley College
Lancaster, California

Rhonda Sansone, MSN, RN
Assistant Professor of Nursing
Community College of Allegheny County, North Campus
Pittsburgh, Pennsylvania

Gwen Scarborough
Assistant Professor of Nursing
University of Tennessee at Martin
Martin, Tennessee

Heather Scarlett-Ferguson, BSP, MDE
Instructor
Grant MacEwan College, Psychiatric Nursing Program
Ponoka, Alberta, Canada

Rosalena Thorpe, PhD, RN
Department Chairperson and Professor
Community College of Allegheny County
Pittsburgh, Pennsylvania

Maureen Tremel, MSN, ARNP
Nursing Professor
Seminole Community College
Sanford, Florida

Michelle Walker, MS, RN
Assistant Professor of Nursing
Norwich University
Northfield, Vermont

Kathy Wheeler, MSN, ARNP
Director, Health Science Programs
Chipola College
Marianna, Florida

Rosemary Wittstadt, EdD, RN
Howard Community College
Columbia, Maryland

Peggy Wyatt, BSN, MSN, RN
Nursing Instructor
British Columbia Institute of Technology
Burnaby, British Columbia, Canada

Preface

Calculation of Medication Dosages: Practical Strategies to Ensure Safety and Accuracy is a new comprehensive medication dosage calculation textbook. It was written for nursing students or other healthcare workers as a reference or review of mathematics and dosage calculations for medication administration. It is intended to be used as a primary textbook in a nursing or other healthcare course, such as "Math for Meds," as a review for nursing students who must meet pre-entrance requirements, or as a supplemental textbook in beginning nursing courses. It provides the fundamental knowledge, concepts, and methods for dosage calculation that all nursing students need for accurate and safe medication administration and for preparing to take the NCLEX-RN.

With a presentation that is inviting and non-threatening to readers, the text approaches dosage calculation in a practical, easy-to-understand way. The chapters integrate critical thinking and decision making into the process of dosage calculation. A nurse–client scenario is woven throughout each chapter to create a "real-world" link between the theory presented and the practice setting. Using the developing case scenario, the text walks readers through the decision-making process of dosage calculation and medication administration. A simple 3-step method—Convert, Compute, and Critically Think—is used to calculate medication dosages.

Content proceeds from simple to complex, with each chapter building on previously-learned information. The text begins with a review of mathematics and an explanation of drug prescriptions and drug labels. Calculation of oral and parenteral medications is then presented, and complex information related to calculation of intravenous solution drip rates, critical care drugs, and pediatric drugs appears at the end of the book.

To better prepare students for nursing practice, the text focuses on application of the information learned. Each chapter concentrates on a different medication type and shows how to calculate medication dosages using the formula or rule method first. Examples and practice problems follow. The second part of each chapter demonstrates dosage calculation using the ratio-proportion method, and provides practice problems for using this method as well. Each chapter also contains a section that focuses on critical thinking

and decision making related to calculations. The final section of each chapter is a practice exam that requires using both methods of dosage calculation to solve problems. At the end of the book, a comprehensive examination covers all the material in the text.

CHAPTER OVERVIEW

Chapter 1, Mathematics Review, provides readers with a review of basic arithmetic. **Chapter 2, Systems of Measurement,** covers the metric, apothecary, and household systems of measurement. Readers will learn the conversion equivalents for each of the measurement systems, along with how to apply each equivalent appropriately and accurately. **Chapter 3, Preparing Equipment and Drugs for Administration,** discusses how to select the correct type of measuring device for oral medications. Additional topics include measuring prescribed liquid medications correctly, selecting the correct syringe for parenteral medications, and measuring prescribed medications correctly in the syringe. **Chapter 4, Drug Orders,** provides information on interpreting prescribed orders for medication, including the key elements of a drug order and standard and accepted abbreviations. **Chapter 5, Medication Labels and Packaging Systems,** covers information nurses need to correctly read a medication label. Information on how medications are supplied and the difference between unit-dose and multi-dose packaging systems are discussed. **Chapter 6, Strategies for Drug Calculation,** teaches a simple 3-step approach—Convert, Compute, and Critically Think—to correctly calculate medication dosages. The formula or rule method and the ratio-proportion method are introduced as ways to set up a dosage calculation. The Six Rights of Medication Administration are also discussed. **Chapter 7, Calculation of Oral Medications,** incorporates the 3-step approach to dosage calculations for oral medications. Calculation of dosages of capsules and tablets, using both the formula and the ratio-proportion methods, is covered. **Chapter 8, Calculation of Parenteral Medications,** uses the 3-step approach to dosage calculations for parenteral medications.

The different parenteral routes are defined and discussed. **Chapter 9, Calculation of Intravenous Rates,** provides information on selection of the correct IV solution and equipment, based on the physician's order. Identification of the drop calibration factor is discussed. Formulas for calculating the amount of solute in intravenous solutions, mL/hour flow rate, and gtt/min are presented. **Chapter 10, Advanced Intravenous Calculations,** gives readers the information needed to safely calculate the dosages and infusion rates of medications ordered in units/hour, mg/hour, mcg/kg/min, mg/min, or mcg/min. **Chapter 11, Pediatric Calculations,** discusses how to safely calculate medication dosages for pediatric patients when the dosage prescribed is based on weight. Safety issues related to dosage calculations for pediatric patients are covered. Finally, the **Appendix** covers calculation of medications using dimensional analysis.

SPECIAL TEXT FEATURES

- **Case Studies.** Each chapter opens with a clinical case study that presents dosage calculation process and content. The case is developed throughout the chapter to highlight key content.
- **Practice Problems.** Plentiful practice problems are interspersed throughout each chapter after each method is presented. These problems give readers the opportunity to immediately apply chapter content, thus increasing the speed at which it is learned.
- **Chapter Review Problems.** Each chapter concludes with review problems that ask readers to demonstrate the skills they learned in that chapter. Problems using both calculation methods are offered.
- **Answers.** Answers to the practice problems and chapter review problems show the problem set up and the steps in solving the problem. This approach promotes learning by allowing readers to analyze the problems and by providing feedback for detection of errors.
- **Safety Alerts.** The Safety Alert feature is incorporated throughout all the chapters. It focuses the readers on key points or concepts that they need to remember to calculate dosages accurately. Information on how to avoid making common errors is also provided.
- **Critical Thinking/Decision Making Exercises.** Critical Thinking/Decision Making Exercises appear at the end of each chapter. These exercises walk the readers through a medication set-up and dosage calculation scenario, guiding them in recognizing potential problems or errors and in correcting the situation. This section gives the readers an opportunity to analyze a client scenario, and then apply their knowledge to correct the situation so that dosage calculation is performed accurately and medications are administered safely.
- **Illustrations.** Illustrations of solutions, tablets, syringes, injectables, and drug labels appear extensively throughout the text, assisting readers to envision a clinically realistic situation when considering dosages to be calculated.
- **Key Terms.** Key words or concepts are highlighted in bold print in the text.
- **Glossary.** A glossary at the end of the text contains key words, concepts, and definitions.
- **Comprehensive Practice Test.** A comprehensive test at the end of the book gives readers additional practice in applying both methods to calculate medication orders.
- **Pocket Card.** A pocket card with common measurements and conversions, along with the basic and advanced dosage calculation formulas from the text, is included. The card is designed so that readers can carry it with them and refer to it as needed while on their clinical units.

ANCILLARY PACKAGE

- **Student Resource CD-ROM.** Found in the front of the textbook, this free CD-ROM includes dosage calculation quizzes, an NCLEX Alternate Item Format tutorial, and videos demonstrating techniques for safe medication administration.
- **thePoint** (http://thePoint.lww.com). This web-based course and content management system provides every resource that instructors and students need in one easy-to-use site. Advanced technology and superior content combine at thePoint to allow instructors to design and deliver on-line and off-line courses, maintain grades and class rosters, and communicate with students. Students can visit thePoint to access supplemental multimedia resources to enhance their learning experience, download content, upload assignments, and join an on-line study group. thePoint . . . where teaching, learning, and technology click!

*thePoint is a trademark of WKHealth.

Contents

CHAPTER 1
Mathematics Review   1

CHAPTER 2
Systems of Measurement   35

CHAPTER 3
Preparing Equipment and Drugs for Administration   49

CHAPTER 4
Drug Orders   73

CHAPTER 5
Medication Labels and Packaging Systems   90

CHAPTER 6
Strategies for Drug Calculation   102

CHAPTER 7
Calculation of Oral Medications   123

CHAPTER 8
Calculation of Parenteral Medications   154

CHAPTER 9
Calculation of Intravenous Rates   188

CHAPTER 10
Advanced Intravenous Calculations   221

CHAPTER 11
Pediatric Calculations   254

Comprehensive Practice Test   287

Answers to Comprehensive Practice Test   293

Appendix: Dimensional Analysis   311

Glossary   315

Index   319

Mathematics Review

This chapter contains content on:

- **Conversion of Arabic Numbers to Roman Numerals**
- **Fractions**
- **Decimals**
- **Ratio and Proportion**

Learning Objectives

Upon completion of Chapter 1, you will be able to:

- Convert Roman numerals and Arabic numbers
- Reduce fractions to lowest common terms
- Convert mixed numbers to improper fractions
- Convert improper fractions to mixed numbers
- Change fractions to decimals
- Set up a ratio and proportion correctly
- Solve ratio and proportion problems
- Determine value of x in simple ratio proportion equations
- Use addition, subtraction, multiplication, and division with fractions, decimals, percents, and ratios

Key Terms

- Arabic numbers
- Complex fraction
- Decimals
- Denominator
- Fraction
- Improper fraction
- Lowest common terms

- Mixed number
- Numerator
- Proper fraction
- Proportion
- Ratio
- Roman numerals

CASE STUDY

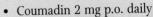

You are the nurse working in a rehabilitation facility. One of your patients is Mr. Boyd who is 60 years old. Mr. Boyd has a history of high blood pressure and five years ago he had a myocardial infarction (MI). After his MI, he developed atrial fibrillation and had a stroke last month. As a result, he has some right-sided weakness and uses a cane when he walks. His current medications include:

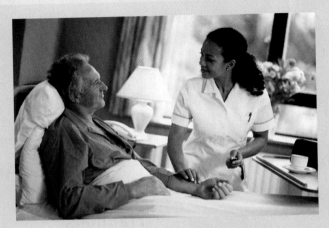

- Coumadin 2 mg p.o. daily
- Digoxin elixir 0.125 mg p.o. daily
- Nitroglycerin transdermal patch 0.4 mg/hour daily to be put on at 0700 and removed at 2100
- Nitroglycerin sublingual tablet 0.3 mg prn as directed for chest pain
- Milk of Magnesia 1/2 ounce daily as needed for constipation

Medication calculations often cause anxiety in nurses. Safe and accurate calculation of medication dosages requires the use of basic arithmetic skills. Careful use of arithmetic knowledge and skills is a way to increase accuracy and safety. Providing nursing care for Mr. Boyd requires you to accurately calculate his dosages of medication using basic math skills. This chapter covers the common skills that are needed to calculate medication dosages. The information presented in this chapter along with other chapters in this book is very important to your success as a nurse!

CONVERSION OF ARABIC NUMBERS TO ROMAN NUMERALS

Medications may be prescribed using both **Arabic numbers** and **Roman numerals**. Arabic numbers are the numbers that you use daily such as 0 to 9. Roman numerals use letters of the alphabet to express numeric values. The most commonly used letters are: I or i (1), V or v (5), and X or x (10). Prescribers often use these numerals when ordering dosages of tablets or capsules. Roman numerals are used in the apothecary system when ordering amounts of medications.

Knowledge of both systems and the ability to change Roman numerals into Arabic numbers is required. Remember the equivalents as shown in the table on p. 3.

Follow these easy, basic rules when converting Roman numerals to Arabic numbers:

- When you have more than one numeral, if the largest valued numeral is on the left and the smallest numeral is on the right, *add* the values.

    Example:
    $$VI = 5 + 1 = 6$$
    $$XII = 10 + 2 = 12$$

- When you have more than one numeral, if the largest valued numeral is on the right and the smallest numeral is on the left, *subtract* the values.

    Example:
    $$IV = 5 - 1 = 4$$
    $$IX = 10 - 1 = 9$$

Equivalents for Roman Numerals and Arabic Numbers

Arabic Number	Roman Numeral
$\frac{1}{2}$	ṡṡ
1	I or i
2	II or ii
3	III or iii
4	IV or iv
5	V or v
6	VI or vi
7	VII or vii
8	VIII or viii
9	IX or ix
10	X or x
20	XX or xx
30	XXX or xxx
50	L
100	C
500	D
1000	M

- Remember that a Roman numeral *will not repeat itself* in sequence more than three times. Once you have a numeral that repeats three times, you must subtract.

Example:

$$3 = \text{III or iii}$$
$$4 = \text{IV or iv} = 5 - 1$$

- When there are three or more numerals and a smaller valued numeral comes between two larger valued numerals, *subtract* the smaller valued numeral from the larger valued numeral that follows it. Then apply the rules of addition for Roman numerals.

Example:

$$\text{XIX} = 10 + (10 - 1) = 19$$
$$\text{XXIV} = 10 + 10 + (5 - 1) = 24$$

⚠ **SAFETY ALERT:** *When using lowercase letters for Roman numerals, a line may be drawn over the letters to identify the letters that are Roman numerals rather than letters in a word or phrase. For lowercase i, dot the i above the line. For example, prescribers may order Tylenol tabs ii.*

PRACTICE PROBLEMS 1-1. Practice Problems for Converting Roman Numerals

DIRECTIONS: Convert the Roman numerals to Arabic numbers. The answers to the problems can be found at the end of the chapter.

1. XXIII _____

2. XLV _____

3. iii ṡṡ _____

4. xvii _____

PRACTICE PROBLEMS 1-2. Practice Problems for Converting Arabic Numbers

DIRECTIONS: Convert the Arabic numbers to Roman numerals. The answers to the problems can be found at the end of the chapter.

1. 33 _____

2. 27 _____

3. 13 _____

4. 6 _____

FRACTIONS

Medications are commonly prescribed and prepared in **fractions**. You need to have an understanding of how to add, subtract, multiply, and divide fractions in order to be able to safely calculate the dosages of these medications. A fraction is a part or piece of the whole that has been divided into equal parts. Fractions are written as $\frac{1}{3}$. The top number is called the **numerator** and the bottom number is the **denominator**. The line between indicates that you can divide the top number by the bottom number to obtain a decimal. For example, $\frac{1}{4}$ can also be written as 0.25, which is what you get by dividing 1 by 4.

For example:

$$\frac{1 \quad \text{Numerator}}{4 \quad \text{Denominator}}$$

Visually, this is shown below.

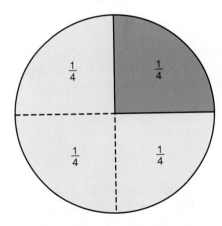

SAFETY ALERT: *Remember, when comparing two fractions, if the numerators of the fractions are the same, the smaller the number in the denominator, the larger the value of the fraction.*

Example: $\frac{1}{3}$ *is larger than* $\frac{1}{4}$ *and* $\frac{1}{4}$ *is larger than* $\frac{1}{8}$

When two fractions have the same denominator but different numerators, the fraction that has the smaller number in the numerator is the smaller fraction.

Example: $\frac{3}{5}$ *is smaller than* $\frac{4}{5}$ *and* $\frac{3}{8}$ *is smaller than* $\frac{5}{8}$

There are four types of fractions:

1. **Proper Fraction**—In this type of fraction, the numerator is smaller than the denominator. This means that the result of dividing the numerator by the denominator is less than 1. For example:

   $\frac{2}{3}$ (read as two thirds)   or $\frac{5}{8}$ (read as five eighths) = less than 1

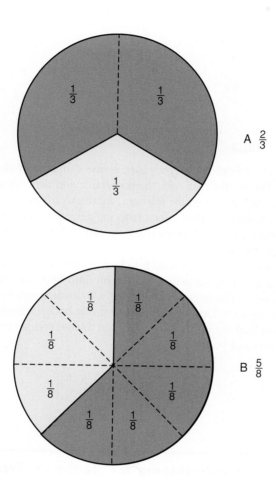

2. **Improper Fraction**—In this type of fraction, the numerator is larger than the denominator. This means that the result of dividing the numerator by the denominator is greater than or equal to 1. For example:

   $\frac{4}{2}$ or $\frac{9}{7}$ = greater than 1

3. **Mixed Number**—In this type of fraction, you have a whole number combined with a proper fraction. This means that the value of this number is always greater than 1. For example:

   $1\frac{7}{8}$ or $2\frac{3}{4}$ = greater than 1

4. **Complex Fraction**—In this type of fraction, the numerator or denominator or both can be a whole number, proper fraction, or mixed number. The value of the fraction can be less than, greater than, or equal to 1. For example:

$$\frac{\frac{1}{2}}{\frac{3}{6}} = \text{equal to } 1$$

$$\frac{\frac{3}{4}}{\frac{3}{8}} = \text{greater than } 1$$

$$\frac{\frac{3}{8}}{2} = \text{less than } 1$$

Reducing Fractions

To make calculating medication dosages easier, always simplify or reduce fractions to their **lowest common terms**. This means that both the numerator and denominator are the lowest numbers possible to still correctly represent the fraction. Numbers such as 2, 3, 5, 7, and 11 are prime numbers and cannot be reduced further. When reducing a fraction to its lowest terms, you are creating an equivalent fraction. In equivalent fractions, the form of the fraction is changed but the value of the fraction remains the same.

The first step in reducing fractions is to look at the numerator and denominator and decide what is the largest number that will divide evenly into both the numerator and denominator. Consider the fraction $\frac{6}{18}$. The largest number that will divide evenly into both 6 and 18 is 6.

The second step to reducing fractions is to divide both the numerator and the denominator by the number identified as the largest number that divides evenly into the numerator and denominator. Using the previous example of $\frac{6}{18}$:

$$\frac{6 \div 6 = 1}{18 \div 6 = 3} \quad \text{or} \quad \frac{10 \div 10 = 1}{20 \div 10 = 2}$$

PRACTICE PROBLEMS 1-3. Practice Problems for Reducing Fractions

DIRECTIONS: Reduce the proper fractions to the lowest terms. The answers to the problems can be found at the end of the chapter.

1. $\frac{30}{48}$ _____

2. $\frac{9}{27}$ _____

3. $\frac{45}{50}$ _____

4. $\frac{60}{100}$ _____

Conversion of Fractions

Another important skill with fractions is the ability to convert different types of fractions. Then you can do your calculations more quickly and easily, reducing your fractions to the lowest common terms.

CONVERTING MIXED NUMBERS TO IMPROPER FRACTIONS

Sometimes you may have dosages that are in mixed numbers such as $2\frac{1}{2}$ and you may need to convert this to an improper fraction. To convert mixed numbers to fractions, multiply the denominator by the whole number and add the numerator to get the numerator of the improper fraction.

The denominator of the improper fraction is the denominator of the fraction that was in the mixed number. For example:

$$2\frac{1}{2} = \frac{(2 \times 2) + 1}{2} = \frac{5}{2}$$

PRACTICE PROBLEMS 1-4. Practice Problems for Converting Mixed Numbers to Improper Fractions

DIRECTIONS: Convert the mixed numbers to improper fractions. Reduce the improper fractions to lowest terms when applicable. The answers to the problems can be found at the end of the chapter.

1. $6\frac{7}{8}$ _____

2. $2\frac{2}{3}$ _____

3. $5\frac{4}{5}$ _____

4. $7\frac{1}{4}$ _____

CONVERTING IMPROPER FRACTIONS TO MIXED NUMBERS

If you have a dosage that is in an improper fraction, you may wish to convert it to a mixed or whole number. To do this conversion, divide the numerator by the denominator. Any remainder is written as the numerator in a proper fraction. Use the denominator of the improper fraction as the denominator for the proper fraction. Then reduce the proper fraction to its lowest terms. For example:

$$\frac{21}{5} = 21 \div 5 = 4\frac{1}{5}$$

$$\frac{15}{6} = 15 \div 6 = 2\frac{3}{6} = 2\frac{1}{2}$$

PRACTICE PROBLEMS 1-5. Practice Problems for Converting Improper Fractions to Mixed Numbers

DIRECTIONS: Convert the improper fraction to a mixed number. Reduce to lowest terms where applicable. The answers to the problems can be found at the end of the chapter.

1. $\frac{10}{7}$ _____

2. $\frac{18}{10}$ _____

3. $\frac{9}{4}$ _____

4. $\frac{25}{8}$ _____

CONVERTING FRACTIONS TO DECIMALS

Fractions can be converted into decimals. Remember the line between the numerator and the denominator is a symbol for division. So to convert a fraction to a decimal, divide the denominator into the numerator using long division and carry the answer out to two or three decimal places.

For example, to convert $\frac{3}{4}$ to a decimal, divide 3 by 4:

$$
\begin{array}{r}
0.75 \\
4\overline{)3.00} \\
\underline{28} \\
20 \\
\underline{20} \\
0
\end{array}
$$

Remember that when looking at decimals, the whole number is to the left of the decimal point and the fraction is to the right of the decimal point.

CASE STUDY

Mr. Boyd is receiving Milk of Magnesia (MOM) $\frac{1}{2}$ ounce for constipation. Through your knowledge of fractions, you know that the dose of MOM, which is ordered as a fraction, can also be written as a decimal. Using your basic math skills, you can convert the fraction to a decimal. To convert $\frac{1}{2}$ to a decimal, divide 1 by 2

$$
\begin{array}{r}
0.5 \\
2\overline{)1.0} \\
\underline{10} \\
0
\end{array}
$$

Based on your division, you can see that Mr. Boyd's dosage of MOM can be written as MOM 0.5 ounces.

PRACTICE PROBLEMS 1-6. Practice Problems for Converting Fractions to Decimals

DIRECTIONS: Convert the fraction to a decimal. The answers to the problems can be found at the end of the chapter.

1. $\frac{4}{5}$

2. $\frac{6}{7}$

3. $\frac{1}{2}$

4. $\frac{7}{9}$

Addition and Subtraction of Fractions

You may at some time have to add or subtract fractions. To add or subtract fractions, the denominators in all the fractions in the equation must be the same. Then you just add or subtract the numbers in the numerator.

- **Step 1:** Convert all the fractions to equivalent fractions that have the least common denominator.
- **Step 2:** Add or subtract the numbers in the numerator. The value that you get becomes the numerator of your answer. Use the least common denominator found in step one as the denominator.
- **Step 3:** Reduce fractions to lowest terms and/or convert improper fractions to mixed numbers.

For example:

$$
\frac{3}{5} + \frac{4}{5}
$$

1. Since the denominators are the same, you do not have to find the least common denominator.
2. Add the numerators.

$$\frac{3 + 4}{5} = \frac{7}{5}$$

3. Now convert the improper fraction to a mixed number.

$$\frac{7}{5} = 7 \div 5 = 1\frac{2}{5}$$

Consider this example:

$$\frac{2}{3} + \frac{4}{5}$$

1. Since the denominators are not the same, you need to find the least common denominator for 3 and 5, which is 15.

   Convert the fractions to fifteenths.

$$\frac{2 \times 5}{3 \times 5} = \frac{10}{15} \quad \text{and} \quad \frac{4 \times 3}{5 \times 3} = \frac{12}{15}$$

2. Now you can add the fractions since the denominators are the same.

$$\frac{10 + 12}{15} = \frac{22}{15}$$

3. Convert the improper fraction to a mixed number.

$$\frac{22}{15} = 22 \div 15 = 1\frac{7}{15}$$

To subtract fractions, follow the same steps. For example:

$$\frac{8}{9} - \frac{4}{9}$$

1. Since the denominators are the same, you do not have to find the least common denominator.
2. Subtract the numerators.

$$\frac{8 - 4}{9} = \frac{4}{9}$$

3. Since your answer is in the lowest common terms, you do not need to reduce.

Consider this example:

$$2\frac{1}{3} - \frac{1}{4}$$

1. Find the least common denominator for 3 and 4. This is 12. Make sure to change the mixed number of $2\frac{1}{3}$ to an improper fraction.

$$2\frac{1}{3} = \frac{(3 \times 2) + 1}{3} = \frac{7}{3} \quad \frac{7 \times 4}{3 \times 4} = \frac{28}{12} \quad \text{and} \quad \frac{1 \times 3}{4 \times 3} = \frac{3}{12}$$

2. Now you can subtract the fractions since the denominators are the same.

$$\frac{28 - 3}{12} = \frac{25}{12}$$

3. Convert the improper fraction to a mixed number.

$$25 \div 12 = 2\frac{1}{12}$$

PRACTICE PROBLEMS 1-7. Practice Problems for Adding Fractions

DIRECTIONS: Add the following fractions. Convert to mixed numbers and/or reduce to lowest terms when applicable. The answers to the problems can be found at the end of the chapter.

1. $\frac{5}{6} + \frac{1}{4}$

2. $\frac{2}{3} + \frac{7}{8}$

3. $\frac{5}{7} + \frac{1}{2}$

4. $\frac{1}{3} + \frac{4}{7}$

PRACTICE PROBLEMS 1-8. Practice Problems for Subtracting Fractions

DIRECTIONS: Subtract the following fractions. Convert to mixed numbers and/or reduce to lowest terms when applicable. The answers to the problems can be found at the end of the chapter.

1. $\frac{11}{13} - \frac{7}{13}$

2. $\frac{7}{8} - \frac{1}{3}$

3. $\frac{2}{3} - \frac{2}{5}$

4. $\frac{7}{9} - \frac{1}{6}$

Multiplication of Fractions

Multiplying two fractions is a simple process. To multiply fractions, first multiply the numerators to get the new numerator. Then multiply the denominators to get the new denominator. Reduce the fractions to lowest terms when possible. Convert improper fractions to mixed numbers if needed. For example:

$$\frac{2}{3} \times \frac{1}{4} = \frac{2}{12}$$

Reduce the fraction to the lowest terms.

$$\frac{2 \div 2}{12 \div 2} = \frac{1}{6}$$

So the answer is $\frac{1}{6}$.

To make the problem simpler, use a process called cancellation. In cancellation, you reduce the numbers in the equation to the lowest terms before you multiply the fractions. After reducing all numbers in the fractions to the lowest terms, multiply new numerators and denominators of the fractions. For example:

$$\frac{2}{3} \times \frac{1}{4}$$

Reduce the numbers before multiplying. You can do this because the numerator of one fraction and the denominator of the other fraction can both be divided by 2.

$$\frac{\overset{1}{2}}{3} \times \frac{1}{\underset{2}{4}} = \frac{1}{6}$$

Apply the same principles if you are multiplying three or more fractions.

Example:
$$\frac{1}{2} \times \frac{3}{4} \times \frac{2}{3} = \frac{6}{24} = \frac{1}{4}$$

Multiplying mixed numbers and fractions also is a simple process. First, convert the mixed number to an improper fraction, then multiply the numerators to get a new numerator and the denominators to get a new denominator. For example:

$$2\frac{2}{3} \times \frac{1}{5}$$

Convert the mixed number and multiply.

$$\frac{8}{3} \times \frac{1}{5} = \frac{8}{15}$$ Your answer is in the lowest terms and cannot be reduced.

For two mixed numbers, follow the same steps. For example:

$$3\frac{1}{2} \times 4\frac{1}{3}$$

Convert both mixed numbers to improper fractions and multiply the numerators and denominators.

$$\frac{7}{2} \times \frac{13}{3} = \frac{91}{6}$$

Convert the answer to a mixed number.

$$91 \div 6 = 15\frac{1}{6}$$

PRACTICE PROBLEMS 1-9. Practice Problems for Multiplying Fractions

DIRECTIONS: Multiply the fractions. Reduce the fractions to lowest terms where appropriate. Convert improper fractions to mixed numbers. The answers to the problems can be found at the end of the chapter.

1. $\frac{5}{6} \times \frac{4}{7}$

2. $\frac{8}{9} \times \frac{2}{5}$

3. $5\frac{2}{3} \times \frac{7}{10}$

4. $3\frac{1}{8} \times 4\frac{1}{2}$

Division of Fractions

At times, you may need to divide fractions to calculate a medication dosage. Dividing fractions is a little more difficult than multiplying fractions, but by following the easy steps you can divide two fractions correctly.

The first step is to set up the problem. Division of fractions can be written in one of two ways. The problems can be written as $\frac{1}{2} \div \frac{1}{4}$ or it may be written as $\frac{\frac{1}{2}}{\frac{1}{4}}$. In both problems, the number you are dividing by, the divisor, is $\frac{1}{4}$.

The second step is to invert the divisor. For this problem, the divisor $\frac{1}{4}$ becomes $\frac{4}{1}$.

Next, multiply the fractions as you did in the previous section. Then reduce your answer to lowest terms and/or convert improper fractions to mixed numbers. The problem would look like this:

$$\frac{1}{2} \times \frac{4}{1} = \frac{4}{2}$$

Finally, convert the improper fraction to a mixed number or reduce to the lowest term. In this example, you need to convert the improper fraction to a mixed number: $4 \div 2 = 2$. The answer to the problem is 2. For example:

$$\frac{3}{4} \div \frac{4}{7}$$

Invert the divisor and multiply:

$$\frac{3}{4} \times \frac{7}{4} = \frac{21}{16}$$

Convert the improper fraction to a mixed number.

$$21 \div 16 = 1\frac{5}{16}$$

The answer to the problem is $1\frac{5}{16}$.

To divide a fraction by a mixed number, convert the mixed number to an improper fraction. Then follow the same three easy steps: set up the problem, invert the divisor, multiply the fractions, then convert to a mixed number, and/or reduce the fraction to the lowest terms.

(!) **SAFETY ALERT:** *Make sure to keep the numerator fraction as the numerator and the denominator fraction as the denominator to ensure that you invert and multiply by the correct fraction.*

PRACTICE PROBLEMS 1-10. Practice Problems for Dividing Fractions

DIRECTIONS: Divide the fractions. Reduce the fractions to lowest terms where appropriate. Convert improper fractions to mixed numbers if needed. The answers to the problems can be found at the end of the chapter.

1. $\frac{4}{5} \div \frac{7}{10}$

2. $\frac{8}{9} \div \frac{1}{2}$

3. $\frac{3}{5} \div \frac{7}{8}$

4. $\frac{1}{2} \div \frac{1}{3}$

PRACTICE PROBLEMS 1-11. Practice Problems for Dividing Fractions and Mixed Numbers

DIRECTIONS: Convert the mixed numbers to improper fractions if needed. Divide the fractions. Reduce the fractions to lowest terms where appropriate. Convert improper fractions to mixed numbers if needed. The answers to the problems can be found at the end of the chapter.

1. $6\frac{3}{4} \div \frac{7}{8}$

2. $\frac{11}{12} \div 3\frac{1}{3}$

3. $3\frac{3}{10} \div 4\frac{4}{5}$

4. $3\frac{1}{8} \div \frac{6}{7}$

DECIMALS

Medication dosages are often ordered in decimals. Being able to correctly add, subtract, multiply, and divide decimals will ensure that you calculate the correct dosage of the medication. **Decimals** are fractions with a denominator that has a value of a multiple of ten. The value of the decimal is determined by the position of the numbers to the right of the decimal point. In a decimal, the value of the numbers to the right of the decimal point is less than one and the value of the numbers to the left of the decimal point is greater than one. The decimal 2.5 is read as two and five tenths and the decimal 4.66 is read as four and sixty-six hundredths.

> **⊘ SAFETY ALERT:** *To avoid medication errors, always add a zero to the left of the decimal point if there is no whole number. An example of this is 0.2 or 0.45. Read decimals from left to right starting with the whole number.*

Remember these points about decimals:

- One position to the right of the decimal point is read as tenths. For example, 0.3 is read as three tenths.
- Two positions to the right of the decimal point is read as hundredths. For example, 0.03 is read as three hundredths.
- Three positions to the right of the decimal point is read as thousandths. For example, 0.003 is read as three thousandths.
- Four positions to the right of the decimal point is read as ten thousandths. For example, 0.0003 is read as three ten-thousandths.

Addition and Subtraction of Decimals

Addition and subtraction of decimals is similar to addition and subtraction of whole numbers. The first step is to align the decimals in a column with the decimal points lined up directly underneath each other. The decimals are then added and subtracted as whole numbers. In the answer, place the decimal point in the exact location as that where it is lined up in the problem.

Consider this example:

Add the decimals: $4.22 + 3.12 + 2.1$

Place the decimals in a column, lining up the decimal points:

$$
\begin{array}{r}
4.22 \\
3.12 \\
+\,2.10 \\
\end{array}
$$

Add the numbers as if they were whole numbers. Adding a zero at the end of a decimal does not change the value of the number. Place the decimal point in the answer directly in line with the decimal points in the problem.

$$
\begin{array}{r}
4.22 \\
3.12 \\
+\,2.10 \\
\hline
9.44
\end{array}
\qquad \text{Answer: 9.44}
$$

Try this example: Add the decimals:

$$21.6 + 1.22 + 0.98$$

Place the decimals in a column, lining up the decimal points:

$$
\begin{array}{r}
21.60 \\
1.22 \\
+\,0.98 \\
\hline
\end{array}
$$

Add the numbers as if they were whole numbers. Adding a zero at the end of a decimal does not change the value of the number. Place the decimal point in the answer directly in line with the decimal points in the problem.

$$
\begin{array}{r}
21.60 \\
1.22 \\
+\,0.98 \\
\hline
23.80
\end{array}
\qquad \text{Answer: 23.8}
$$

Now subtract decimals. For example, subtract the decimals

$$5.24 - 2.16$$

Place the decimals in a column lining up the decimal points.

$$
\begin{array}{r}
5.24 \\
-\,2.16 \\
\hline
\end{array}
$$

Subtract the numbers as if they were whole numbers. Place the decimal point in the answer directly in line with the decimal points in the problem.

$$
\begin{array}{r}
5.24 \\
-\,2.16 \\
\hline
3.08
\end{array}
\qquad \text{Answer: 3.08}
$$

Consider this example: Subtract the decimals:

$$18.54 - 3.66$$

Place the decimals in a column lining up the decimal points.

$$
\begin{array}{r}
18.54 \\
-\,3.66 \\
\hline
\end{array}
$$

Subtract the numbers as if they were whole numbers. Place the decimal point in the answer directly in line with the decimal points in the problem.

$$
\begin{array}{r}
18.54 \\
-\,3.66 \\
\hline
14.88
\end{array}
\qquad \text{Answer: 14.88}
$$

CASE STUDY

Mr. Boyd calls you to his room to tell you that he is experiencing chest pain. Mr. Boyd rates his chest pain as 6, on a scale of 0 to 10. You give Mr. Boyd a nitroglycerin sublingual tablet 0.3 mg as ordered for chest pain. Five minutes later, Mr. Boyd is still having chest pain rated at 3, on a scale of 0 to 10. You give him a second nitroglycerin sublingual tablet 0.3 mg. In three minutes, Mr. Boyd tells you that his chest pain has disappeared.

Using your knowledge of basic math skills, you know that Mr. Boyd received a total dosage of 0.6 mg of sublingual nitroglycerin. By adding the two dosages in decimals, you obtain the total dosage.

$$\begin{array}{r} 0.3 \\ + 0.3 \\ \hline 0.6 \end{array}$$

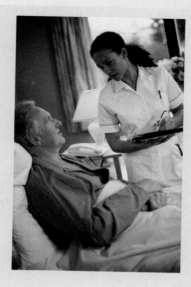

PRACTICE PROBLEMS 1-12. Practice Problems for Adding Decimals

DIRECTIONS: Add the decimals. The answers to the problems can be found at the end of the chapter.

1. 12.567 + 8.453

2. 2.148 + 5.657

3. 2.03 + 0.678 + 1.508

4. 0.67 + 1.82

PRACTICE PROBLEMS 1-13. Practice Problems for Subtracting Decimals

DIRECTIONS: Subtract the following decimals. The answers to the problems can be found at the end of the chapter.

1. 5.48 − 2.78

2. 1.896 − 0.522

3. 3.45 − 3.23

4. 0.951 − 0.788

Multiplication of Decimals

You may have to multiply decimals to calculate a drug dosage. Multiplying decimals is the same as multiplying whole numbers except the decimal point in the product must be correctly placed. Following these steps will help you correctly multiply decimals.

- First, set up the problem like you were multiplying whole numbers.
- Second, multiply the numbers as if they were whole numbers. At this point, do not place a decimal point in the product.

- Finally, place the decimal point in the product, deciding its placement by counting the number of decimal places to the right of the decimal in the two numbers being multiplied. Then count off this number of places in the product, starting at the right moving left, and place the decimal point.

Here is an example showing each of the steps:

Multiply: $\qquad 1.2 \times 2.3$

First, set up the problem like you would with whole numbers.

$$
\begin{array}{r}
1.2 \\
\times\,2.3 \\
\end{array}
$$

Next, multiply the numbers like whole numbers.

$$
\begin{array}{r}
1.2 \\
\times\,2.3 \\
\hline
36 \\
24 \\
\hline
276 \\
\end{array}
$$

Count the number of decimal places to right in the two numbers being multiplied.

$$
\begin{array}{r}
1.2 \\
\times\,2.3 \\
\hline
\end{array}
$$

One place to the right
One place to the right
For a total of two places

Place the decimal point two places to the right in the product

$$
\begin{array}{r}
1.2 \\
\times\,2.3 \\
\hline
36 \\
24 \\
\hline
2.76 \\
\end{array}
$$

The decimal point is placed two places to the right.

The correct answer is 2.76

When multiplying decimals by 10, 100, or 1000, use this quick and easy method. Look at the number of zeros in the number by which you are multiplying. Then move the decimal point to the right the same number of places as there are numbers of zeros. For example, if you were multiplying a decimal by 10, there is one zero in 10. You would then move the decimal point, one place to the right. Review this example:

$$1.55 \times 10 \qquad \text{There is one zero in 10.}$$

Move the decimal point one place to the right.

$$1.55 = 1.55 = 15.5 \qquad \text{The answer is 15.5.}$$

Consider this example: $\quad 2.43 \times 100 \qquad$ There are two zeros in 100.

Move the decimal point two places to the right.

$$2.43 = 2.43 = 243$$

PRACTICE PROBLEMS 1-14. Practice Problems for Multiplying Decimals

DIRECTIONS: Multiply these decimals. The answers to the problems can be found at the end of the chapter.

1. 2.8×4.6

2. 1.5×5.6

3. 1.45×0.78

4. 6.3×2.1

Division of Decimals

Some medication dosage calculations may require you to divide decimals to obtain the amount of medication you need to give to the patient. Dividing decimals uses the same process of division as dividing whole numbers. The challenge in dividing decimals is to know what to do with the decimal point in the divisor, dividend, and quotient. It is important to remember that when setting up a division problem with two decimals, the decimal in the quotient is placed directly above the decimal point in the dividend. For example:

$$\text{(divisor)} \quad 3\overline{)99.9} \quad \text{(dividend)} \qquad \text{or} \qquad \text{(divisor)} \quad 6\overline{)42.6} \quad \text{(dividend)}$$

with quotients 33.3 and 7.1 respectively.

The first step in dividing decimals is to make the decimal number in the divisor into a whole number. To do this, move the decimal point to the right the number of places that are in the decimal number. For example, to work the problem $0.75 \div 1.5$, identify the divisor of the problem, which is 1.5. Move the decimal point one place to the right to make the divisor 15. If the divisor of the problem is 2.66, you move the decimal point two places to the right to make the divisor 266.

The second step in dividing decimals is to move the decimal point in the dividend the same number of places to the right that you moved the decimal point in the divisor. In the above problem, the dividend is 0.75. You moved the decimal point in the divisor (1.5) one place to the right; therefore, you need to move the decimal point in the dividend one place to the right. The dividend of 0.75 would become 7.5.

The next step is to place the decimal point in the quotient directly above the decimal point in the dividend. Then divide 7.5 by 15. In our example, the division problem would be set up as follows:

$$1.5\overline{)0.75}$$

Move the decimal point in the divisor one place to the right (Step 1).

$$15\overline{)0.75}$$

Then you need to move the decimal point in the dividend one place to the right (Step 2).

$$15\overline{)7.5}$$

Then put the decimal point in the quotient directly above the decimal point in the dividend and divide the numbers (Step 3).

$$\begin{array}{r} 0.5 \\ 15\overline{)7.5} \\ \underline{75} \\ 0 \end{array} \qquad \text{The answer is 0.5}$$

Dividing by multiples of 10 such as 10, 100, or 1000 is quite easy. Move the decimal point to the left the same number of places that there are zeros in the divisor. For example, when solving this problem:

$$5.55 \div 10$$

Move the decimal point one place to the left because there is one zero in 10. The answer is 0.555.

$$5.55 = 5.55 = 0.555$$

SAFETY ALERT: *Be extremely careful with the placement of the decimal point. An error in the placement of the decimal point can lead to a critical medication error.*

PRACTICE PROBLEMS 1-15. Practice Problems for Dividing Decimals

DIRECTIONS: Divide these decimals. The answers to the problems can be found at the end of the chapter.

1. 3.64 ÷ 4

2. 1.59 ÷ 0.3

3. 0.666 ÷ 0.03

4. 0.028 ÷ 0.07

RATIO AND PROPORTION

Ratio and proportion are two important concepts often used to calculate medication dosages safely. The relationship between two units or quantities is expressed as a **ratio**. To write ratios use the symbols of a slash (/) or colon (:) between the numbers. The slash or colon is read as "is to" or "per." The ratio 4/5 is read as "4 is to 5." The symbols indicate that division of the two numbers should be done. Fractions are ratios.

When setting up a ratio, the numerator of the fraction is to the left of the slash or colon and the denominator is to the right of the slash or colon. For example, a ratio of 3 is to 1 can be written 3/1 or 3:1.

In medication administration, ratios are used to express the quantity or weight of a medication in a solution. For example, the medication is 15 mg/5 mL. This means that there is 15 mg (weight) of the drug in 5 mL of liquid (solution).

Proportions are a statement that two ratios are equal. Proportions can be written in an equivalent fraction form or in a form that uses colons to express the equality. A proportion using the fraction form would be written as: $\frac{2}{3} = \frac{6}{9}$. The equal sign is read as "as." You would read this proportion as "2 is to 3 as 6 is to 9". You can verify that the fractions are equal by multiplying the numerator of each fraction by the opposite denominator. The products should be equal. In this example, $2 \times 9 = 18$ and $3 \times 6 = 18$. The products are equal, showing that the ratios in the proportion are equivalent.

When writing a proportion in the colon form, a double colon is used in place of the = sign and is read as "as". Proportions using the colon form are written: 2:3::6:9. This is read as "2 is to 3 as 6 is to 9". In the colon form, the two outside numbers are called the *extremes* and the two middle numbers are called the *means*. In the above example, 2 and 9 are the extremes and 3 and 6 are the means. When you multiply the two extremes and then multiply the two means, the products from each multiplication will be equal. In this example, $2 \times 9 = 18$ (extremes) and $3 \times 6 = 18$ (means). This shows that the ratios in this proportion are equivalent.

Ratio and Proportion: Solving for *x*

A common problem when working with ratio and proportion is to be given one ratio and have an unknown in the other ratio. The unknown is represented by the symbol x. This requires the use of mathematical skills to determine the value of x in the proportion and solve the problem. In the problem $\frac{1}{2} = \frac{x}{4}$, x is unknown. To solve this problem and find the value of x, cross multiply the numerator in each ratio with the denominator in the other ratio.

$$2 \times x = 1 \times 4$$
$$2x = 4$$

Then divide each side of the equation by the number before the x.

$\frac{2x}{2} = \frac{4}{2}$ Because the numerator and denominator of the ratio with x are the same, they will cancel each other out leaving x alone.

Divide the other side of the equation $x = \frac{4}{2}$

This reduces to $x = 2$.

Solving for x using ratio and proportion is a common method to calculate medication dosages when the dosage ordered is not the same as how the medication is supplied. The process of calculating medication dosages using this method will be reviewed in much greater detail in Chapter 6 in this book.

CASE STUDY

Mr. Boyd has a history of mild heart failure and atrial fibrillation since his MI. He is receiving digoxin (Lanoxin) elixir for this. The prescribed dose is digoxin 0.125 mg to be given by mouth every morning. The medication is supplied as digoxin elixir 0.05 mg/mL. To do this calculation use your knowledge of decimals, fractions, and ratio-proportion to solve for x. You would solve the problem like this:

$$\frac{0.05 \text{ mg}}{1 \text{ mL}} = \frac{0.125 \text{ mg}}{x}$$

Cross multiply: 0.05 mg x = 0.125 mg/mL

Divide both sides of the equation to isolate x. Since mg is in the numerator and denominator, they cancel each other out and you are left with mL as the volume of medication.

$$\frac{0.05 \text{ mg } x}{0.05 \text{ mg}} = \frac{0.125 \text{ mg/mL}}{0.05 \text{ mg}}$$

Perform the math: $x = \dfrac{0.125 \text{ mL}}{0.05}$

Solve for x: $x = 2.5 \text{ mL}$

PRACTICE PROBLEMS 1-16. Practice Problems for Ratio and Proportion: Solving for *x*

DIRECTIONS: Solve for the unknown *x* in the proportions. The answers to the problems can be found at the end of the chapter.

1. $\dfrac{10}{20} = \dfrac{x}{5}$

2. $\dfrac{1}{3} = \dfrac{x}{18}$

3. $\dfrac{x}{24} = \dfrac{5}{12}$

4. $\dfrac{x}{40} = \dfrac{5}{8}$

Critical Thinking/Decision Making Exercise

Correct dosage calculation is a critical component of safe medication administration by nurses. Your knowledge of basic math skills will help you correctly calculate medication dosages for your patients. Consider the following situation.

Mr. Harris is 42 years old. He visited his doctor complaining of fatigue, having no energy, weight gain, and being cold all the time. The doctor diagnosed Mr. Harris with hypothyroidism and started him on levothyroxine sodium (Synthroid). His initial dose of medication is levothyroxine sodium 0.05 mg daily for the first week. He is to increase his dose 0.025 mg each week until he reaches a maintenance dose of 0.150 mg.

How much levothyroxine sodium should Mr. Harris take at the start of week 4 of the medication? To find the answer to this problem, use your knowledge of basic math skills to calculate his dosage for week 4. You know that weeks 2 through 4 total 3 weeks. Use your knowledge of multiplication of decimals to find how much medication Mr. Harris would get each week. Remember the order was to increase his dosage 0.025 mg each week. Set up and solve the problem:

$$\begin{array}{r} 0.025 \text{ mg} \\ \times\ 3 \\ \hline 0.075 \text{ mg} \end{array}$$

Increasing Mr. Harris's medication by 0.025 mg each week means that weeks 2 through 4, you will increase his medication by 0.075 mg. If you use addition of decimals, you take the starting dose of 0.05 mg and add 0.075 mg. Set up and solve the problem like this:

$$\begin{array}{r} 0.050 \text{ mg} \\ +0.075 \text{ mg} \\ \hline 0.125 \text{ mg} \end{array}$$

In using your math skills, according to the physician's medication order, you determine that Mr. Harris needs to receive levothyroxine sodium 0.125 mg starting week 4. Your knowledge of math skills provides you the ability to calculate the correct dosage of medication for Mr. Harris.

CHAPTER REVIEW PROBLEMS

The answers to the problems can be found at the end of the chapter.

Review Problems 1-1. Convert the Roman numerals to Arabic numbers.

1. XIX

2. VIII

3. XIV

4. XXVI

Review Problems 1-2. Convert the Arabic numbers to Roman numerals.

1. 13

2. 4

3. 23

4. 31

Review Problems 1-3. Convert the improper fractions to mixed numbers.

1. $\frac{9}{5}$

2. $\frac{5}{3}$

3. $\frac{7}{2}$

4. $\frac{13}{4}$

Review Problems 1-4. Convert the mixed numbers to improper fractions.

1. $4\frac{1}{2}$

2. $5\frac{1}{3}$

3. $2\frac{7}{8}$

4. $3\frac{5}{6}$

Review Problems 1-5. Add the fractions. Convert to improper fractions as needed. Reduce to lowest terms.

1. $\dfrac{1}{8} + 2\dfrac{1}{4}$

2. $\dfrac{3}{5} + \dfrac{3}{10}$

3. $\dfrac{1}{4} + \dfrac{2}{3}$

4. $\dfrac{6}{9} + \dfrac{5}{6}$

Review Problems 1-6. Subtract the fractions. Reduce to lowest terms.

1. $\dfrac{7}{8} - \dfrac{1}{4}$

2. $\dfrac{4}{5} - \dfrac{1}{2}$

3. $\dfrac{7}{9} - \dfrac{2}{6}$

4. $\dfrac{1}{3} - \dfrac{2}{9}$

Review Problems 1-7.. Multiply the fractions. Convert to mixed numbers as needed. Reduce to lowest terms.

1. $\dfrac{5}{6} \times \dfrac{4}{7}$

2. $\dfrac{2}{3} \times \dfrac{3}{8}$

3. $\dfrac{5}{9} \times \dfrac{1}{2}$

4. $\dfrac{7}{10} \times \dfrac{1}{3}$

Review Problems 1-8. Divide the fractions. Convert to improper fractions as needed. Reduce to lowest terms.

1. $\dfrac{6}{7} \div \dfrac{1}{5}$

2. $\dfrac{2}{3} \div \dfrac{1}{4}$

3. $\dfrac{5}{6} \div \dfrac{1}{2}$

4. $\dfrac{3}{7} \div \dfrac{2}{5}$

Review Problems 1-9. Add the decimals.

1. $2.67 + 4.89$
2. $5.168 + 1.801$
3. $6.811 + 3.01$
4. $2.44 + 1.92$

Review Problems 1-10. Subtract the decimals.

1. $8.66 - 2.01$
2. $5.926 - 3.234$
3. $1.894 - 0.762$
4. $7.54 - 2.82$

Review Problems 1-11. Multiply the decimals.

1. 4.8×2.1
2. 3.4×4.2
3. 11.3×3.4
4. 8.2×1.6

Review Problems 1-12. Divide the decimals.

1. $7.2 \div 1.5$
2. $4.65 \div 3.1$
3. $8.88 \div 2.22$
4. $81.7 \div 1.9$

Review Problems 1-13. Solve for x.

1. $\dfrac{x}{5} = \dfrac{7}{10}$

2. $\dfrac{4}{8} = \dfrac{x}{4}$

3. $\dfrac{x}{6} = \dfrac{3}{4}$

4. $\dfrac{2}{3} = \dfrac{x}{18}$

Answers to Practice Problems

Practice Problem Answers 1-1

1. $XXIII = 10 + 10 + 1 + 1 + 1 = 23$

2. $XLV = (50 - 10) + 5 = 45$

3. $iii \, \dot{s}\dot{s} = 1 + 1 + 1 + \dfrac{1}{2} = 3\dfrac{1}{2}$

4. $xvii = 10 + 5 + 1 + 1 = 17$

Practice Problem Answers 1-2

1. 33   XXXIII

2. 27   XXVII

3. 13   XIII

4. 6   VI

Practice Problem Answers 1-3

1. $\dfrac{30 \div 6 = 5}{48 \div 6 = 8}$

2. $\dfrac{9 \div 9 = 1}{27 \div 9 = 3}$

3. $\dfrac{45 \div 5 = 9}{50 \div 5 = 10}$

4. $\dfrac{60 \div 20 = 3}{100 \div 20 = 5}$

Practice Problem Answers 1-4

1. $6\dfrac{7}{8} = \dfrac{(8 \times 6) + 7}{8} = \dfrac{55}{8}$

2. $2\dfrac{2}{3} = \dfrac{(2 \times 3) + 2}{3} = \dfrac{8}{3}$

3. $5\dfrac{4}{5} = \dfrac{(5 \times 5) + 4}{5} = \dfrac{29}{5}$

4. $7\dfrac{1}{4} = \dfrac{(4 \times 7) + 1}{4} = \dfrac{29}{4}$

Practice Problem Answers 1-5

1. $\dfrac{10}{7} = 10 \div 7 = 1\dfrac{3}{7}$

2. $\dfrac{18}{10} = 18 \div 10 = 1\dfrac{8}{10} = 1\dfrac{4}{5}$

3. $\dfrac{9}{4} = 9 \div 4 = 2\dfrac{1}{4}$

4. $\dfrac{25}{8} = 25 \div 8 = 3\dfrac{1}{8}$

Practice Problem Answers 1-6

1.
$$\begin{array}{r} 0.80 \\ 5\overline{)4.00} \\ \underline{40} \\ 0 \end{array}$$

3.
$$\begin{array}{r} 0.5 \\ 2\overline{)1.0} \\ \underline{10} \\ 0 \end{array}$$

2.
$$\begin{array}{r} 0.857 \\ 7\overline{)6.000} \\ \underline{56} \\ 40 \\ \underline{35} \\ 50 \\ \underline{49} \\ 1 \end{array}$$
You can round 0.857 to 0.86

4.
$$\begin{array}{r} 0.777 \\ 9\overline{)7.000} \\ \underline{63} \\ 70 \\ \underline{63} \\ 70 \\ \underline{70} \\ 7 \end{array}$$
You can round 0.777 to 0.78

Practice Problem Answers 1-7

1. $\dfrac{5}{6} + \dfrac{1}{4}$ Since the denominators are not the same, you need to find the least common denominator for 6 and 4. Remember this is the smallest number that each denominator goes into.

Convert the fractions to twelfths $\dfrac{5}{6} = \dfrac{10}{12}$ and $\dfrac{1}{4} = \dfrac{3}{12}$

Add the numerators since the denominators are now the same. $\dfrac{10 + 3}{12} = \dfrac{13}{12}$

Convert the improper fraction to a mixed number. $13 \div 12 = 1\dfrac{1}{12}$

2. $\dfrac{2}{3} + \dfrac{7}{8}$ Since the denominators are not the same, you need find the least common denominator for 3 and 8. Remember this is the smallest number into which each denominator goes.

Convert the fractions to twenty-fourths. $\dfrac{2}{3} = \dfrac{16}{24}$ and $\dfrac{7}{8} = \dfrac{21}{24}$

Add only the numerators since the denominators are now the same. $\dfrac{16 + 21}{24} = \dfrac{37}{24}$

Convert the improper fraction to a mixed number. $37 \div 24 = 1\dfrac{13}{24}$

3. $\dfrac{5}{7} + \dfrac{1}{2}$ Since the denominators are not the same, you need to find the least common denominator for 7 and 2.

Convert the fractions to fourteenths. $\dfrac{5}{7} = \dfrac{10}{14}$ and $\dfrac{1}{2} = \dfrac{7}{14}$

Add the numerators since the denominators are now the same. $\dfrac{10 + 7}{14} = \dfrac{17}{14}$

Convert the improper fraction to a mixed number. $17 \div 14 = 1\dfrac{3}{14}$

4. $\dfrac{1}{3} + \dfrac{4}{7}$ Since the denominators are not the same, you need to find the least common denominator for 3 and 7.

Convert the fractions to twenty-firsts. $\dfrac{1}{3} = \dfrac{7}{21}$ and $\dfrac{4}{7} = \dfrac{12}{21}$

Add the numerators since the denominators are now the same. $\dfrac{7 + 12}{21} = \dfrac{19}{21}$

No further steps are needed since the fraction is in the lowest common terms.

Practice Problem Answers 1-8

1. $\dfrac{11}{13} - \dfrac{7}{13}$ Since the denominators are not the same, you do not have to find the least common donominator.

Subtract the numerators since the denominator is the same. $\dfrac{11 - 7}{13} = \dfrac{4}{13}$

No further steps are needed since the fraction is in the lowest common terms.

2. $\dfrac{7}{8} - \dfrac{1}{3}$ Since the denominators are not the same, you need to find the least common denominator for 8 and 3. Remember this is the smallest number into which the denominator goes.

Convert the fractions to twenty-fourths. $\dfrac{7}{8} = \dfrac{21}{24}$ and $\dfrac{1}{3} = \dfrac{8}{24}$

Subtract the numerators since the denominators are now the same. $\dfrac{21 - 8}{24} = \dfrac{13}{24}$

No further steps are needed since the fraction is in the lowest common terms.

3. $\dfrac{2}{3} - \dfrac{2}{5}$ Since the denominators are not the same, you need to find the least common denominator for 3 and 5.

Convert the fractions to fifteenths. $\dfrac{2}{3} = \dfrac{10}{15}$ and $\dfrac{2}{5} = \dfrac{6}{15}$

Subtract the numerators since the denominators are now the same. $\dfrac{10 - 6}{15} = \dfrac{4}{15}$

No further steps are needed since the fraction is in the lowest common terms.

4. $\dfrac{7}{9} - \dfrac{1}{6}$ Since the denominators are not the same, you need to find the least common denominator for 9 and 6.

Convert the fractions to eighteenths. $\dfrac{7}{9} = \dfrac{14}{18}$ and $\dfrac{1}{6} = \dfrac{3}{18}$

Subtract the numerators since the denominators are now the same. $\dfrac{14 - 3}{18} = \dfrac{11}{18}$

No further steps are needed since the fraction is in the lowest common terms.

Practice Problem Answers 1-9

1. $\dfrac{5}{6} \times \dfrac{4}{7} = \dfrac{20}{42}$ Reduce to lowest terms $\dfrac{20}{42} = \dfrac{10}{21}$

2. $\dfrac{8}{9} \times \dfrac{2}{5} = \dfrac{16}{45}$ Does not reduce

3. $5\dfrac{2}{3} \times \dfrac{7}{10} = \dfrac{17}{3} \times \dfrac{7}{10} = \dfrac{119}{30}$

   Convert to a mixed number $119 \div 30 = 3\dfrac{29}{30}$

4. $3\dfrac{1}{8} \times 4\dfrac{1}{2} = \dfrac{25}{8} \times \dfrac{9}{8} = \dfrac{225}{64}$

   Convert to a mixed number $225 \div 64 = 3\dfrac{33}{64}$

Practice Problem Answers 1-10

1. $\dfrac{4}{5} \div \dfrac{7}{10}$

   Invert the divisor and multiply $\dfrac{4}{5} \times \dfrac{10}{7} = \dfrac{40}{35}$

   Convert the improper fraction to a mixed number and reduce the fraction by dividing the numerator and denominator by 5.

   $$\dfrac{40}{35} = \dfrac{8}{7} = 1\dfrac{1}{7}$$

2. $\dfrac{8}{9} \div \dfrac{1}{2}$

   Invert the divisor and multiply $\dfrac{8}{9} \times \dfrac{2}{1} = \dfrac{16}{9}$

   Convert the improper fraction to a mixed number $\dfrac{16}{9} = 1\dfrac{7}{9}$

3. $\dfrac{3}{5} \div \dfrac{7}{8}$

   Invert the divisor and multiply $\dfrac{3}{5} \times \dfrac{8}{7} = \dfrac{24}{35}$

   This fraction cannot be reduced.

4. $\dfrac{1}{2} \div \dfrac{1}{3}$

Invert the divisor and multiply $\dfrac{1}{2} \times \dfrac{3}{1} = \dfrac{3}{2}$

Convert the improper fraction to a mixed number. $\dfrac{3}{2} = 1\dfrac{1}{2}$

Practice Problem Answers 1-11

1. $6\dfrac{3}{4} \div \dfrac{7}{8}$

   Convert the mixed number to an improper fraction $\dfrac{27}{4} \div \dfrac{7}{8}$

   Invert the divisor and multiply $\dfrac{27}{4} \times \dfrac{8}{7} = \dfrac{216}{28}$

   Convert the improper fraction to a mixed number and reduce by dividing the numerator and denominator by 4.

   $$\dfrac{216}{28} = 7\dfrac{20}{28} \div \dfrac{\div\ 4}{\div\ 4} = 7\dfrac{5}{7}$$

2. $\dfrac{11}{12} \div 3\dfrac{1}{3}$

   Convert the mixed number to an improper fraction $\dfrac{11}{12} \div \dfrac{10}{3}$

   Invert the divisor and multiply $\dfrac{11}{12} \times \dfrac{3}{10} = \dfrac{33}{120}$

   Reduce the fraction by dividing the numerator and denominator by 3.

   $$\dfrac{33 \div 3}{120 \div 3} = \dfrac{11}{40}$$

3. $3\dfrac{3}{10} \div 4\dfrac{4}{5}$

   Convert the mixed number to an improper fraction $\dfrac{33}{10} \div \dfrac{24}{5}$

   Invert the divisor and multiply $\dfrac{33}{10} \times \dfrac{5}{24} = \dfrac{165}{240}$

   Reduce the fraction by dividing the numerator and denominator by 15.

   $$\dfrac{165 \div 15}{240 \div 15} = \dfrac{11}{16}$$

4. $3\dfrac{1}{8} \div \dfrac{6}{7}$

Convert the mixed number to an improper fraction $\dfrac{25}{8} \div \dfrac{6}{7}$

Invert the divisor and multiply $\dfrac{25}{8} \times \dfrac{7}{6} = \dfrac{175}{48}$

Convert the improper fraction to a mixed number. $\dfrac{175}{48} = 3\dfrac{31}{48}$

Practice Problem Answers 1-12

1. 12.567
    +8.453
    ─────
    21.020

2. 2.148
    +5.657
    ─────
    7.805

3. 2.03
    0.678
    +1.508
    ─────
    4.216

4. 0.67
    +1.82
    ─────
    2.49

Practice Problem Answers 1-13

1. 5.48
    −2.78
    ─────
    2.70

2. 1.896
    −0.522
    ─────
    1.374

3. 3.45
    −3.23
    ─────
    0.22

4. 0.951
    −0.788
    ─────
    0.163

Practice Problem Answers 1-14

1. 2.8
    × 4.6
    ─────
    168
    112
    ─────
    12.88

2. 1.5
    × 5.6
    ─────
    90
    75
    ─────
    8.40

3. 1.45
    × 0.78
    ─────
    1160
    1015
    ─────
    1.1310

4. 6.3
    × 2.1
    ─────
    63
    126
    ─────
    13.23

Practice Problem Answers 1-15

1. $3.64 \div 4$

   Set up problem. $4\overline{)3.64}$

   The divisor is a whole number; you do not need to move the decimal point.

   Place decimal point in quotient directly above decimal point in dividend. Divide.

$$\begin{array}{r} 0.91 \\ 4\overline{)3.64} \\ \underline{36} \\ 04 \\ \underline{04} \\ 0 \end{array}$$ Answer: 0.91

2. $1.59 \div 0.3$

   Set up the problem. $0.3\overline{)1.59}$

   Move the decimal point to the right one place in the divisor and the dividend. Place the decimal point in the quotient directly above the decimal point in the dividend. Divide.

$$\begin{array}{r} 5.3 \\ 3\overline{)15.9} \\ \underline{15} \\ 09 \\ \underline{9} \\ 0 \end{array}$$ Answer: 5.3

3. $0.666 \div 0.03$

   Set up the problem. $0.03\overline{)0.666}$

   Move the decimal point to the right two places in the divisor and the dividend. Place the decimal point in the quotient directly above the decimal point in the dividend. Divide.

$$\begin{array}{r} 22.2 \\ 3\overline{)66.6} \\ \underline{6} \\ 06 \\ \underline{6} \\ 06 \\ \underline{6} \\ 0 \end{array}$$ Answer: 22.2

4. $0.028 \div 0.07$

   Set up the problem. $0.07\overline{)0.028}$

   Move the decimal point to the right two places in the divisor and the dividend. Place the decimal point in the quotient directly above the decimal point in the dividend. Divide.

$$\begin{array}{r} 0.4 \\ 7\overline{)2.8} \\ \underline{28} \\ 0 \end{array}$$ Answer: 0.4

Practice Problem Answers 1-16

1. $\dfrac{10}{20} = \dfrac{x}{5}$

   Cross multiply $20x = 50$

   Divide each side of the equation by the number in front of the x.

   $$\dfrac{20x}{20} = \dfrac{50}{20} \qquad x = \dfrac{50}{20}$$

   Reduce $x = 2.5$ Answer is 2.5

2. $\dfrac{1}{3} = \dfrac{x}{18}$

   Cross multiply $3x = 18$

   Divide each side of the equation by the number in front of the x.

   $$\dfrac{3x}{3} = \dfrac{18}{3} \qquad x = \dfrac{18}{3}$$

   Reduce $x = 6$ Answer is 6

3. $\dfrac{x}{24} = \dfrac{5}{12}$

   Cross multiply $12x = 120$

   Divide each side of the equation by the number in front of the x.

   $$\dfrac{12x}{12} = \dfrac{120}{12} \qquad x = \dfrac{120}{12}$$

   Reduce $x = 10$ Answer is 10

4. $\dfrac{x}{40} = \dfrac{5}{8}$

   Cross multiply $8x = 200$

   Divide each side of the equation by the number in front of the x.

   $$\dfrac{8x}{8} = \dfrac{200}{8} \qquad x = \dfrac{200}{8}$$

   Reduce $x = 25$ Answer is 25

Answers to Chapter Review Problems

Chapter Review Problem Answers 1-1

1. XIX = 19

2. VIII = 8

3. XIV = 14

4. XXVI = 26

Chapter Review Problem Answers 1-2

1. $13 = XIII$

2. $4 = IV$

3. $23 = XXIII$

4. $31 = XXXI$

Chapter Review Problem Answers 1-3

1. $\dfrac{9}{5} = 1\dfrac{4}{5}$

2. $\dfrac{5}{3} = 1\dfrac{2}{3}$

3. $\dfrac{7}{2} = 3\dfrac{1}{2}$

4. $\dfrac{13}{4} = 3\dfrac{1}{4}$

Chapter Review Problem Answers 1-4

1. $4\dfrac{1}{2} = \dfrac{(4 \times 2) + 1}{2} = \dfrac{9}{2}$

2. $5\dfrac{1}{3} = \dfrac{(5 \times 3) + 1}{3} = \dfrac{16}{3}$

3. $2\dfrac{7}{8} = \dfrac{(2 \times 8) + 7}{8} = \dfrac{23}{8}$

4. $3\dfrac{5}{6} = \dfrac{(3 \times 6) + 5}{6} = \dfrac{23}{6}$

Chapter Review Problem Answers 1-5

1. $\dfrac{1}{8} + 2\dfrac{1}{4}$

   $\dfrac{1}{8} + \dfrac{9}{4} = \dfrac{1}{8} + \dfrac{18}{8} = \dfrac{19}{8}$ or $2\dfrac{3}{8}$

2. $\dfrac{3}{5} + \dfrac{3}{10}$

   $\dfrac{6}{10} + \dfrac{3}{10} = \dfrac{9}{10}$

3. $\dfrac{1}{4} + \dfrac{2}{3}$

   $\dfrac{3}{12} + \dfrac{8}{12} = \dfrac{11}{12}$

4. $\dfrac{6}{9} + \dfrac{5}{6}$

   $\dfrac{12}{18} + \dfrac{15}{18} = \dfrac{27}{18} = 1\dfrac{9}{18} = 1\dfrac{1}{2}$

Chapter Review Problem Answers 1-6

1. $\dfrac{7}{8} - \dfrac{1}{4}$

   $\dfrac{7}{8} - \dfrac{2}{8} = \dfrac{5}{8}$

2. $\dfrac{4}{5} - \dfrac{1}{2}$

   $\dfrac{8}{10} - \dfrac{5}{10} = \dfrac{3}{10}$

3. $\dfrac{7}{9} - \dfrac{2}{6}$

   $\dfrac{14}{18} - \dfrac{6}{18} = \dfrac{8}{18} = \dfrac{4}{9}$

4. $\dfrac{1}{3} - \dfrac{2}{9}$

   $\dfrac{3}{9} - \dfrac{2}{9} = \dfrac{1}{9}$

Chapter Review Problem Answers 1-7

1. $\dfrac{5}{6} \times \dfrac{4}{7} = \dfrac{20}{42}$ or $\dfrac{10}{21}$

2. $\dfrac{2}{3} \times \dfrac{3}{8} = \dfrac{6}{24}$ or $\dfrac{1}{4}$

3. $\dfrac{5}{9} \times \dfrac{1}{2} = \dfrac{5}{18}$

4. $\dfrac{7}{10} \times \dfrac{1}{3} = \dfrac{7}{30}$

Chapter Review Problem Answers 1-8

1. $\dfrac{6}{7} \div \dfrac{1}{5}$

$\dfrac{6}{7} \times \dfrac{5}{1} = \dfrac{30}{7} = 4\dfrac{2}{7}$

2. $\dfrac{2}{3} \div \dfrac{1}{4}$

$\dfrac{2}{3} \times \dfrac{4}{1} = \dfrac{8}{3} = 2\dfrac{2}{3}$

3. $\dfrac{5}{6} \div \dfrac{1}{2}$

$\dfrac{5}{6} \times \dfrac{2}{1} = \dfrac{10}{6} = 1\dfrac{4}{6}$ or $1\dfrac{2}{3}$

4. $\dfrac{3}{7} \div \dfrac{2}{5}$

$\dfrac{3}{7} \times \dfrac{5}{2} = \dfrac{15}{14} = 1\dfrac{1}{14}$

Chapter Review Problem Answers 1-9

1. $2.67 + 4.89$

```
  2.67
+ 4.89
  7.56
```

2. $5.168 + 1.801$

```
  5.168
+ 1.801
  6.969
```

3. $6.811 + 3.01$

```
  6.811
+ 3.01
  9.821
```

4. $2.44 + 1.92$

```
  2.44
+ 1.92
  4.36
```

Chapter Review Problem Answers 1-10

1. $8.66 - 2.01$

```
  8.66
- 2.01
  6.65
```

2. $5.926 - 3.234$

```
  5.926
- 3.234
  2.692
```

3. $1.894 - 0.762$

```
  1.894
- 0.762
  1.132
```

4. $7.54 - 2.82$

```
  7.54
- 2.82
- 2.82
```

Chapter Review Problem Answers 1-11

1. 4.8×2.1

```
   4.8
×  2.1
    48
   96
 10.08
```

2. 3.4×4.2

```
   3.4
×  4.2
    68
  136
 14.28
```

3. 11.3 × 3.4

$$\begin{array}{r}11.3\\ \times\ 3.4\\ \hline 452\\ 339\\ \hline 38.42\end{array}$$

4. 8.2 × 1.6

$$\begin{array}{r}8.2\\ \times\ 1.6\\ \hline 492\\ 82\\ \hline 13.12\end{array}$$

Chapter Review Problem Answers 1-12

1. 7.2 ÷ 1.5

$1.5\overline{)7.2}$ → $15\overline{)72.0}$ →

$$\begin{array}{r}4.8\\ 15\overline{)72.0}\\ 60\\ \hline 120\\ 120\\ \hline 0\end{array}$$

3. 8.88 ÷ 2.22

$2.22\overline{)8.88}$ → $222\overline{)888}$ →

$$\begin{array}{r}4\\ 222\overline{)888}\\ 888\\ \hline 0\end{array}$$

2. 4.65 ÷ 3.1

$3.1\overline{)4.65}$ → $31\overline{)46.5}$ →

$$\begin{array}{r}1.5\\ 31\overline{)465}\\ 31\\ \hline 155\\ 155\\ \hline 0\end{array}$$

4. 81.7 ÷ 1.9

$1.9\overline{)81.7}$ → $19\overline{)817}$ →

$$\begin{array}{r}43\\ 19\overline{)817}\\ 76\\ \hline 57\\ 57\\ \hline 0\end{array}$$

Chapter Review Problem Answers 1-13

1. $\frac{x}{5}=\frac{7}{10}$ $10x=35$ $\frac{10x}{10}=\frac{35}{10}=3\frac{1}{2}$

3. $\frac{x}{6}=\frac{3}{4}$ $4x=18$ $\frac{4x}{4}=\frac{18}{4}=4\frac{1}{2}$

2. $\frac{4}{8}=\frac{x}{4}$ $8x=16$ $\frac{8x}{8}=\frac{16}{8}=2$

4. $\frac{2}{3}=\frac{x}{18}$ $3x=36$ $\frac{3x}{3}=\frac{36}{3}=12$

Systems of Measurement

This chapter contains content on:

- **Metric System**
- **Apothecary System**
- **Household Measurement System**

Learning Objectives

Upon completion of Chapter 2, you will be able to:

- Identify the conversion equivalents for metric, household, and apothecary measurements.
- Apply the metric, household, and apothecary equivalents appropriately and accurately.
- Discuss milligrams and milliliters as appropriate in dosage calculations.

Key Terms

- Apothecary system
- Household measurement system
- International System of Units
- Metric system
- Milligrams

CASE STUDY

Mrs. Sawyer, a 72-year-old woman, is receiving home care nursing services following coronary artery bypass surgery. Mrs. Sawyer has a history of diabetes mellitus, hypertension, and mild heart failure. Her daughter is visiting this morning. Mrs. Sawyer is on the following medications:

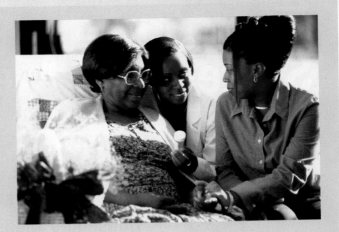

- Milk of Magnesia $\frac{1}{2}$ ounce as needed for constipation
- Digoxin (Lanoxin) 0.25 milligrams p.o. q A.M.
- Enalapril (Vasotec) 10 mg p.o. q A.M.
- Robitussin syrup 2 teaspoons every 4 hours as needed for cough

When you ask Mrs. Sawyer about her medications, she says, "Sometimes I get confused, because the two pills say 'milligrams' and the liquid says 'ounces.'"

Medication doses may vary, based on the manner in which the medication is prepared, such as in a liquid or according to the weight or amount of medication in a tablet or capsule. Thus dosage orders may be written in one measurement system, while the drug company supplies the medication using a different system. The nurse is responsible for recognizing and interpreting the different systems of measurements used to express medication doses.

Three common systems of measurement are used for drug dosages. These are the metric, household, and apothecary measurement systems. Your goal is to accurately convert dosages from one system to the other.

The drug companies and many prescribers use the metric system. However, in the home setting, families commonly use household measurements, due to the availability of common utensils or containers such as a teaspoon or a measuring cup. On rare occasions, medication dosages may be prescribed using the apothecary system, if the prescriber is more familiar with that dosage or if it is an older drug product.

Three terms related to measurement must be understood: weight, volume, and length. Weight of the medication, the most common measurement, is expressed in metric terms such as milligrams or grams. Volume, the total amount of liquid, also relates to the quantity of medication in the liquid, and to the concentration. Volume is expressed in terms such as milliliters, liters, or ounces. Length is rarely used as a measurement; however, when used, it relates to height, or to the circumference of an infant's head. Length may be used when a topical paste or ointment is ordered and the unit of measurement is millimeters or centimeters.

THE METRIC SYSTEM

The **metric system** is an international system of weights and measures that uses meter, liter, and gram as the units of measurement, and is based on multiples of 10. The metric system is used exclusively in the *United States Pharmacopeia* and is a common system used worldwide. In 1960, the **International System of Units (SI)** (SI stands for the French Système International d'Unités) was adopted as the standard system of abbreviations for the metric units of measurement. Use of the metric system is being encouraged worldwide in the hopes that it will become the only measurement system used.

The information presented in Chapter 1 related to decimals and Arabic numbers applies when using the metric system. When converting from larger to smaller units in the metric system, move the decimal point to the right one place for every increment of ten. When converting from smaller to larger units, move the decimal point to the left for every increment of 10. For example, when changing milliliters to liters you need to move the decimal point three places to the left—

$$100 \text{ mL} = 0.1 \text{ L}.$$

When changing liters to milliliters, you need to move the decimal point three places, but to the right—

$$1.5 \text{ L} = 1500 \text{ mL}.$$

In the metric system, length is expressed in meters, weight is expressed in grams, and volume is expressed in liters. Prefixes are used to denote the exact measurement. Important ones to remember include:

- micro, meaning one millionth, or 0.000001, or $\frac{1}{1,000,000}$
- milli, meaning one thousandth, or 0.001, or $\frac{1}{1000}$
- centi, meaning one hundredth, or 0.01, or $\frac{1}{100}$
- deci, meaning one tenth, or 0.1, or $\frac{1}{10}$
- kilo, meaning one thousand, or 1000, times the unit

Abbreviations in SI units and equivalents that you will need to remember for the metric system are listed below.

	Unit	Abbreviation	Equivalents
Weight	gram	g	1 g = 1000 mg
	milligram	mg	1 mg = 1000 mcg = 0.001 g
	microgram	mcg	1 mcg = 0.001 mg = 0.000001 g
	kilogram	kg	1 kg = 1000 g
Volume	liter	L	1 L = 1000 mL
	milliliter	mL	1 mL = 0.001 L = 1 cc
	cubic centimeter	cc	1 cc = 1 mL = 0.001 L
Length	meter	m	1 m = 100 cm = 1000 mm
	centimeter	cm	1 cm = 0.01 m = 10 mm
	millimeter	mm	1 mm = 0.001 m = 0.1 cm

 SAFETY ALERT: *Do not confuse weight, volume, and length units that have similar names. Milligram is a weight unit, milliliter is a volume unit, and millimeter is a length unit.*

Remember these basic rules when working with the metric system:

- Arabic numbers come before the metric abbreviation. Example: 0.4 mL or 5 kg.
- Abbreviations are always written with lowercase letters except for liter or the L in milliliter—these are capitalized. Example: mg = milligram; mL = milliliter.
- Fractions are not used. Fractions are written as decimals. Example: write 0.25 mL rather than $\frac{1}{4}$ mL.
- A leading zero is always added to the left of the decimal point if there is no whole number. Do not add a trailing zero to the right of the decimal point. Example: write 0.3 mL rather than .3 mL. Write 1 mg rather than 1.0 mg.

SAFETY ALERT: *As part of the National Patient Safety Goals, the Joint Commission on Accreditation of Healthcare Organizations has set up specific guidelines for the use of leading and trailing zeroes. The rule in the metric system is critical to preventing confusion and medication errors. Always use this rule correctly. Double check the placement of the decimal and the zero.*

CASE STUDY

You review Mrs. Sawyer's medications with her, explaining the difference between ounces and milligrams. You explain to Mrs. Sawyer that milligrams are part of the metric system and are a measure of weight. Many medication dosages are in milligrams.

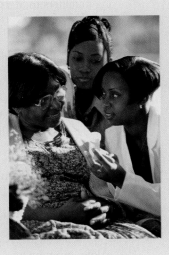

PRACTICE PROBLEMS 2-1. Practice Problems for Converting Metric Weights

DIRECTIONS: Convert the following weights by moving the decimal point. The answers to the problems can be found at the end of the chapter.

1. 0.5 g = _____ mg
2. 4 kg = _____ g
3. 225 mg = _____ g
4. 1,555 mcg = _____ mg

5. 0.125 mg = _____ mcg
6. 0.008 g = _____ mg
7. 0.1 mg = _____ mcg
8. 0.02 g = _____ mg

PRACTICE PROBLEMS 2-2. Practice Problems for Converting Metric Volumes

DIRECTIONS: Convert the following volumes by moving the decimal point. The answers to the problems can be found at the end of the chapter.

1. 3,000 mL = _____ L
2. 0.15 L = _____ mL
3. 100 mL = _____ L

4. 2.5 L = _____ mL
5. 775 mL = _____ L
6. 0.6 L = _____ mL

THE APOTHECARY SYSTEM

Prescribers seldom use the **apothecary system** today when ordering dosages of medications. However, some older medications, such as aspirin, or liquid medications, such as laxatives, are still ordered using this system.

The two basic units of measurement in the apothecary system are weight and volume. The basic unit for weight is grains. Volume is expressed in minim, dram, or ounce.

Important abbreviations and terms that you need to remember when working with the apothecary system are highlighted below.

Unit	Term	Abbreviation
Weight	Grain	gr
Volume	Minim	m
	Dram	dr or ʒ
	Ounce	oz or ℥

Remember these basic rules when using the apothecary system:

- The apothecary abbreviation goes before the quantity of the medication. For example, gr x.
- Lowercase Roman numerals are used to indicate smaller quantities. For example, aspirin gr v is ordered. The Roman numeral for one (i) will usually have a dot over it such as viï (to prevent making a mistake or to avoid confusion).
- Fractions are used when ordering quantities less than one. The exception is $\frac{1}{2}$, which is written as ss̈.
- When larger quantities are ordered, either Roman numerals or Arabic numbers can be used.

Conversion of Weight Units

At times, you may need to convert weight units from the apothecary system to the metric system. Use the following table for conversions:

Apothecary and Metric Equivalents

Grain	Milligram	Gram	Microgram
gr $\frac{1}{200}$	0.3 mg		300 mcg
gr $\frac{1}{100}$	0.6 mg		600 mcg
gr $\frac{1}{6}$	10 mg	0.01 g	
gr $\frac{1}{4}$	15 mg	0.015 g	
gr ss̈	30 mg	0.03 g	
gr i	60 mg	0.06 g	
gr i ss̈	100 mg	0.1 g	
gr iii	200 mg	0.2 g	
gr v	300 mg	0.3 g	
gr x	600 mg	0.6 g	
gr xv	1000 mg	1 g	

 SAFETY ALERT: *Remember, when converting from the apothecary to the metric system, equivalents are not exact.*

You may notice that one aspirin is equivalent to 325 mg or gr v. However, you note on the table that gr v is equivalent to 300 mg. The difference occurs because you are trying to convert from the apothecary system to the metric system and this conversion is not exact. When solving dosage problems requiring conversion from one system to another, use the equivalent that is closer. For example, if the prescriber orders aspirin gr v and the label reads aspirin 325 mg per tablet, you will administer the entire tablet because the dosage is close. This inaccuracy in conversion is one of the reasons that the apothecary system is seldom used.

 CASE STUDY

As you continue to review Mrs. Sawyer's medications with her, you provide teaching on Milk of Magnesia. You explain that it is a liquid medication that has been ordered in ounces. Ounces are part of the apothecary system and are a measure of volume of a liquid.

PRACTICE PROBLEMS 2-3. Practice Problems for Converting Apothecary and Metric Weight Measures

DIRECTIONS: Convert the following apothecary and metric measures. The answers to the problems can be found at the end of the chapter.

1. gr vss̄ = _____ mg

2. gr viiss̄ = _____ g

3. 300 mg = gr _____

4. gr $\frac{1}{150}$ = _____ mg

5. 90 mg = gr _____

6. 400 mcg = gr _____

Conversion of Liquid Measurements

When you need to convert from the apothecary to the metric equivalents for liquids, use the following conversion table:

Apothecary and Metric Equivalents for Liquid Measures

Unit	Abbreviation	Volume	Metric Equivalent
Drop	gtt	15	1 mL
Minim	min, m, *m*, or mx	15–16	1 mL
Dram	dr or ʒ	1	4 mL
Ounce	oz or ℥	1	30 mL
Dram	dr or ʒ	8	1 oz
Pint	pt	16 oz	500 mL
Quart	qt	32 oz	1000 mL
Gallon	gal	4 qts	4000 mL

Note that the symbol for ounce may have a line through the top or it may have two top loops, whereas the dram symbol has only one top loop. Because of the similarity of these two symbols and the risk of misinterpretation, many physicians avoid using them. However, as a nurse, you must remember the difference.

 SAFETY ALERT: *Be careful to accurately interpret the ounce and dram symbols. If you misread the dram symbol for an ounce, it results in a mistake of 8 times the amount ordered.*

PRACTICE PROBLEMS 2-4. Practice Problems for Converting Apothecary and Metric Liquid Measures

DIRECTIONS: Convert the following apothecary and metric liquid measures. The answers to the problems can be found at the end of the chapter.

1. dr 2 = _____ mL

2. 3 oz = dr _____

3. 1.5 mL = m _____

4. gtt 10 = _____ mL

5. $\frac{1}{4}$ oz = dr _____

6. m 4 = _____ mL

Apothecary to Metric Conversions

When it is necessary to change from the apothecary to the metric systems, be sure to follow this guide:

- Look up the system and its equivalent values, such as when you are trying to determine how many ounces there are in 24 drams. You determine there are 8 drams in 1 ounce.
- Use the fraction or ratio format:

$$\frac{8 \text{ drams}}{1 \text{ ounce}} \quad \text{or} \quad 8 \text{ drams:1 ounce}$$

- Remember the numerators and denominators must be in the same system and you must solve for the unknown, *x*:

$$\frac{8 \text{ drams}}{1 \text{ ounce}} : \frac{24 \text{ drams}}{x} \quad \text{or} \quad 8 \text{ drams:1 ounce::24 drams:} x \text{ ounces}$$

Cross multiply, dropping the measurement terms.

$$8 \text{ drams} \times x \text{ ounces} = 24 \text{ drams} \times 1 \text{ ounce}$$
$$8x = 24$$

- Then solve for *x* by dividing both sides by the number in front of the *x*, which in this case is 8.

$$\frac{8x}{8} = \frac{24}{8} \qquad \frac{1}{1}\frac{\cancel{8}x}{\cancel{8}} = \frac{\cancel{24}}{\cancel{8}}\frac{3}{1} \qquad x = 3 \text{ ounces}$$

If you need this amount in a metric system unit, recall that 1 ounce = 30 mL. Therefore, you will administer

$$30 \text{ mL} \times 3 \text{ ounces} = 90 \text{ mL.}$$

HOUSEHOLD MEASUREMENT SYSTEM

The **household measurement system** uses as units such items as a teaspoon, tablespoon, cup, pint, quart, and even a medicine dropper. This system is convenient when preparing dosages since it involves common containers found in the home. This system of measurement is important to understand because nurses play a major role in teaching patients exactly what dose to use at home. This commonly involves converting from the metric or apothecary system to the household equivalent. However, remember that the household system is the least accurate system, because containers vary in shape, capacity, and design. For example, some containers are a solid, nontransparent color, making it difficult to see the exact measurement. Always use a clear measuring cup and use the teaspoon, tablespoon, and other measuring utensils used for baking or cooking, to be as accurate as possible. Today many suppliers are providing measuring spoons, droppers, and ounce cups to assist people taking medicine at home.

> **⚠ SAFETY ALERT:** *Remember the household system requires that you use household utensils that are marked or calibrated to ensure accurate doses. Always remember to review the household abbreviations and equivalents, and be extremely careful not to confuse the abbreviations for teaspoon (t) and tablespoon (T). Since 1 teaspoon equals 5 mL and 1 tablespoon equals 15 mL, a mistake could mean the patient receives 3 times the prescribed dose of medication.*

When you need to convert from the household to the metric system, use the following table for conversions:

Household Measurements and Metric Equivalents

Unit of Measure	Abbreviation	Household	Metric Equivalent
Drop*	gtt	15 gtts	1 mL
Teaspoon	tsp or t	60 gtts	4–5 mL
Tablespoon	T, tbs, or tbsp	3 teaspoons	15 mL
Ounce	oz	2 tablespoons	30 mL
Cup	C	6 ounces**	180 mL
Glass or cup	gl	8 ounces	240 mL
Pint	pt	16 ounces	480 mL (approx 500 mL)
Quart	qt	2 pints	1000 mL

*Remember: A drop is always equal to 1 drop regardless if the liquid is thick or thin.
**Refers to a tea cup.

When you need to change from the metric to the household system, follow these guidelines:

- For safety and accuracy, look up the system and its equivalent values such as if you were trying to determine how many ounces are in 6 tablespoons. You determine the equivalent value of 2 tablespoons is 1 ounce.

- Use the fraction or ratio format such as:

$$\frac{2 \text{ tbs}}{1 \text{ oz}} \quad \text{or} \quad 2 \text{ tbs:1 oz.}$$

- Determine the desired quantity by solving for x in a ratio or a fraction format, keeping the desired unit of measurement in mind, in this example, ounces. Remember that the numerator and denominator have to be in the same measurement system. Therefore, the setup will look like:

$$\frac{2 \text{ tbs}}{1 \text{ oz}} : \frac{6 \text{ tbs}}{x}$$

- Next you will cross multiply, then solve for x:

$$2 \text{ tbs} \times x = 6 \text{ tbs} \times 1 \text{ oz}$$
$$2x = 6$$

- Then solve for x by placing the number before the x on both sides of the equation. In this case you use the number 2.

$$\frac{2x}{2} = \frac{6}{2}$$

- Now simply reduce the equation and in this case $x = 3$. Therefore, the correct answer is 3 ounces.

$$\frac{1 \, \cancel{2}x}{1 \, \cancel{2}} = \frac{\cancel{6}^{\,3}}{\cancel{2}^{\,1}} \qquad x = 3$$

PRACTICE PROBLEMS 2-5. Practice Problems for Converting Household Measurements

DIRECTIONS: Convert the following household equivalents. The answers to the problems can be found at the end of the chapter.

1. 2 tsp = _____ drops

2. $\frac{1}{2}$ cup = _____ tablespoons

3. 10 ounces = _____ cup/gl

4. 4 tbsp = _____ ounces

5. $1\frac{1}{2}$ tbsp = _____ teaspoons

6. $1\frac{3}{4}$ pint = _____ cup/gl

Critical Thinking/Decision Making Exercise

One of the patients assigned to Susan, a nurse on the surgical floor, is Mr. Stoneman. Mr. Stoneman is 65 years old and had abdominal surgery yesterday. Mr. Stoneman has a history of diabetes for 15 years. Mr. Stoneman has an order for nothing by mouth and therefore requires insulin to keep his blood sugar down. As Susan checks Mr. Stoneman's orders she sees that the physician has given the following order:

Physician's Orders

Page 1 of 1

1. Imprint set at top. Insert in chart.
2. After each medication order, remove Pharmacy Copy and send to Pharmacy.

DRUG SENSITIVITY AND PERTINENT DIAGNOSIS

DATE	TIME	PHYSICIAN'S ORDERS	REASON	READ BACK	NURSE INITIALS
10/24/07	0845	*Humulin Regular Insulin, 2.0 units subq*			

PLEASE USE BALLPOINT PEN

DATE: *10/24/07*   PHYSICIAN SIGNATURE: *Dr. Perry*   NARCOTIC NUMBER:

PHYSICIAN'S ORDERS   **CHART COPY**

Susan obtains the Humulin Regular Insulin from the refrigerator and draws up 20 units in the insulin syringe. Per institution policy, prior to giving the insulin Susan has another nurse verify the dosage and medication. The nurse checks the order in the chart and then the insulin Susan has drawn up. She questions why Susan has drawn up 20 units of insulin when it looks to her like the physician has ordered 2 units. What should Susan's action be at this time?

The Next Action

Susan holds the insulin for now, and double checks the written order. Because there is a question of the dosage that was ordered, Susan contacts Dr. Perry to verify the correct dosage of insulin. Dr. Perry tells Susan that he wants Mr. Stoneman to receive 2 units of insulin.

Prevention

How could this situation have been prevented?

The problem in this situation initially arose because Dr. Perry used a decimal point and trailing zero when writing his order. If Dr. Perry had followed the National Patient Safety Goals by the Joint Commission on Accreditation of Healthcare Organizations, which states that trailing zeroes should not be used, this problem would have been prevented. Also, Susan should have called Dr. Perry and clarified the insulin order before drawing up the medication. She should have recognized that 20 units of regular insulin is a significant dose and questioned if that was correct. By following the institution's policy on having insulin dosages checked by a second nurse, Susan did avoid making a serious medication error.

 CASE STUDY

After completely reviewing Mrs. Sawyer's medications with her, she thanks you and says, "Now I understand why the dosage for each of the medications is different." You complete the visit, assessing her suture line, which is well approximated and without any drainage or redness, and her nutritional status.

Mrs. Sawyer tells you that she is enjoying her time in the outpatient cardiac rehabilitation program walking with other people who have had heart surgery. On her next visit, you plan to reassess Mrs. Sawyer's understanding of her medications and dosages.

CHAPTER REVIEW PROBLEMS

The answers to the problems can be found at the end of the chapter.

Review Problems 2-1. Convert the following metric weights by moving the decimal point.

1. 0.3 g = _____ mg

2. 0.002 g = _____ mg

3. 0.3 mg = _____ mcg

4. 125 mg = _____ g

5. 12 kg = _____ g

6. 0.01 g = _____ mg

Review Problems 2-2. Convert the following metric volumes by moving the decimal points.

1. 400 mL = _____ L

2. 0.75 L = _____ mL

3. 8000 mL = _____ L

4. 150 mL = _____ L

5. 4.8 L = _____ mL

6. 0.2 L = _____ mL

Review Problems 2-3. Convert the following apothecary and metric weight measures.

1. 30 mg = gr _____

2. gr 4 = _____ mg

3. 150 mg = gr _____

4. gr $\frac{1}{100}$ = _____ mg

5. gr x = _____ g

6. 200 mcg = gr _____

Review Problems 2-4. Convert the following apothecary and metric liquid measures.

1. 30 gtt = _____ mL

2. $\frac{1}{2}$ oz = dr _____

3. dr 6 = _____ mL

4. 0.75 mL = m _____

5. 8 oz = dr _____

6. m 45 = _____ mL

Review Problems 2-5. Convert the following to household measurements.

1. $\frac{3}{4}$ gl/cup = _____ ounces

2. 4 ounces = _____ gl/cup

3. $\frac{1}{4}$ pint = _____ ounces

4. 6 teaspoons = _____ tbs

5. 2 teaspoons = gtt _____

6. $\frac{1}{2}$ ounce = _____ tbs

Answers to Practice Problems

Practice Problem Answers 2-1

1. 0.5 g = 500 mg

2. 4 kg = 4000 g

3. 225 mg = 0.225 g

4. 1555 mcg = 1.555 mg

5. 0.125 mg = 125 mcg

6. 0.008 g = 8 mg

7. 0.1 mg = 100 mcg

8. 0.02 g = 20 mg

Practice Problem Answers 2-2

1. 3000 mL = 3 L

2. 0.15 L = 150 mL

3. 100 mL = 0.1 L

4. 2.5 L = 2500 mL

5. 775 mL = 0.775 L

6. 0.6 L = 600 mL

Practice Problem Answers 2-3

1. gr v$\dot{s}\dot{s}$ = 330 mg

2. gr vii$\dot{s}\dot{s}$ = 0.5 g

3. 300 mg = gr v

4. gr $\dfrac{1}{150}$ = 0.4 mg

5. 90 mg = gr i$\dot{s}\dot{s}$

6. 400 mcg = gr $\dfrac{1}{150}$

Practice Problem Answers 2-4

1. dr 2 = 8 mL

2. 3 oz = dr 24

3. 1.5 mL = m 24 (1 mL = 16 m)

4. gtt 10 = 0.67 mL

5. $\dfrac{1}{4}$ oz = dr 2

6. m 4 = 0.25 mL

Practice Problem Answers 2-5

1. 2 tsp = 120 drops

2. $\dfrac{1}{2}$ cup = 8 tablespoons

3. 10 ounces = $1\dfrac{1}{4}$ cup (gl)

4. 4 tbsp = 2 ounces

5. $1\dfrac{1}{2}$ tbsp = 4.5 teaspoons

6. $1\dfrac{3}{4}$ pint = 3.5 cups

Answers to Chapter Review Problems

Chapter Review Problem Answers 2-1

1. 300 mg
2. 2 mg
3. 300 mcg

4. 0.125 g
5. 12,000 g
6. 10 mg

Chapter Review Problem Answers 2-2

1. 0.4 L
2. 750 mL
3. 8 L

4. 0.15 L
5. 4,800 mL
6. 200 mL

Chapter Review Problem Answers 2-3

1. gr ṡṡ
2. 240 mg
3. gr ii ṡṡ

4. 0.6 mg
5. 0.6 g
6. gr $\dfrac{1}{300}$

Chapter Review Problem Answers 2-4

1. 2 mL
2. dr 4
3. 24 mL

4. m 12 (1 mL = 16 m)
5. dr 60
6. 3 mL

Chapter Review Problem Answers 2-5

1. 6 ounces
2. $\dfrac{1}{2}$ cup (gl)
3. 4 ounces

4. 2 tbs
5. gtts 120
6. 1 tbs

Preparing Equipment and Drugs for Administration

This chapter contains content on:

- **Equipment for Liquid Oral Medications**
- **Syringes**

Learning Objectives

Upon completion of Chapter 3, you will be able to:

- Select the correct type of measuring device for administering oral medications.
- Measure the amount of prescribed liquid medication correctly.
- Select the correct type of syringe to administer parenteral medications.
- Measure the prescribed amount of medication correctly in a syringe.

Key Terms

- Calibrated medication dropper
- Insulin syringe
- Medication spoon
- Medication syringe
- Medicine cup
- Meniscus
- Tuberculin syringe

CASE STUDY

As the nurse on a medical floor working first shift, you are getting ready to set up your 0900 medications for Mrs. Henson. Mrs. Henson was admitted two days ago for treatment of a severe respiratory infection with a persistent productive cough. Periodically, Mrs. Henson is able to cough up small amounts of white mucus. When you auscultate her lungs you hear bibasilar crackles anterior and posterior. She also has a history of constipation, which she treats at home with Milk of Magnesia. She has two oral liquid medications to be given at 0900: Robitussin syrup 2 TSP and Milk of Magnesia 30 mL. Mrs. Henson also is to receive a subcutaneous injection of 5,000 units of heparin for prevention of deep vein thrombosis.

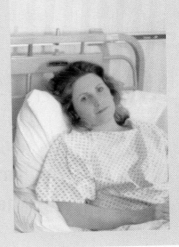

Before you administer the medications, you must be sure to select the correct equipment to set up your medications. Once you have selected the appropriate equipment, you must accurately measure the amount of prescribed medication. Both of these steps are critical to the safe administration of medications. This chapter provides you with the knowledge and skills to do both.

Many oral liquid medication orders require pouring a prescribed amount of liquid medication from a bottle containing a larger volume. Oral liquid medications are usually measured in a medicine cup, a calibrated dropper, or devices made especially for pediatric oral medications. Once the proper amount is measured, the oral liquid can be administered.

Parenteral medications are measured and administered using the appropriate syringe. The type of syringe selected is determined by the medication being administered and the amount prescribed. The most common syringes used for parenteral medication administration include: insulin syringes, 3-mL syringes, tuberculin syringes in 0.5 and 1 mL size, safety syringes, and larger-volume intravenous syringes. Some parenteral medications also come in prefilled syringes.

EQUIPMENT FOR LIQUID ORAL MEDICATIONS

Liquid oral medications are given using a medicine cup, calibrated syringe, or special devices for administering doses of medication to children and calibrated droppers for use with children and specialized medications. When using these devices for oral medications, always measure to a line on the device while holding the device at eye level to measure the liquid. Pour the liquid so that the base or lower edge of the **meniscus** (the natural curve that the liquid makes when poured) is level with the line on the device. This ensures that you pour the accurate dosage of prescribed medication (see Figure 3-1).

Medicine Cup

The **medicine cup** is used to measure most liquid oral medications. As the name implies, it is a disposable plastic cup that holds 30 milliliters, or one ounce, of liquid (see Figure 3-2). Each medicine cup provides measurement units in the metric, apothecary, and household measurement

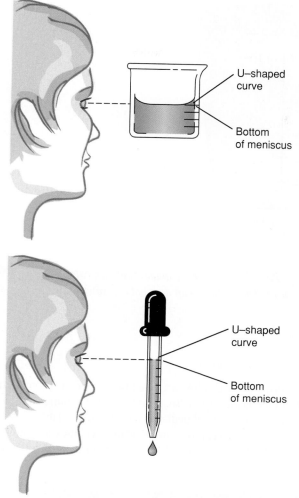

Figure 3-1. The meniscus.

systems. The equivalent measurements on the cup are in milliliters (mL), teaspoon (TSP), tablespoon (TBSP), ounces (OZ), and drams.

To administer the prescribed medication, pour the liquid into the medicine cup up to the marking that corresponds to the ordered dosage. Figure 3-3 shows an ordered medication dosage of 15 mL poured into a medicine cup.

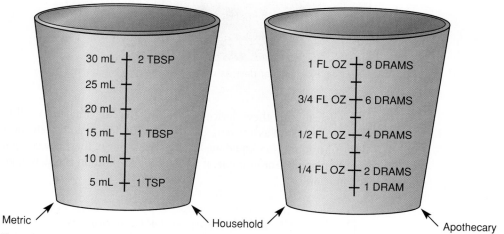

Figure 3-2. Medicine cup showing measurement systems.

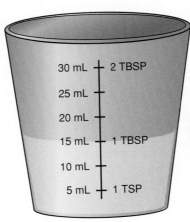

Figure 3-3. Medication dose of 15 mL.

> **SAFETY ALERT:** *To measure amounts of medication less than 2.5 mL, another device should be used. The medicine cup does not accurately measure amounts of medications less than 2.5 mL.*

Special Pediatric Devices

Oral medication dosages for children are often prescribed in amounts that are too small to be accurately measured in medicine cups. Also, infants and very young children are not able to drink from medicine cups. As a result, special pediatric devices are available to administer oral medications to children. The devices are special oral **medication syringes** and **measuring spoons** made especially for liquid medications. Figure 3-4 shows some of the devices available.

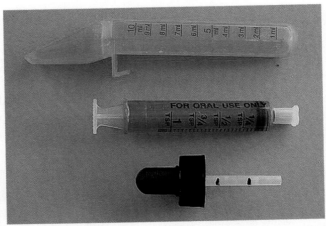

Figure 3-4. Examples of devices used for measuring liquid medications.

When using these devices, make sure that the adult who will be administering the medication at home, such as a parent, has been taught how to accurately measure the medication with the device. To administer liquid medications using one of these devices, pour the medication to the prescribed amount. For example, if 5 mL of the medication is ordered, pour to the 5 mL mark on the spoon handle.

> **SAFETY ALERT:** *Always use a pediatric measuring device when measuring small amounts of medication for infants and children. Household teaspoons and tablespoons vary in size and can be inaccurate when measuring medication dosages.*

Calibrated Medication Dropper

A **calibrated medication dropper** can be used to accurately measure and administer small dosages of liquid medications (see Figure 3-5). A dropper can also be used to give pediatric formulations of liquid medications to children. Droppers are calibrated according to the liquid medication with which they are supplied. Each dropper is specific to the medication so that the correct dosage of the prescribed medication will be given. You cannot change droppers between different types of medications because doing so can lead to a serious medication error.

To use a calibrated dropper, draw up the medication to the prescribed amount on the dropper (see Figure 3-6).

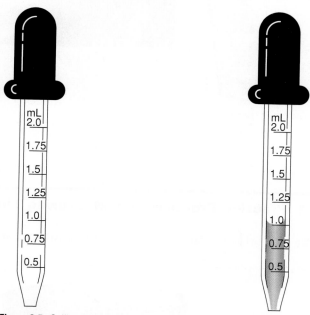

Figure 3-5. Calibrated medication dropper. **Figure 3-6.** Calibrated dropper with 1 mL of medication.

> **⚠ SAFETY ALERT:** *Use the dropper that comes with a medication for that medication only. The droppers are calibrated to deliver correct dosages of the medications with which they are supplied. Interchanging droppers between medications can result in inaccurate medication dosages and potential harm to the patient.*

CASE STUDY

You prepare the Robitussin syrup and Milk of
Magnesia in individual medication cups for
Mrs. Henson. Your medications, after being poured,
would look like this:

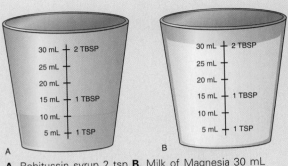

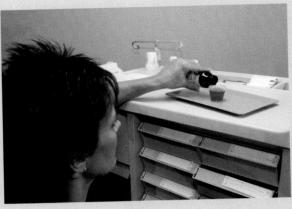

Photo by Rick Brady.

A. Robitussin syrup 2 tsp **B.** Milk of Magnesia 30 mL

PRACTICE PROBLEMS 3-1. Practice Problems for Measuring Liquid Medications

DIRECTIONS: Mark each medication cup at the prescribed level of medication. The answers to the problems can be found at the end of the chapter.

1. 10 mL

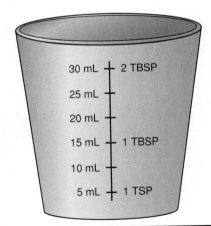

2. 2 tsp

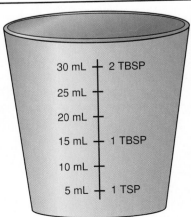

3. 25 mL

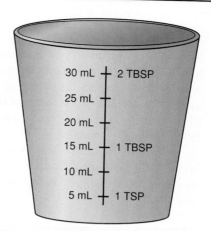

4. $\frac{1}{4}$ ounce

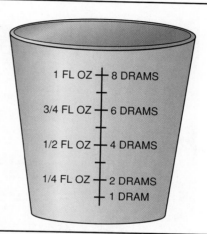

5. dr 6

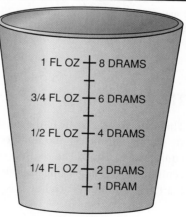

6. 1 tbsp

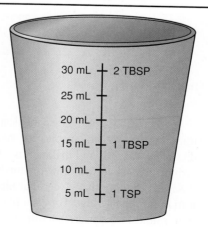

SYRINGES

Syringes are used to accurately measure and administer prescribed amounts of parenteral medications. Parenteral medications are those medications that are given via injection. There are a variety of syringes available for parenteral medications. The type of medication, amount of prescribed medication, and the type of injection required to administer the medication are factors to consider when selecting a syringe. Choosing the correct syringe is important for accurate medication preparation and administration.

The most common syringes used include the 3-mL syringe, 1 mL tuberculin syringe, and insulin syringes, available in sizes of 100 units/mL and 50 units/0.5mL (see Figure 3-7). Syringes also come in 5-mL, 10-mL, 20-mL, and 60-mL sizes. Only the most common syringes are discussed here.

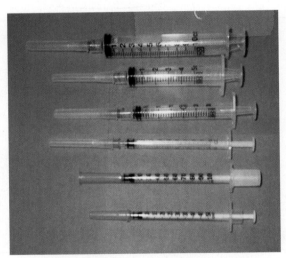

Figure 3-7. Syringes (top to bottom): 10-mL syringe, 5-mL syringe, 3-mL syringe, 1-mL syringe, insulin 100-unit syringe, and insulin 50-unit syringe.

The 3-mL Syringe

The 3-mL syringe is one of the most common syringes used. The syringe is marked with both metric (cubic centimeter) and apothecary (minim) systems (see Figure 3-8). Remember that 1 cc is equivalent to 1 mL. The cc (mL) side of the syringe has line markings for each tenth (0.1) cubic centimeter. The larger line indicates each 0.5 cubic centimeter up to 3 mL. The opposite side has marking in minims. Each line is equivalent to 1 minim.

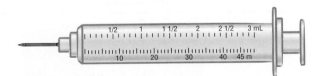

Figure 3-8. A 3-mL syringe.

To accurately measure a medication in a syringe, insert the needle of the syringe into the medication vial. Invert the medication vial with the needle inserted, holding the syringe with the needle facing upwards and maintaining the needle in the medication solution. Then, pull back on the syringe plunger to withdraw the medication from the container into the syringe. If the calculated dosage is more than 1 decimal place, round to the nearest tenth before withdrawing the medication into the syringe. For example, if you calculated that you would need 2.35 mL of a medication, round to the nearest tenth, 2.4, and draw up 2.4 mL of medication. Make sure to draw the medication to the line reading from the top of the black ring on the plunger. Always check to make sure that the syringe is full of medication and does not contain air. Air in the syringe will lead to inaccurate medication dosages.

> ⊘ **SAFETY ALERT:** *Do not use the bottom of the plunger or the middle raised section of the plunger to measure the medication. This will result in an inaccurate amount of medication being withdrawn into the syringe.*

PRACTICE PROBLEMS 3-2. Practice Problems for Using a 3-mL Syringe

DIRECTIONS: Mark each syringe at the prescribed level of medication. Round to the appropriate amount as needed. The answers to the problems can be found at the end of the chapter.

1. 1.4 mL

2. 0.7 mL

3. 2.3 mL

4. 1.65 mL

5. 2.75 mL

6. 0.25 mL

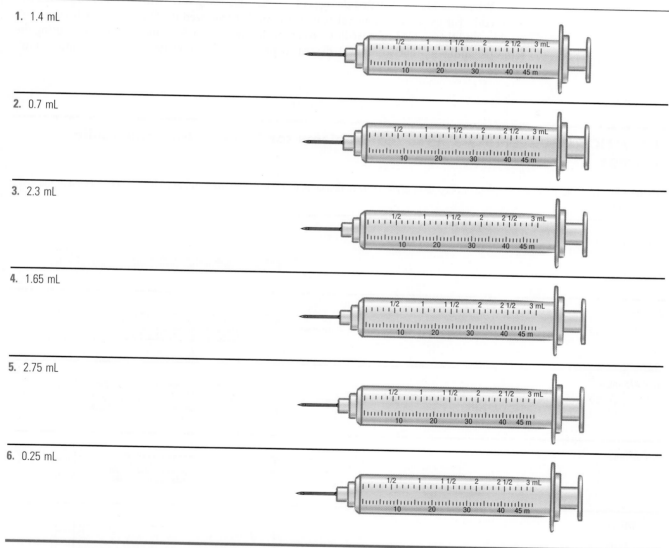

1-mL Tuberculin Syringe

The 1-mL **tuberculin syringe** is a syringe for use in measuring a small dosage of medication, typically those less than 1 mL, and for subcutaneous injections (see Figure 3-9). This type of syringe generally comes with an attached 25-gauge, $\frac{1}{2}$-inch needle.

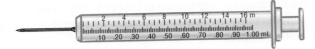

Figure 3-9. Tuberculin or 1-mL syringe.

Note that the lines on a tuberculin syringe are marked in hundredths (0.01) of a milliliter with each 0.1 tenth printed on the syringe. There are apothecary markings of minims on the other side. The markings of 0.01 mL allow very precise measurements of medications.

> **(!) SAFETY ALERT:** *Make sure to use this syringe when the dosage of medication is unusually small and needs to be very precise, such as when administering to children.*

When rounding calculated dosages of medications using this syringe, round to the nearest hundredth. For example, if your calculation shows that you need 0.427 mL of a medication, you would round that to 0.43 mL. Medications are withdrawn into a 1-mL tuberculin syringe using the same technique as that which was described previously for drawing medications into a 3-mL syringe.

PRACTICE PROBLEMS 3-3. Practice Problems for Using a 1-mL Tuberculin Syringe

DIRECTIONS: Mark each syringe at the prescribed level of medication. Round as needed. The answers to the problems can be found at the end of the chapter.

1. 0.15 mL

2. 0.76 mL

3. 0.475 mL

4. 0.82 mL

5. 0.325 mL

6. 0.28 mL

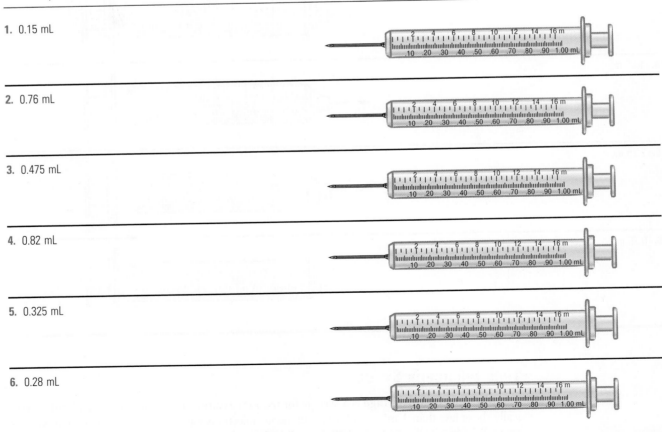

CASE STUDY

You are ready to prepare the subcutaneous injection of heparin for Mrs. Henson. After doing the calculation for the dosage, you know that you need to give her 0.5 mL of heparin solution. Because the dosage is less than 1 mL, you select the 1-mL tuberculin syringe with the 25-gauge, $\frac{1}{2}$-inch needle. After you have drawn up the heparin in the syringe it will look like this:

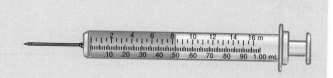

Insulin Syringe

Insulin syringes are used only for the accurate measurement and administration of insulin. The syringe is marked in units rather than in milliliters or minims. The standard insulin syringe is the U-100 syringe that holds 100 units of U-100 insulin, which is equal to 1 mL (see Figure 3-10A). The U-100 syringe should only be used to measure U-100 insulin. For smaller prescribed doses of insulin, a U-100 syringe is available that is marked in units up to 50 units per 0.5 mL. Every 5 units are labeled (see Figure 3-10B).

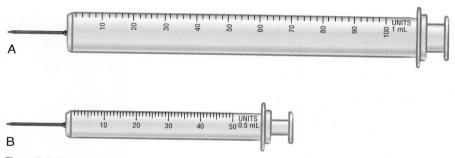

Figure 3-10. Insulin syringes. **A.** 100-unit syringe. **B.** Low-dose or 50-unit syringe.

(!) **SAFETY ALERT:** *For safety and accuracy, always use an insulin syringe when administering insulin.*

PRACTICE PROBLEMS 3-4. Practice Problems for Using a U-100 Insulin Syringe

DIRECTIONS: Mark each syringe at the prescribed level of medication. Round as needed. The answers to the problems can be found at the end of the chapter.

1. 15 units

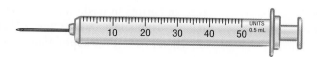

2. 66 units

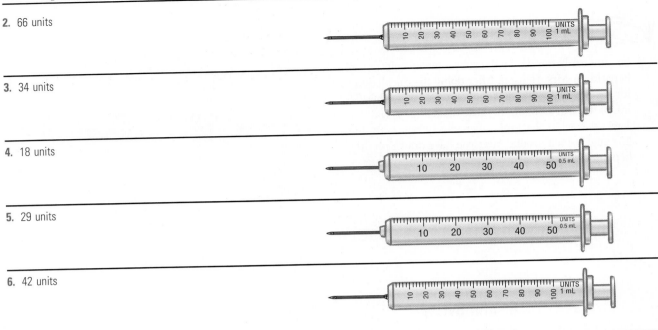

3. 34 units

4. 18 units

5. 29 units

6. 42 units

CASE STUDY

At the end of your shift, you stop by to see if Mrs. Henson is resting comfortably. She says, "My doctor told me that I can go home tomorrow, but I'm worried about my constipation problem at home." You talk with her about ways to increase her fiber and water intake, and arrange for the dietician to discuss foods that will help Mrs. Henson with her problem. Mrs. Henson is discharged home after seeing the dietician with a referral for home care follow up.

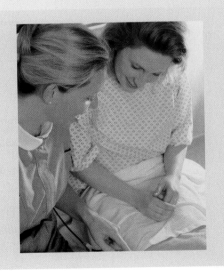

Critical Thinking/Decision Making Exercise

Selecting the incorrect measuring device for oral liquid or parenteral medications leads to inaccuracy and errors in medication dosages. These inaccuracies can result in serious problems for the patient. Thinking about the type and amount of medication prescribed will steer you in the right direction to select the appropriate measuring device.

A patient has the following medication orders:

Regular insulin 4 units (U-100 Insulin) subcutaneously.
Amoxicillin 100 mg. It comes in amoxicillin 250 mg/5 mL.

The nurse calculates that the volume of amoxicillin liquid needed to deliver 100 mg is 2 mL. The nurse sets up the medications like this:

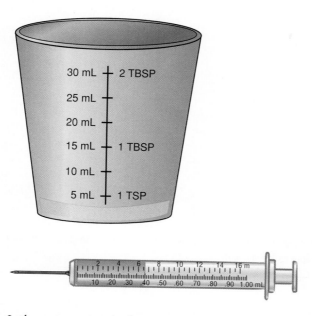

Is the nurse correct in the measurement of the prescribed dosages of the two medications?

Correct Way to Measure Medications

The nurse made two critical errors in selecting measuring devices that would result in the administration of inaccurate medication dosages. The first mistake was selecting a medicine cup to measure the 2 mL of medication. Notice that the first marking on the medicine cup is 5 mL. The medicine cup is inaccurate in measuring dosages of medications less than this amount. The nurse should have used an appropriately calibrated dropper or a medicine spoon or syringe to measure the 2 mL. These devices will accurately measure small volumes of medications.

The second mistake was choosing the incorrect syringe to administer the insulin. Insulin syringes should always be used to accurately measure and administer insulin. Because the regular insulin is U-100 type, a U-100 syringe, most likely a low-dose (50-unit) 0.5 mL syringe is the correct choice. The nurse should have selected this syringe:

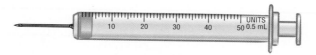

The nurse mistakenly thought that the 0.40 line on the tuberculin syringe was equal to 4 units on the U-100 insulin syringe. If administered, the nurse would have given the patient more insulin than was ordered, possibly resulting in serious adverse effects for the patient.

Prevention

These two serious medication errors could have been prevented if the nurse had reviewed the devices available for preparing oral liquid and parenteral medications. Thinking critically about the type and volume of medication ordered, the nurse would then select the correct measuring device. This would lead to the patient receiving the correct dosage of the prescribed medication.

CHAPTER REVIEW PROBLEMS

The answers to the problems can be found at the end of the chapter.

Review Problems 3-1. Write the letter of the appropriate device that you would use to measure the volume of medication most accurately.

A. Medicine cup
B. Pediatric medication syringe

_____ **1.** 2 tbsp

_____ **2.** $\frac{1}{2}$ tsp

_____ **3.** 1 mL

_____ **4.** dr 4

_____ **5.** 20 mL

_____ **6.** $\frac{3}{4}$ oz

_____ **7.** 0.5 mL

_____ **8.** dr 8

Review Problems 3-2. Using a 3-mL syringe to administer each of the following volumes of medication, mark the syringe at the correct amount (round the calculated volume to the appropriate amount).

1. 2.08 mL

2. 0.99 mL

3. 1.68 mL

4. 0.55 mL

5. 1.23 mL

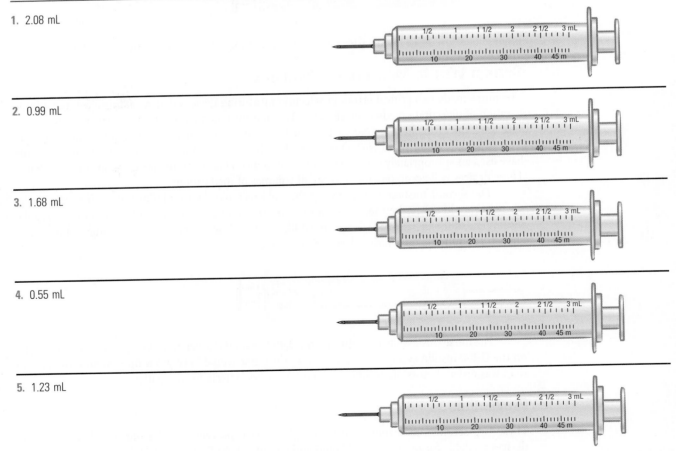

6. 2.11 mL

7. 1.76 mL

8. 0.43 mL

Review Problems 3-3. Using a 1-mL tuberculin syringe to administer each of the following volumes of medication, mark the syringe at the correct amount (round the calculated volume to the appropriate amount).

1. 0.623 mL

2. 0.141 mL

3. 0.899 mL

4. 0.501 mL

5. 0.929 mL

6. 0.722 mL

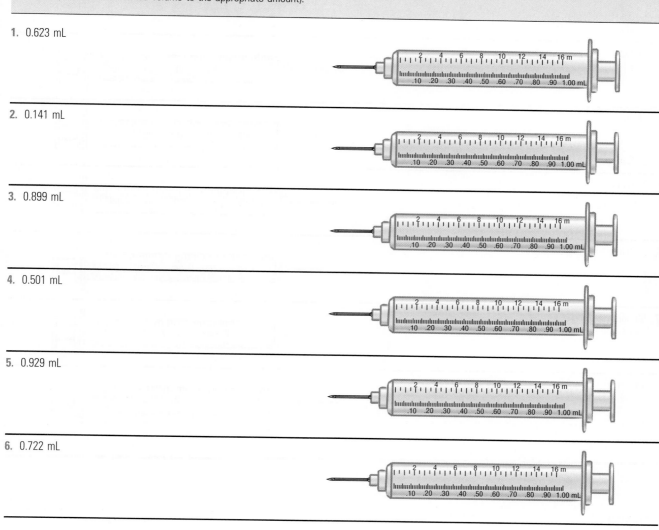

7. 0.366 mL

8. 0.488 mL

Review Problems 3-4. Mark the U-100 insulin syringes for the prescribed amount of insulin.

1. 12 units

2. 46 units

3. 8 units

4. 17 units

5. 33 units

6. 22 units

7. 65 units

8. 74 units

Answers to Practice Problems

Practice Problem Answers 3-1

1.   10 mL

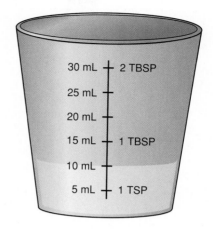

2.   2 tsp

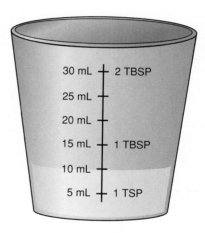

3.   25 mL

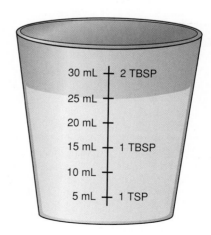

4. $\frac{1}{4}$ ounce

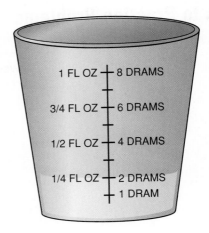

5. dr 6

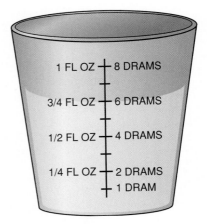

6. 1 tbs

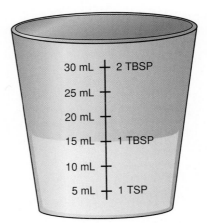

Practice Problem Answers 3-2

1. 1.4 mL

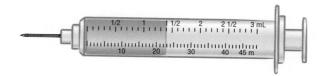

2. 0.7 mL

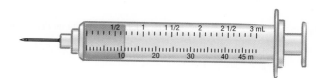

3. 2.3 mL

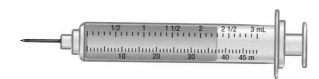

4. 1.65 mL (Round and show at 1.7 mL)

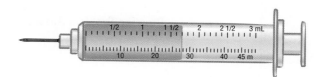

5. 2.75 mL (Round and show at 2.8 mL)

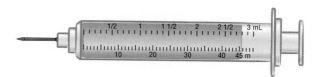

6. 0.25 mL (Round and show at 0.3 mL)

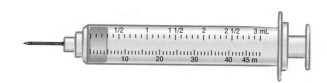

Practice Problem Answers 3-3

1. 0.15 mL

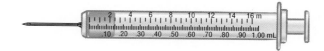

2. 0.76 mL

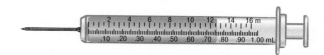

3. 0.475 mL (Round and show at 0.48 mL)

4. 0.82 mL

5. 0.325 mL (Round and show at 0.33 mL)

6. 0.28 mL

Practice Problem Answers 3-4

1. 15 units

2. 66 units

3. 34 units

4. 18 units

5. 29 units

6. 42 units

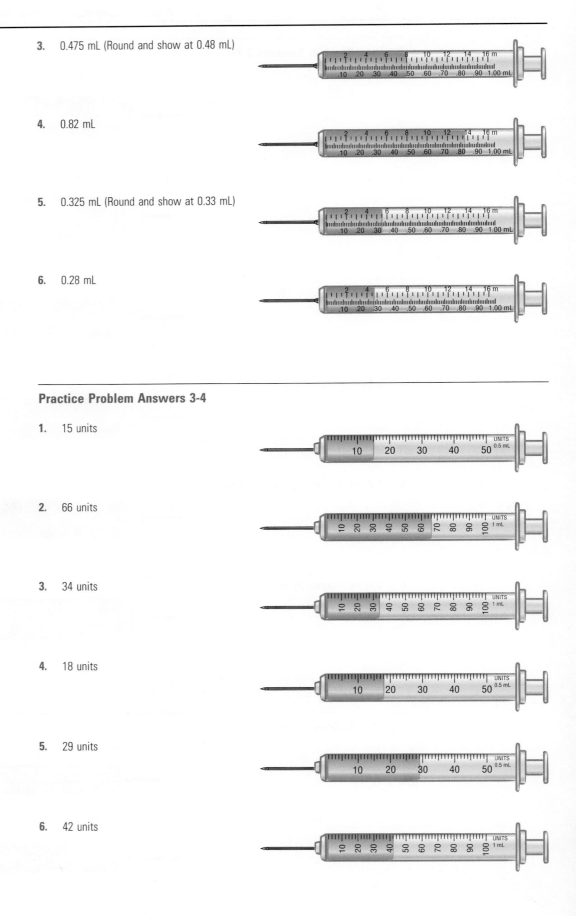

Answers to Chapter Review Problems

Chapter Review Problem Answers 3-1

A.   Medicine cup

B.   Pediatric medication syringe

    __A__   **1.** 2 tbsp

    __B__   **2.** $\frac{1}{2}$ tsp

    __B__   **3.** 1 mL

    __A__   **4.** dr 4

    __A__   **5.** 20 mL

    __A__   **6.** $\frac{3}{4}$ oz

    __B__   **7.** 0.5 mL

    __A__   **8.** dr 8

Chapter Review Problem Answers 3-2

1.   2.08 mL (Round and show at 2.1 mL)

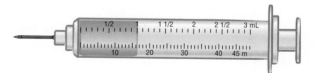

2.   0.99 mL (Round and show at 1.0 mL)

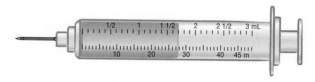

3.   1.68 mL (Round and show at 1.7 mL)

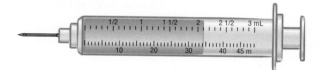

4.   0.55 mL (Round and show at 0.6 mL)

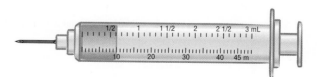

5. 1.23 mL (Round and show at 1.2 mL)

6. 2.11 mL (Round and show at 2.1 mL)

7. 1.76 mL (Round and show at 1.8 mL)

8. 0.43 mL (Round and show at 0.4 mL)

Chapter Review Problem Answers 3-3

1. 0.623 mL (Round and show at 0.62 mL)

2. 0.141 mL (Round and show at 0.14 mL)

3. 0.899 mL (Round and show at 0.90 mL)

4. 0.501 mL (Round and show at 0.50 mL)

5. 0.929 mL (Round and show at 0.93 mL)

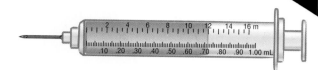

6. 0.722 mL (Round and show at 0.72 mL)

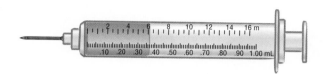

7. 0.366 mL (Round and show at 0.37 mL)

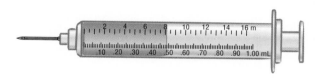

8. 0.488 mL (Round and show at 0.49 mL)

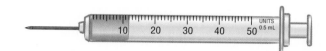

Chapter Review Problem Answers 3-4

1. 12 units

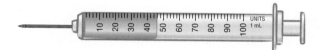

2. 46 units

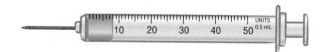

3. 8 units

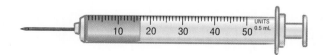

4. 17 units

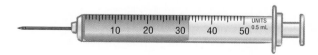

5. 33 units

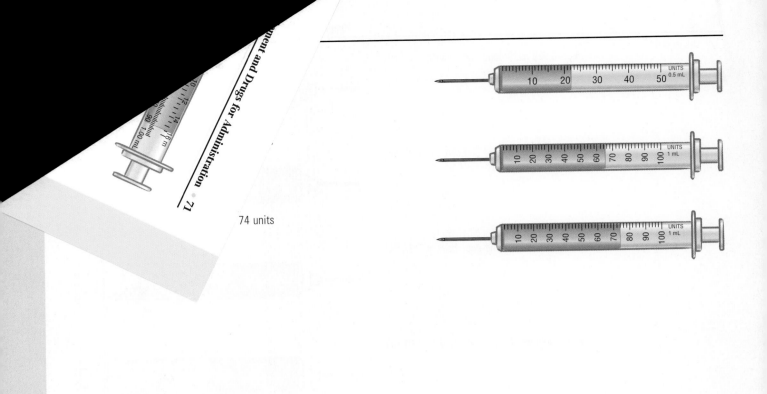

74 units

Drug Orders

This chapter contains content on:

- **Medication Orders**
- **Abbreviations Used in Medication Orders**
- **Medication Administration Record**

Learning Objectives

Upon completion of Chapter 4, you will be able to:

- Interpret prescriber orders for medications.
- Recognize the seven key elements of a drug order.
- Use standard medical abbreviations related to medications.
- Identify the components of the medication administration record.

Key Terms

- Drug order
- Medication administration record

CASE STUDY

While you are working the 3 to 11 shift on the surgical unit, your patient, Mrs. Baker, age 65, returns from surgery following her abdominal hysterectomy and bilateral salpingo-oophorectomy. She is awake, her vital signs are stable, and she has an indwelling urinary catheter draining clear yellow urine. Intravenous fluid, 1000 mL of Lactated Ringer's, is infusing at 125 mL/hour. Her husband is at the bedside with her.

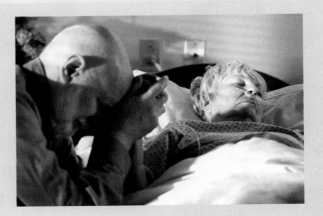

Nurses are responsible for reading and interpreting medication orders, calculating dosages of medications, and administering prescribed medications. Preventing medication errors and safely carrying out these tasks are crucial. In order to be able to prepare and administer medications safely, you must be able to read and interpret the medication order correctly. As the nurse, you must have knowledge of all the components of a medication order and abbreviations used in medication orders. After safely administering the correct dosage of the medication, you also are responsible for documenting the administration of the medication.

MEDICATION ORDERS

CASE STUDY

After settling Mrs. Baker into her room and completing your assessment, you review her postoperative orders which are as follows:

4/28/07   1600   Clear liquids post nausea and advance diet as tolerated
                       Simethicone 80 mg chewable tablet after each meal
                       Vicodin 1 tab p.o. q 4 hrs p.r.n. for pain
                       Aspirin 81 mg p.o. daily
                       Tylenol 650 mg p.o. q 4 hrs p.r.n. for headache
                       Dangle tonight, OOB to chair three times a day starting tomorrow
                       Dr. Wallace

Medication orders, or **drug orders**, should be received from the authorized prescriber in a written form. In the hospital setting, medication orders are written on the appropriate order form (Figure 4-1). The written medication order should be legible. If the order is not legible or is incomplete, **DO NOT GUESS**. It is the responsibility of the nurse to call the prescriber and clarify illegible or incomplete medication orders. This is very important in preventing medication errors.

Physician's Orders

Page 1 of 1

1. Imprint set at top. Insert in chart.
2. After each medication order, remove Pharmacy Copy and send to Pharmacy.

PLEASE USE BALLPOINT PEN

DRUG SENSITIVITY AND PERTINENT DIAGNOSIS

DATE	TIME	PHYSICIAN'S ORDERS	REASON	READ BACK	NURSE INITIALS

PLEASE USE BALLPOINT PEN

DATE: PHYSICIAN SIGNATURE: NARCOTIC NUMBER:

PHYSICIANS ORDERS   **CHART COPY**

Figure 4-1. Physician's order form.

The medication order should contain the following parts:

- Date and time of medication order
- Patient name
- Medication name
- Dosage of medication
- Route of administration of the medication
- Frequency or time of medication administration
- Signature of authorized prescriber

An example of a written drug order is:

Susan Dodson

4/4/07   1100   Lanoxin 0.125 mg p.o. daily

Dr. Thomas

The nurse interprets this medication order to be that the patient should be given 0.125 milligrams of Lanoxin by mouth every day. You can see that this order contains all the required components:

- Date and time of medication order: 4/4/07, 1100
- Patient name: Susan Dodson
- Medication name: Lanoxin
- Dosage of medication: 0.125 mg
- Route of administration of the medication: p.o.
- Frequency or time of medication administration: daily
- Signature of authorized prescriber: *Dr. Thomas*

(!) SAFETY ALERT: *In some situations, a physician may give an order to a nurse verbally rather than in written form. It is best to accept verbal medication orders only in an emergency. If you accept a verbal order, be sure to repeat the order back to the prescriber, write it down, and read it back to the prescriber. If you are unsure of the medication, spell the medication back to the prescriber. Using these steps will help decrease the chance of making a medication error.*

CASE STUDY

Applying knowledge about the components of a medication order, you examine the medication orders for Mrs. Baker and find that all the required parts to a medication order are present. You then correctly interpret the medication orders to be:

- 80 milligrams of Simethicone to be given in a chewable tablet after each meal

- One Vicodin tablet to be given by mouth every 4 hours as needed for pain
- 81 milligrams of aspirin to be given by mouth every day
- 650 milligrams of Tylenol to be given by mouth every four hours as needed for a headache

PRACTICE PROBLEMS 4-1. Practice Problems for Medication Orders

DIRECTIONS: Study each of the following medication orders and identify the component that is missing and needs clarification by the nurse before the prescribed medication can be given. The answers to the problems can be found at the end of the chapter.

1. Tom Hardy

2/4/07   1000   Amoxicillin 250 mg 4 times a day

Nancy Clark RN, NP

2. Mary Thompson

6/10/07   0900   Vitamin K IM today

Dr. Carlson

3. 1/4/07 1300 Ibuprofen 800 mg p.o. t.i.d.
Dr. Hall

4. Stanley Fromm
7/21/07 1500 Furosemide 40 mg IV
Dr. Harris

5. Sally Nelson
Synthroid 50 mcg p.o. daily
Dr. Larsen

6. Danielle Taylor
4/21/07 0800 Estradiol 0.5 mg p.o. HS
Erin Malloy RN, NP

7. George Dillon
11/31/07 1200 Aspirin p.o. daily
Dr. Polly

8. Casey Johnson
6/5/07 0900 Zantac 150 mg BID
Dr. Carter

ABBREVIATIONS USED IN MEDICATION ORDERS

CASE STUDY

The next day you continue to care for Mrs. Baker on the 3 to 11 shift. Assessment reveals that her indwelling urinary catheter has been removed and she has voided 800 mL of clear urine without any burning. She is taking in full liquids without nausea and asked if she could have "real food" for breakfast. Mrs. Baker rates her abdominal pain as 6 out of 10 on the pain scale. After reviewing the Medication Administration Record, you find that Mrs. Baker received pain medication at 1100. Her pain medication orders are:

Vicodin 1 tab po q 4h p.r.n. for pain

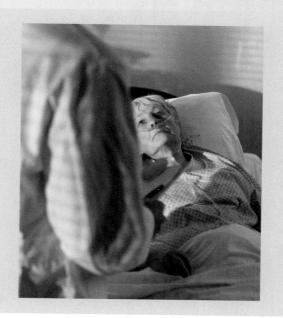

Prescribers often use abbreviations when writing medication orders. The abbreviations are often related to route of administration, drug preparation, or timing of medication. Common abbreviations and their meanings are listed in Box 4-1. You need to memorize the abbreviations.

Box 4-1. COMMON ABBREVIATIONS

Time

h	hour
min	minute
noc	night
q	every
q.h.	every hour
q 2h	every 2 hours
q 4h	every 4 hours
q 8h	every 8 hours
b.i.d.	two times a day
t.i.d.	three times a day
q.i.d.	four times a day
a.c.	before meals
p.c.	after meals
p.r.n.	as needed
ad lib.	as desired
stat	immediately

Route

GT	gastrostomy tube
ID	intradermal
IM	intramuscular
IV	intravenous
IVP	intravenous push
IVPB	intravenous piggyback
MDI	metered dose inhaler
NG	nasogastric tube
NJ	nasojejunal tube
O.D.	right eye
O.S.	left eye
O.U.	both eyes
PO or p.o.	by mouth, oral
PR or p.r.	per rectum
SubQ	subcutaneous
SL	sublingual, under the tongue

Drug Preparation

tab	tablet
cap	capsule
el, elix	elixir
gtt	drop
susp	suspension
supp	suppository
syr	syrup
tr, tinct.	tincture
ung, oint.	ointment
Sp	spirit
EC	enteric coated
CR	controlled release
SR	sustained release
SA	sustained action
LA	long acting
DS	double strength

Other Abbreviations

NPO	nothing by mouth
$\dot{s}\dot{s}$	one half
$\bar{c}$	with
$\bar{s}$	without
$\bar{a}$	before
$\bar{p}$	after

The misinterpretation of certain abbreviations in written medication orders has caused medication errors. The National Patient Safety Goals established by the Joint Commission on Accreditation of Healthcare Organizations has identified specific abbreviations that should not be used when writing medication orders or medication related documentation. Box 4-2 lists the abbreviations that should not be used. Some healthcare institutions prohibit use of additional abbreviations. Always check the institutional policy on use of abbreviations.

Box 4-2. ABBREVIATIONS THAT SHOULD NOT BE USED

Abbreviation	What You Should Write
U	Unit
IU	International Unit
QD, qd	Daily
QOD, qod	Every other day
MS, MSO_4, $MgSO_4$	Morphine sulfate
	Magnesium sulfate
H.S. or hs	Half-strength, bedtime
SC or SQ	SubQ or subcutaneous
D/C	Discharge
cc	mL
AD, AS, AU	Right ear, left ear, both ears
μg	mcg or microgram
.X mg	0.X mg (leading zero)
X.0 mg	X mg (no trailing zero)

⊘ SAFETY ALERT: *Be careful of abbreviations! They can be a source of medication error. Always follow the National Patient Safety Goals on abbreviations that should not be used. Check the policy at your institution for accepted abbreviations and use of abbreviations when ordering medications. For example, to avoid medication errors, prescribers need to write out right ear or left ear rather than using the abbreviation AD or AS.*

CASE STUDY

When reviewing the medication orders for Mrs. Baker, you interpret the abbreviations as follows:

- tab   to mean tablet
- p.o.   to mean by mouth or orally

- q   to mean every
- p.r.n. to mean as needed

PRACTICE PROBLEMS 4-2. Practice Problems for Abbreviations Used in Medication Orders

DIRECTIONS: Write the correct abbreviations for the following terms used in medication prescriptions. The answers to the problems can be found at the end of the chapter.

1. by mouth _____

2. right eye _____

3. three times a day _____

4. every 8 hours _____

5. tablet _____

6. intramuscular _____

7. after meals _____

8. night _____

PRACTICE PROBLEMS 4-3. Practice Problems for Abbreviations Used in Medication Orders

DIRECTIONS: Write the correct term(s) for the abbreviations used in medication prescriptions. The answers to the problems can be found at the end of the chapter.

1. SubQ _____
2. a.c. _____
3. p.r.n. _____
4. ad lib. _____

5. q 2h _____
6. stat _____
7. h _____
8. SL _____

MEDICATION ADMINISTRATION RECORD

The **Medication Administration Record (MAR)** is the form that the nurse uses to document administration of medications (Figure 4-2). The form may either be computer generated or hand written by the nurse. The date, patient's name, and other pertinent data such as hospital identification number and physician name should be on the form. The form typically has a section that lists the patient's allergies. Each drug order containing the seven parts of the order previously discussed will be on the form.

MARs frequently contain recommendations for administration times and codes to use when completing the form. There also is an area on the form for the complete signature of the nurse administering the medication.

The MAR is a permanent part of the patient's medical record. Each institution has its own policies related to documentation and usage of the MAR form. This will include information on procedures to add new medications, discontinue medications, document one-time or stat medications, what to do if a medication is held or a patient refuses a medication, or how to correct an error in entry on the form.

 SAFETY ALERT: *It is very important that you document promptly and accurately any medication given on the MAR. This will help prevent medication errors.*

 CASE STUDY

After giving Mrs. Baker the prescribed Vicodin, you document the medication administration on the Medication Administration Record, including the exact time that the medication was given. When you check back with Mrs. Baker one hour after giving her the Vicodin, she rates her pain as a 2 out of 10 on the pain scale and indicates that the rating of 2 is acceptable.

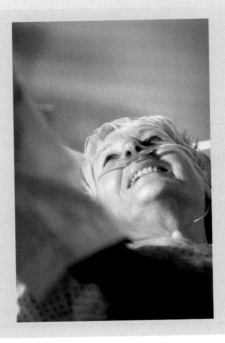

Medication Administration Record

Form No. 113-0686 (3/98) *MS*

Dates: _____ To _____ ADE/Non Drug Allergies _____

MEDICATION	DOSE	ROUTE	0800	0900	1000	1100	1200	1300	1400	1500	1600	1700	1800	1900	2000	2100	2200	2300	2400	0100	0200	0300	0400	0500	0600	0700

CIRCLE = DOSE NOT GIVEN
INITIALS = DOSE GIVEN
DELTOID = R.D., L.D.
VASTUS LATERALIS = R.V.L., LV.L.
LOWER ABDOMINAL = R. L. A., L.L.A.
ANTERIOR GLUTEAL = R.A.G., L.A.G.
POSTERIOR GLUTEAL = R.P.G., L.P.G.

0800	0900	1000	1100	1200	1300	1400	1500	1600	1700	1800	1900	2000	2100	2200	2300	2400	0100	0200	0300	0400	0500	0600	0700

INITIALS AND SIGNATURE | INITIALS AND SIGNATURE | INITIALS AND SIGNATURE

INITIALS AND SIGNATURE | INITIALS AND SIGNATURE | INITIALS AND SIGNATURE

INITIALS AND SIGNATURE | INITIALS AND SIGNATURE | INITIALS AND SIGNATURE

Figure 4-2. Computerized medication administration record.

PRACTICE PROBLEMS 4-4. Practice Problems for the Medication Administration Record

DIRECTIONS: Refer to the Computerized Medication Administration Record in Figure 4-2. Answer the questions on the following page based on your interpretation of the MAR. The answers to the problems can be found at the end of the chapter.

Medication Administration Record

Form No. 113-0686 (3/98) *MS*

Dates: __4/7/2007__ To __4/8/2007__   ADE/Non Drug Allergies __Codeine, adhesive tape, nuts__

MEDICATION	DOSE	ROUTE	0800	0900	1000	1100	1200	1300	1400	1500	1600	1700	1800	1900	2000	2100	2200	2300	2400	0100	0200	0300	0400	0500	0600	0700
Warfarin sodium (Coumadin) 3 mg p.o. daily										X MAS															
Aspirin EC 81 mg p.o. daily			X MAS																						
Furosemide (Lasix) 40 mg IVP daily			X MAS																						
Ampicillin 500 mg p.o. q.i.d.			X MAS			X MAS			X TER			X TER													
Metoclopramide 10 mg IVP every 6 hours for 4 doses			X MAS				X MAS			X TER								X						
Milk of magnesia 30 mL at bedtime p.r.n. for constipation																									

CIRCLE = DOSE NOT GIVEN
INITIALS = DOSE GIVEN.
DELTOID = R.D., L.D.
VASTUS LATERALIS = R.V.L., LV.L.
LOWER ABDOMINAL = R. L. A., L.L.A.
ANTERIOR GLUTEAL = R.A.G., L.A.G.
POSTERIOR GLUTEAL = R.P.G., L.P.G.

0800	0900	1000	1100	1200	1300	1400	1500	1600	1700	1800	1900	2000	2100	2200	2300	2400	0100	0200	0300	0400	0500	0600	0700

INITIALS AND SIGNATURE
MAS *M.A. Salkins, RN*

INITIALS AND SIGNATURE
TER *T.E. Resnick, RN*

INITIALS AND SIGNATURE

INITIALS AND SIGNATURE

INITIALS AND SIGNATURE

INITIALS AND SIGNATURE

INITIALS AND SIGNATURE

INITIALS AND SIGNATURE

1. By what route was the ampicillin given?

2. What medication allergies does the patient have?

3. At what time was the Coumadin given to the patient?

4. What dosage of aspirin did the patient receive?

5. What frequency is the metoclopramide to be given?

6. What time was the furosemide given?

7. What medication is ordered p.r.n?

8. What nurse administered the medications on the 3 to 11 shift?

CASE STUDY

Mrs. Baker is discharged without complications on postoperative day 4. Her discharge instructions include teaching on the pain medication that was prescribed for her to use at home. She also received instruction on activity, diet, wound care, and signs and symptoms of infection.

Critical Thinking/Decision Making Exercise

You are caring for a patient who is NPO after abdominal surgery. When checking the physician's order sheet for the patient, you note the following orders:

May 23, 2007   Furosemide 40 mg stat and then start daily
                      Digoxin 0.25 mg stat and then start daily
                                                    Dr. Bowers

You go to the medication-dispensing unit on the nursing floor and take out one furosemide 40 mg tablet and one digoxin 0.25 mg tablet. You prepare to give the two tablets to the patient. As you go to give the medications to the patient, you realize that the patient does not have a water cup because of being NPO.

How Did This Medication Error Almost Occur?

This medication error almost occurred because, in seeing that the medications were ordered stat, you wrote down the medications on the MAR but did not notice that one of the seven required parts of medication orders was not in the order. The physician neglected to write the route of administration for the medication.

How Could the Error Have Been Prevented?

This situation could have been prevented by carefully reviewing the medication order for all of the required components. In doing so, you would have noted that the route of administration was missing from the written order. As a result, you would need to contact the prescriber to clarify the route of administration. Do not assume that all medications are to be given by mouth. In this case, the patient is NPO. Subsequently, when you called the physician, he ordered both of the medications to be given by the intravenous (IV) route.

CHAPTER REVIEW PROBLEMS

The answers to the problems can be found at the end of the chapter.

Review Problems 4-1. Examine each of the drug orders. Indicate which part of the drug order is missing.

1. 4/16/07
   Heparin 5000 units SubQ q12h
   Dr. Wallach

2. 3/26/07
   Susan Smithson
   Digoxin 0.125 mg daily
   Dr. Jensen

3. February 22, 2007
   Thomas Allen
   Lovenox SubQ daily
   Dr. Bailey

4. Kathy Dodd
   Synthroid 100 mcg p.o. every A.M
   Dr. Potts

5. July 2, 2007
   Kristen Fischer
   Compazine 10 mg q 6h p.r.n. for nausea
   Dr. Larson

6. August 15, 2007
   Mark Wills
   Lopressor 50 mg p.o. every A.M

7. September 4, 2007
   William Martin
   Coumadin 5 mg p.o.
   Dr. Sandstrom

8. 1/6/07
   Sandy Williams
   Milk of Magnesia p.o. daily p.r.n. for constipation
   Dr. Allen

Review Problems 4-2. Give the correct term for each of the abbreviations used in medication orders.

1. IV

2. NG

3. b.i.d.

4. OS

5. EC

6. gtt

7. q 4h

8. ss̄

Review Problems 4-3. Give the abbreviation for the term used in medication orders.

1. four times a day

2. sustained-release

3. ointment

4. suppository

5. every 6 hours

6. intravenous push

7. nothing by mouth

8. metered dose inhaler

Review Problems 4-4. Examine the MAR shown on the next page. Answer the following questions based on your interpretation of the MAR.

1. What is the name of the nurse who administered the medications on the 7 to 3 shift?

2. What medication allergies does the patient have?

3. At what time was the digoxin given?

4. What medication is ordered to be given at 1000?

5. What medication(s) is ordered to be given p.r.n.?

6. What is the ordered dosage of potassium?

7. What frequency is the Keflex to be given?

8. At what time was the Synthroid given?

Medication Administration Record

Form No. 113-0686 (3/98) *MS*

Dates: __5/12/07__ To __5/13/07__   **ADE/Non Drug Allergies** ___Penicillin, Erythromycin___

MEDICATION / DOSE / ROUTE	0800	0900	1000	1100	1200	1300	1400	1500	1600	1700	1800	1900	2000	2100	2200	2300	2400	0100	0200	0300	0400	0500	0600	0700
Digoxin 0.25 mg IVP daily — Hold if heartrate less than 60		X PAS																						
Keflex (cephalexin) 500 mg p.o. three times per day		X PAS						X						X										
Synthroid (levothyroxine) 100 mcg p.o. every morning	X PAS																							
Furosemide (Lasix) 40 mg IVP daily	X PAS																							
Potassium chloride 20 mEq p.o. BID	X PAS													X										
Tylenol (acetaminophen) 650 mg p.o. every 4 hours prn for headache					X PAS																			
Toradol (ketorolac) 15 mg IVP every 6 hours for four doses			X PAS						X						X						X			
Milk of magnesia 30 mL p.o. daily prn for constipation																								

CIRCLE = DOSE NOT GIVEN
INITIALS = DOSE GIVEN
DELTOID = R.D., L.D.
VASTUS LATERALIS = R.V.L., LV.L.
LOWER ABDOMINAL = R. L. A., L.L.A.
ANTERIOR GLUTEAL = R.A.G., L.A.G.
POSTERIOR GLUTEAL = R.P.G., L.P.G.

INITIALS AND SIGNATURE	INITIALS AND SIGNATURE	INITIALS AND SIGNATURE
PAS *P.A. Sheldon, RN*		
INITIALS AND SIGNATURE	INITIALS AND SIGNATURE	INITIALS AND SIGNATURE
INITIALS AND SIGNATURE	INITIALS AND SIGNATURE	INITIALS AND SIGNATURE

Answers to Practice Problems

Practice Problem Answers 4-1

1. Route of administration
2. Dosage of medication
3. Patient name
4. Frequency or time of medication administration
5. Date and time of order
6. Frequency or time of medication administration
7. Dosage of medication
8. Route of administration

Practice Problem Answers 4-2

1. by mouth – p.o.
2. right eye – OD
3. three times a day – t.i.d.
4. every 8 hours – q 8h
5. tablet – tab
6. intramuscular – IM
7. after meals – p.c.
8. night – noc

Practice Problem Answers 4-3

1. SubQ – subcutaneous
2. a.c. – before meals
3. p.r.n. – as needed
4. ad lib. – as desired
5. q 2h – every 2 hours
6. stat – immediately
7. h – hour
8. SL – sublingual

Practice Problem Answers 4-4

1. Ampicillin is given p.o., which means orally
2. Codeine
3. Coumadin was administered at 1500
4. 81 mg
5. Every 6 hours for 4 doses
6. Furosemide was given at 0900
7. Milk of Magnesia 30 mL
8. T. E. Resnick, RN

Answers to Chapter Review Problems

Chapter Review Problem Answers 4-1

1. Patient name

2. Route of administration

3. Dosage of medication

4. Date of medication order

5. Route of administration

6. Signature of authorized prescriber

7. Frequency of administration

8. Dosage of medication

Chapter Review Problem Answers 4-2

1. IV – intravenous

2. NG – nasogastric

3. b.i.d. – two times a day

4. O.S. – left eye

5. EC – enteric coated

6. gtt – drop

7. q 4h – every 4 hours

8. ṡṡ – one half

Chapter Review Problem Answers 4-3

1. four times a day – q.i.d.

2. sustained-release – SR

3. ointment – ung or oint

4. suppository – supp

5. every 6 hours – q 6h

6. intravenous push – IVP

7. nothing by mouth – NPO

8. metered dose inhaler – MDI

Chapter Review Problem Answers 4-4

1. What is the name of the nurse who administered the medications on the 7 to 3 shift?

   P.A. Sheldon

2. What medication allergies does the patient have?

   Penicillin, erythromycin

3. At what time was the digoxin given?

   0900

4. What medication is ordered to be given at 1000?

   Toradol 15 mg IVP

5. What medication(s) is ordered to be given p.r.n.?

   Tylenol and MOM

6. What is the ordered dosage of potassium?

   20 mEq

7. What frequency is the Keflex to be given?

   TID at 0900,1500, and 2100

8. At what time was the Synthroid given?

   0800

Medication Labels and Packaging Systems

This chapter contains content on:

- **Medication Labels**
- **Medication Packaging**

Learning Objectives

Upon completion of Chapter 5, you will be able to:

- Identify pertinent information on a medication label.
- Recognize information on how medications are supplied.
- Discuss the difference between unit-dose and multi-dose packaging systems.

Key Terms

- Brand name
- Expiration date
- Generic name
- Lot number
- Medication label
- Multi-dose packaging

- NDC number
- Precautions
- Proprietary name
- Storage
- Trade name
- Unit-dose packaging

CASE STUDY

Mrs. Tilton is a 60-year-old woman who was diagnosed with diabetes 15 years ago and is now admitted for treatment of a diabetic ulcer and infection on her right foot that has not responded to treatment at home. Over the last several months she has been having trouble keeping her blood sugar at an acceptable level because of repeated infections in the ulcer on her right foot. These infections have prevented the ulcer from healing. She also has a history of primary hypertension that is controlled by diet, exercise, and medication. Mrs. Tilton is 75 pounds over the weight her physician would like her to maintain. Mrs. Tilton's medication orders include:

- Heparin 5000 units SubQ q 12h
- NPH Insulin 15 units SubQ q A.M.
- Regular Insulin 10 units SubQ q A.M.
- Hydrochlorothiazide 50 mg PO q A.M.

You are preparing to set up the medications that Mrs. Tilton is to receive.

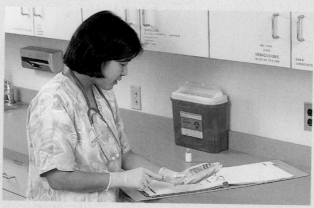

Photo: B. Proud.

MEDICATION LABELS

Having an understanding of medication labels is essential for safe medication administration. Nurses must be knowledgbable and skillful in reading the medication labels correctly and in understanding the difference between the packaging of medications (Figure 5-1).

All medications come in packages with labels. The medication labels provide you with information about the medications so that you can safely calculate the correct dosage and administer the medication appropriately. Medication labels contain the following information:

- Brand, trade, or proprietary name of medication
- Generic name of medication
- Medication strength
- Medication quantity
- Medication form
- Usual medication dosage
- Storage
- Precautions
- Manufacturer's name
- Expiration date
- Lot number
- NDC number

However, in cases where the medication label is small in size, some information may be omitted due to lack of space.

Brand, Trade, or Proprietary Name of Medication

The **brand name, trade name, or proprietary name** of the medication is the name given to the medication by the manufacturer. The brand name has the symbol ® or ™ after it, which indicates a registered trademark. The brand or trade name either starts with an uppercase letter or is in all uppercase letters on the label. It is generally the largest printed information on the label (Figure 5-2). If the same drug is manufactured by several different companies, it will be sold under several brand names because each company gives the drug a proprietary name.

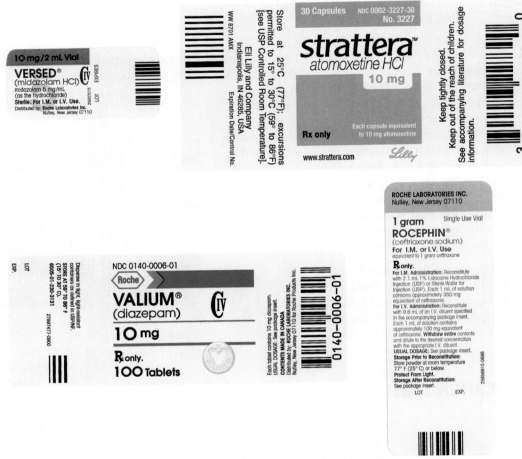

Figure 5-1. Medication labels. (Copyright Eli Lilly and Company. Used with permission. Copyright Hoffmann-La Roche, Inc. Used with permission.)

Generic Name of Medication

The **generic name,** or nonproprietary name, of the medication is the official name of the medication that is listed in the *United States Pharmacopeia* (USP). Each medication has only one generic name. The generic name is usually found under the brand or trade name. The generic name is in lowercase letters. The prescriber may order the medication using the generic or trade name.

The initials USP (*United States Pharmacopeia*) or NF (National Formulary) are found after the generic name of the medication. In the United States, the official national lists of approved drugs are the USP and NF. Guidelines are given to manufacturers related to the use and placement of these initials on medication labels (Figure 5-3).

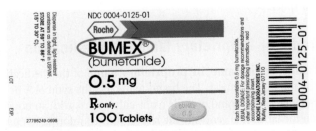

Figure 5-2. Brand name. (Hoffmann-La Roche, Inc. Used with permission.)

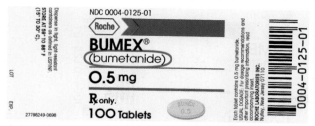

Figure 5-3. Generic name. (Hoffmann-La Roche, Inc. Used with permission.)

Medication Strength

The **medication strength** is the amount of medication provided. The metric system is the unit of measurement used for medications that come in a solid form. For medications that come in a liquid form, the strength is indicated as the solution of the medication in the solvent (Figure 5-4).

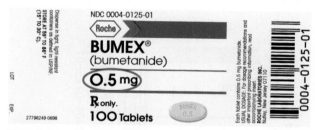

Figure 5-4. Medication strength. (Hoffmann-La Roche, Inc. Used with permission.)

Medication Quantity

The **medication quantity** is the total amount of medication found in the package, ampule, vial, or bottle. For example, if the medication is in tablets, this number will tell you how many tablets are in the bottle. For a liquid medication, the number will tell you the total volume in the bottle, vial, or ampule. This number is generally found at the top of the label on the right or left side or at the bottom of the label (Figure 5-5).

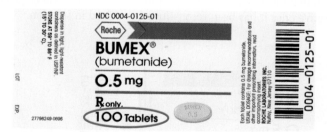

Figure 5-5. Medication quantity. (Hoffmann-La Roche, Inc. Used with permission.)

Medication Form

The **medication form** refers to the type of medication that is in the package. Solid medications generally come in tablet or capsule form. Liquid medications may be in the form of solutions, suspensions, emulsions, syrups, elixirs, or tinctures. Some medications for oral use come in powder or granule form that requires the drug to be mixed with food or liquids before administration. Medications for injection can come in solution form or in a powder form that requires the addition of the appropriate liquid for reconstitution. Other medication forms include suppositories, ointments, or patches (Figure 5-6).

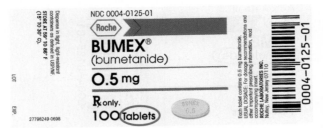

Figure 5-6. Medication form. (Hoffmann-La Roche, Inc. Used with permission.)

Usual Medication Dosage

The **usual medication dosage** tells how much medication is given in a single dosage or over a 24-hour period. Because this information is often longer than what would fit on the label itself, the label often refers to reading the package insert for complete information (Figure 5-7).

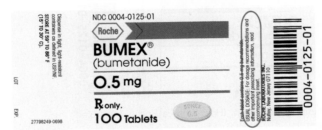

Figure 5-7. Usual dosage. (Hoffmann-La Roche, Inc. Used with permission.)

Storage

The **storage** section of the label provides information related to how the medication should be stored to prevent the drug from losing its potency or effectiveness. The information here is often related to the temperature at which the drug should be stored (Figure 5-8). If the drug comes in a powder form that must be reconstituted, storage information will be given indicating how long the drug is effective once it has been reconstituted or mixed in solution.

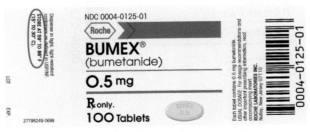

Figure 5-8. Storage. (Hoffmann-La Roche, Inc. Used with permission.)

Precautions

Many labels contain warnings, alerts, or **precautions** from the manufacturer of the medication. These precautions or warnings provide information related to medication safety, effectiveness, or administration. Some medications may come with precautions labeled by the dispensing pharmacy. Always read and follow the instructions given by manufacturers or pharmacies.

Examples of precautions, warnings, or alerts that might appear on medication labels include the following:

- Keep medication refrigerated.
- Medication may cause drowsiness. Do not drive or operate heavy machinery.
- Shake well before using.

Manufacturer's Name

All medication labels contain the name of the company that manufactured the medication (Figure 5-9). This provides you with an information source if you have questions about the medication.

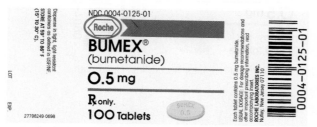

Figure 5-9. Manufacturer. (Hoffmann-La Roche, Inc. Used with permission.)

Expiration Date

Each medication label will have an **expiration date**—the date after which the medication cannot be used (Figure 5-10). This date typically appears as the month/year such that the medication is no longer usable after the last day of the month stated. In the acute care setting, medications that have expired should be returned to the pharmacy.

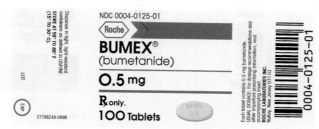

Figure 5-10. Expiration date. (Hoffmann-La Roche, Inc. Used with permission.)

Lot Number

The **lot number** is a label component that is required by federal law. This number refers to the batch of medication from which this medication came (Figure 5-11). This number is used to identify medication if it needs to be recalled by the manufacturer for any reason.

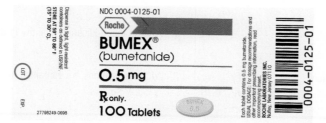

Figure 5-11. Lot number. (Hoffmann-La Roche, Inc. Used with permission.)

National Drug Code (NDC) Number

NDC stands for National Drug Code. The **NDC number** is required by federal law to be given to all prescription medications and must appear on the manufacturer's label (Figure 5-12). Each medication has its own unique NDC number. The NDC number consists of NDC followed by three groups of numbers.

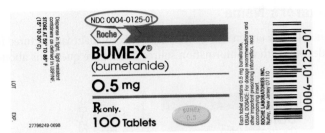

Figure 5-12. NDC number. (Hoffmann-La Roche, Inc. Used with permission.)

PRACTICE PROBLEMS 5-1. Practice Problems for Medication Labels

DIRECTIONS: Use the medication labels provided to answer the questions. The answers to the problems can be found at the end of the chapter.

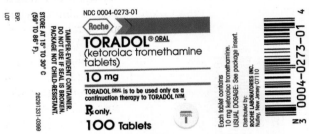

Hoffmann-La Roche, Inc. Used with permission.

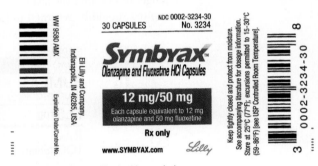

Eli Lilly and Company. Used with permission

Use the label above to answer questions 1–4.

1. Who is the manufacturer of the medication?

2. What is the generic name of the medication?

3. What is the dosage of the medication?

4. What is the NDC number of the medication?

Use the label above to answer questions 5-8.

5. What information related to storage is provided?

6. Are there any precautions, warnings, or alerts given? If yes, what are they?

7. What is the medication quantity in the package?

8. What medications are contained in the product?

CASE STUDY

It is time for Mrs. Tilton's daily dose of insulin. Her blood glucose level this morning was 105 mg/dL; yesterday her levels ranged from 90 to 118 mg/dL, indicating that control of her sugars is improving. Today she is to receive the same combination dosage of NPH and regular insulin—NPH insulin 15 units and regular insulin 10 units. The insulin comes in multi-dose bottles.

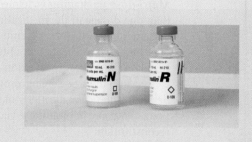

MEDICATION PACKAGING

Medications are typically packaged as one of two types: unit-dose or multi-dose. Oral, parenteral, and topical medications can be supplied as either type. Most healthcare institutions will purchase some medications in unit-dose packaging and some medications in multi-dose packaging. The nurse is responsible for ensuring that the prescribed medication is given correctly to the patient.

Unit-dose Packaging

Unit-dose packaging is defined as the packaging and labeling of each individual dosage of medication. A single capsule, tablet, or liquid dosage of medication is sealed in an individual package. Unit-dose parenteral medications come in bottles, vials, pre-filled syringes, or ampules that contain one dosage of the prescribed medication. Topical medications in unit-dose packaging can include individually packaged and labeled transdermal patches, suppositories, and tubes of ointments and creams. In healthcare institutions that use unit-dose packaging, a 24-hour supply of individual medication packages are sent to the nursing units each day.

Not all prescribed dosages of medications come prepared in a unit-dose package. The nurse must carefully read the label of each medication package to make sure that the right medication and dosage is being prepared for the patient. For example, the prescriber may order metoprolol (Lopressor) 50 mg every morning. The unit dosage of the medication is metoprolol (Lopressor) 25 mg. Therefore, the nurse, after calculating correctly, recognizes that 2 packages of the medication must be used to obtain the correct prescribed dosage.

CASE STUDY

Mrs. Tilton is to receive hydrochlorothiazide 50 mg orally each day. The healthcare facility supplies medication in a unit-dose package. When you check her medication drawer, you note that there are two pills in the package. Checking the label, you see that each tablet is 25 mg. Therefore, you would need to give two tablets.

(!) **SAFETY ALERT:** *Read the medication labels carefully to avoid medication errors. Many medication names are similar in sound and spelling. You may need to do a medication calculation to obtain the correct dosage of medication using the unit-dose packaging.*

Multi-dose Packaging

Multi-dose packaging is defined as the packaging of medications in containers that contain more than one dosage of the medication. The medications may be part of the floor stock of medications that are sent to the nursing unit. When the nurse needs a prescribed dosage of medication, the correct dosage of medication is obtained from the multi-dose container. Often times, the nurse must calculate the correct medication dosage before obtaining the medication from the stock container.

Multi-dose packaging provides enough medication for several days. Tablets, capsules, powders, and liquid medications may be supplied in stock bottles for dispensing. Parenteral medications may come in multi-dose vials that often contain the medication in a powder form that requires reconstitution.

 CASE STUDY

Remember, Mrs. Tilton is to receive NPH and regular insulin. These are supplied in multi-dose packaging systems. To administer the insulin correctly, you draw up both types of insulin using the same insulin syringe, remembering to draw up the regular rapid-acting (clear) insulin first. When finished, there should be a total of 25 units of insulin in the syringe.

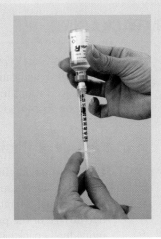

> (!) **SAFETY ALERT:** *When reconstituting multi-dose vials of parenteral medications, make sure to write the date and time of reconstitution on the label. It is crucial to follow the manufacturer's instructions for reconstitution, storage, and expiration of the medication.*

Multi-dose tubes, jars of creams and ointments, and bottles of eye and ear drops are frequently prescribed for patients. When removing cream or ointment from a multiple use jar, use a sterile tongue blade or glove to prevent contaminating the remaining medication.

When administering medications with a dropper, be careful not to touch the dropper to the patient. This contaminates the dropper and the remaining medication. Remember from Chapter 3 to use the dropper that comes with the prescribed medication because it is calibrated specifically for that medication—this ensures that the dosage of medication you draw into the dropper is accurately measured.

 CASE STUDY

The facility Diabetes Educator has worked out a plan with Mrs. Tilton so she will check her blood sugars more frequently and follow her diet as prescribed. Mrs. Tilton has been taught how to change the dressing on her ulcer and to report any signs of infection in the wound. A referral for home care visits, initially three times a week, has been made to ensure that Mrs. Tilton is able to do her dressing change and follow her diet.

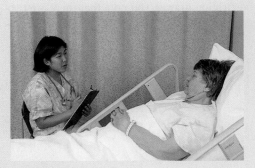

Photo: B. Proud.

Critical Thinking/Decision Making Exercise

A responsibility of the nurse is to use proper administration techniques based on the type of medication being given. Using the wrong technique can put the patient at risk for development of complications from the medication administration. Consider the following case.

The nurse is caring for a client who sustained first- and second-degree burns on the left hand from a kitchen fire. The physician has ordered dressing changes on the burned area twice a day with the application of mafenide (Sulfamylon) cream to the burn area with each dressing change. The cream is supplied by the pharmacy in a multi-dose jar. Each jar supplies enough medication for six dressing changes.

When performing the dressing change, the nurse removes the old dressing and then performs hand washing. To apply the mafenide (Sulfamylon), the nurse scoops out the cream using the three middle fingers. Using the same fingers that scooped out the cream, the nurse then smoothes the cream over the burn. Additional cream is needed to cover the entire burned area so the nurse again scoops some from the jar using the three middle fingers. After the entire burned area is covered with cream, the nurse wraps the patient's fingers and hand in gauze.

What Error Has Occurred?

The nurse used incorrect technique when removing the cream from a multi-dose jar. Because the nurse used an ungloved hand to remove the cream from the jar, the remaining medication in the jar was contaminated. This contamination of medication could lead to infection in the burned area for the patient. The nurse also applied the cream to the burned area with an ungloved hand potentially contaminating the wound.

What Should the Nurse Have Done?

Proper technique for removing cream from a multi-dose jar requires the nurse to use a sterile glove or sterile tongue depressor. This ensures that the remaining cream remains sterile and reduces the risk of infection from contaminated medication. Using a sterile glove or tongue depressor to apply the sterile cream decreases the risk of wound infection at the burn site. Properly applying the cream also reduces the risk of further complications for the patient.

CHAPTER REVIEW PROBLEMS

The answers to the problems can be found at the end of the chapter.

Review Problems 5-1. Examine the medication label below. Using the medication label, correctly identify each part of the medication label.

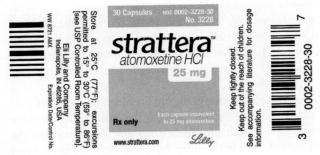

Eli Lilly and Company. Used with permission.

1. Brand name
2. Generic name
3. Manufacturer's name
4. Medication strength
5. Medication quantity
6. Medication form
7. Usual medication dosage
8. Storage
9. Precautions

Review Problems 5-2. Examine the medication label below. Using the medication label, correctly identify each part of the medication label.

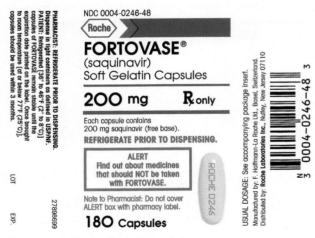

Hoffmann-La Roche, Inc. Used with permission.

1. Brand name
2. Generic name
3. Manufacturer's name
4. Medication strength
5. Medication quantity
6. Medication form
7. Usual medication dosage
8. Storage
9. Precautions

Answers to Practice Problems

Practice Problem Answers 5-1

1. Roche

2. Ketorolac tromethamine

3. 10 mg

4. 0004-0273-01

5. Store at 25°C (77°F); 15° to 30°C (59° to 86°F) permitted

6. Keep tightly closed and protect from moisture.

7. 30 capsules

8. olanzapine 12 mg and fluoxetine HCl 50 mg

Answers to Chapter Review Problems

Chapter Review Problem Answers 5-1

1. Brand name – Strattera

2. Generic name – atomoxetine HCl

3. Manufacturer's name – Lilly

4. Medication strength – 25 mg

5. Medication quantity – 30

6. Medication form – capsules

7. Usual medication dosage – 25 mg

8. Storage – 25°C (77°F)

9. Precautions – Keep tightly closed. Keep out of reach of children.

Chapter Review Problem Answers 5-2

1. Brand name – Fortovase

2. Generic name – saquinavir

3. Manufacturer's name – Roche

4. Medication strength – 200 mg

5. Medication quantity – 180

6. Medication form – capsules

7. Usual medication dosage – Instructed to see accompanying package insert

8. Storage – Refrigerate prior to dispensing

9. Precautions – Find out about medicines that should not be taken with Fortovase

Strategies for Drug Calculation

This chapter contains content on:

- **The 3-Step Approach**
- **Formula Method**
- **Ratio-Proportion Method**
- **Six Rights of Medication Administration**

Learning Objectives

Upon completion of Chapter 6, you will be able to:

- Use the 3-Step Approach—Convert, Compute, and Critically Think—to correctly calculate medication dosages.
- Use the formula method to set up a medication dosage calculation.
- Use the ratio-proportion method to set up a medication dosage calculation.
- Determine when to use the formula versus the ratio-proportion method for calculation of medication dosages.
- Apply the Six Rights of Medication Administration when administering medications.
- Critically evaluate the calculation process and accuracy of answers.

Key Terms

- Compute
- Convert
- Critically Think
- Formula method
- Ratio-proportion method
- Six Rights of Medication Administration

CASE STUDY

Mr. Dodson, a 63-year-old patient, is transferred from the cardiac care unit to the cardiac step down unit while recovering from coronary artery bypass surgery. Mr. Dodson has a history of gastro-esophageal reflux disease and osteoarthritis. His medication orders include the following:

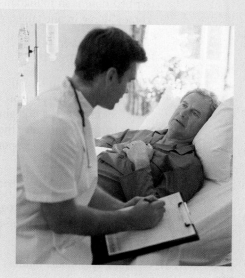

- Pepcid 20 mg oral suspension p.o. b.i.d.
- Toradol 30 mg IVP daily for 2 days
- Aspirin 81 mg p.o. daily

While reviewing the medications, you find that you need to calculate medication doses for two of the medications: Pepcid oral suspension, supplied as a suspension containing 40 mg/5mL and Toradol injection supplied as a solution containing 15 mg/mL.

Nurses need to be skilled in setting up and calculating doses of medication to ensure patient safety. Using the 3-Step Approach is a valuable way to accomplish this task. Nurses can use either the Formula Method or the Ratio-Proportion Method to calculate medication dosages. It is recommended that you select one of these methods and stick with that method of calculation to decrease the risk of making errors. In addition, adhering to the Six Rights of Medication Administration further ensures that medications ordered for your patient are administered correctly and safely.

THE 3-STEP APPROACH

When preparing to calculate medication doses, you need an easy way to correctly work through the problems and find the right answer. One easy approach to correctly solve your medication dosage problems is the 3-Step Approach. The three steps are:

- Convert
- Compute
- Critically Think

Following, this simple 3-step approach each time you calculate medication doses will enable you to calculate the medication dose accurately.

Step 1: Convert

The first step in the approach is to convert. **Converting** requires you to make sure that the medication dose ordered is in the same system of measurement and measurement unit as the medication available. If either the system of measurement or the unit of measurement in the prescribed medication or available medication is different, you need to convert to a like measurement. For example, if a medication was ordered in grams and the medication is available in milligrams, you need to convert the ordered medication dosage to milligrams. Or if the medication is ordered in ounces (apothecary system) and it is available in milliliters (metric system) you would need to convert the ordered medication dosage to milliliters.

For example, the physician orders codeine gr. ss p.o. every 4 hours. The medication is supplied as codeine 30 mg per tablet. Because the system of measurement for the ordered medication differs from what is supplied, you must convert one of them to the other system. Converting to the metric system is recommended because this is the most commonly used system of measurement.

Recall from Chapter 2 that 1 grain = 60 mg. Therefore gr. $\text{ss} = \frac{60\,mg}{2} = 30$ mg. Now the prescribed dose is in milligrams and the medication available is in milligrams. Because the Codeine comes 30 mg in one tablet, you would then give one tablet as the prescribed dose.

Step 2: Compute

The second step in the approach is to compute. **Computing** requires you to determine the data needed to solve the dose problem, to set up the problem correctly, and to calculate an answer. This step requires the use of higher-level thinking skills to determine the data needed, select the correct formula to use, and solve the mathematical problem. When computing, you can use either the formula method or ratio-proportion method. These are both discussed later in this chapter.

Step 3: Critically Think

The final step in this approach is to critically think. **Critical thinking** requires you to ask yourself if the answer you obtained seems correct, logical, and plausible. Evaluate your answer by asking yourself these questions:

- Is it a reasonable number of tablets or capsules or amount of liquid to administer orally or parenterally?
- Does the dose seem unusually large or small for a safe dose?

When first learning how to do calculations, it might be advisable to have your instructor check your math calculations.

> **SAFETY ALERT:** *Always double check your math. It is often during simple tasks and calculations that mistakes are made due to rushing or lack of caution. Even with simple problems, stop and double check your math. Always ask yourself if the dose is reasonable and correct.*

FORMULA METHOD

The **formula method** or rule method is one method for calculating medication doses. It uses a standard formula equation to set up the calculation of the medication dose. This method is helpful when the dosage of medication prescribed is different from the dosage available.

In the formula or rule method:

$$\frac{D}{H} \times V = A$$

Where: D = desired or prescribed dosage of the medication

H = dosage of medication available or on hand

V = volume that the medication is available in, such as one tablet or milliliters

A = amount of medication to administer

For example, the physician prescribes 100 mg of a medication. The medication is available in 50-mg tablets. Using the formula or rule method, set up the problem like this:

$$\frac{100\,mg}{50\,mg} \times 1\ \text{tablet}$$

D = prescribed dosage of 100 mg

H = available medication dosage of 50 mg

V = volume of medication of one tablet

You get the answer by solving the equation:

$$\frac{100 \text{ mg}}{50 \text{ mg}} \times 1 \text{ tablet}$$

In this problem, because mg appears in both the numerator and denominator, mg is cancelled out and you are left with tablet as the volume of medication in the answer.

$$\frac{100 \text{ mg}}{50 \text{ mg}} \times 1 \text{ tablet} = 2 \text{ tablets}$$

Therefore, you would administer 2 tablets.

CASE STUDY

Recall Mr. Dodson, who is ordered to receive Pepcid. You have the following information:

Medication ordered: Pepcid 20 mg oral suspension p.o. b.i.d.
Medication available: Pepcid oral suspension 40 mg/5 mL

Using the formula method, you calculate the dosage of Pepcid that you need to give Mr. Dodson. Set up the problem using the formula to look like this:

$$\frac{D}{H} \times V = A$$

$$\frac{20 \text{ mg}}{40 \text{ mg}} \times 5 \text{ mL}$$

Again, in this problem because mg appears in both the numerator and denominator, mg is cancelled out and you are left with mL as the volume of medication in the answer.

$$\frac{20 \text{ mg}}{40 \text{ mg}} \times 5 \text{ mL} = 2.5 \text{ mL}$$

Therefore, you would administer 2.5 mL of Pepcid to Mr. Dodson.

PRACTICE PROBLEMS 6-1. Using the Formula Method

DIRECTIONS: Solve the following medication dosage problems using the formula method. The answers to the problems can be found at the end of the chapter.

1. **Medication Ordered:** Erythromycin 750 mg
   Medication Available: Erythromycin 250 mg tablets

Calculation:

Dispense in a USP tight container.
Keep tightly closed.
Store below 86°F (30°C).

NDC 0074-6326-53
500 Tablets

ERYTHROMYCIN
Base Filmtab®

ERYTHROMYCIN
TABLETS, USP

250 mg Erythromycin, USP

Do not accept if seal over bottle opening is broken or missing.

Each tablet contains:
Erythromycin, USP
..................250 mg

Usual adult dose: One tablet every six hours. See enclosure for full prescribing information.

Filmtab — Film-sealed tablets, Abbott

©Abbott

℞ only

Abbott Laboratories
North Chicago, IL 60064, U.S.A.

Abbott Laboratories. Used with permission.

2. Medication Ordered: Biaxin 250 mg

Medication Available: Biaxin 500 mg tablets

Calculation:

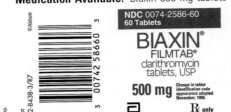

6505-01-354-8581
Store tablets at 20° to 25°C (68° to 77°F).
Do not accept if seal over bottle opening is broken or missing.
Dispense in a USP tight container.
Each tablet contains:
500 mg clarithromycin.
See enclosure for full prescribing information.
Filmtab – Film-sealed tablets, Abbott.

Abbott Laboratories
North Chicago, IL60064, U.S.A.

Abbott Laboratories. Used with permission.

3. Medication Ordered: Furosemide 60 mg

Medication Available: Furosemide 100 mg/mL

Calculation:

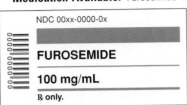

4. Medication Ordered: Digoxin 0.125 mg

Medication Available: Digoxin 0.05 mg/mL

Calculation:

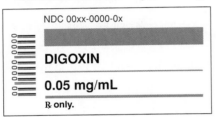

5. Medication Ordered: Gantrisin 1.5 g

Medication Available: Gantrisin 0.5 g per tablet

Calculation:

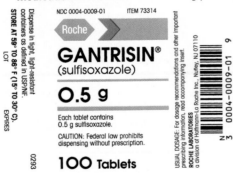

Hoffmann-La Roche Inc. Used with permission.

6. Medication Ordered: Versed 4 mg

Medication Available: Versed 10 mg/2 mL

Calculation:

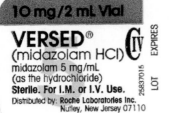

Hoffmann-La Roche Inc. Used with permission.

RATIO-PROPORTION METHOD

The **ratio-proportion method** is a second method that can be used to calculate medication doses. It is useful when the medication dosage prescribed is different from the dosage of the medication available and it is only necessary to find one unknown quantity.

Recall from Chapter 1 that a ratio expresses the relationship between two units or quantities. A proportion is a statement that two ratios are equal. This formula expresses the proportion as two equivalent fractions. The first fraction represents the equivalent of the medication that you have on hand. The second fraction is the desired dose and the unknown x or amount of medication to administer. When using this method, you are solving for an unknown x (the amount of medication to administer) in the equation.

The first step in using this method is to set up the equivalent equation. The equation for the ratio-proportion method is:

$$\frac{\text{Dosage on hand (D)}}{\text{Amount on hand (H)}} = \frac{\text{Dosage prescribed (Q)}}{x \ \text{Amount desired}}$$

The second step is to cross multiply.

$$\frac{\text{Dosage on hand (D)}}{\text{Amount on hand (H)}} \quad \diagdown\!\!\!\diagup \quad \frac{\text{Dosage prescribed (Q)}}{x \ \text{Amount desired}}$$

$$Dx = HQ$$

The next step is to isolate x on one side of the equation. Do this by dividing both sides of the equation by D (dosage on hand).

$$\frac{Dx}{D} = \frac{HQ}{D}$$

You then solve for x.

$$\frac{\cancel{D}x}{\cancel{D}} = \frac{HQ}{D}$$

$$x = \frac{HQ}{D}$$

As in the example for the formula method, the physician orders 100 mg of a medication that is available in 50-mg tablets. Using the ratio-proportion method, set up the problem like this:

$$\frac{50 \text{ mg}}{1 \text{ tablet}} = \frac{100 \text{ mg}}{x}$$

Cross multiply.

$$\frac{50 \text{ mg}}{1 \text{ tablet}} \quad \diagdown\!\!\!\diagup \quad \frac{100 \text{ mg}}{x}$$

$$50 \text{ mg } x = 100 \text{ mg} \times 1 \text{ tablet}$$

Isolate the x by dividing both sides by 50 mg. Milligrams (mg) in the numerator and denominator cancel each other out, and you are left with tablet as the volume of medication in the answer.

$$\frac{\cancel{50 \text{ mg}} \, x}{\cancel{50 \text{ mg}}} = \frac{100 \cancel{\text{ mg}} \times 1 \text{ tablet}}{50 \cancel{\text{ mg}}}$$

Solve for x.

$$x = \frac{100 \text{ tablets}}{50} = 2 \text{ tablets}$$

Therefore, the answer to the problem is 2 tablets.

CASE STUDY

Mr. Dodson is to receive his Toradol. You have the following information:

Medication ordered: Toradol 30 mg IVP daily for 2 days

Medication available: Toradol injectable solution 15 mg/mL

Calculate the dosage of Toradol using the ratio-proportion method. Remember the ratio-proportion method uses this equation:

$$\frac{\text{Dosage on hand (D)}}{\text{Amount on hand (H)}} = \frac{\text{Dosage prescribed (Q)}}{x \text{ Amount desired}}$$

Using the equation, set up your problem:

$$\frac{15 \text{ mg}}{1 \text{ mL}} = \frac{30 \text{ mg}}{x}$$

Cross multiply to get:

$$15 \text{ mg } x = 30 \text{ mg} \times \text{mL}$$

Isolate x by dividing both sides by 15 mg:

$$\frac{15 \text{ mg } x}{15 \text{ mg}} = \frac{30 \text{ mg} \times \text{mL}}{15 \text{ mg}}$$

Milligrams (mg) in the numerator and denominator cancel each other out and you are left with mL as the volume of medication in the answer.

Solve for x:

$$x = \frac{30 \text{ mg} \times \text{mL}}{15 \text{ mg}} = 2 \text{ mL}$$

Therefore, Mr. Dodson should receive 2 mL of Toradol as the correct dose.

PRACTICE PROBLEMS 6-2. Using the Ratio-Proportion Method

DIRECTIONS: Set up and solve the medication dosage problems in the previous exercise using the ratio-proportion method. The answers to the problems can be found at the end of the chapter.

1. **Medication Ordered:** Erythromycin 750 mg
   Medication Available: Erythromycin 250 mg tablets

Calculation:

Dispense in a USP tight container.
Keep tightly closed.
Store below 86°F (30°C).

NDC 0074-6326-53
500 Tablets
ERYTHROMYCIN
Base Filmtab®
ERYTHROMYCIN
TABLETS, USP
250 mg Erythromycin, USP

⅃ ℞ only

Do not accept if seal over bottle opening is broken or missing.

Each tablet contains:
Erythromycin, USP
.............................250 mg

Usual adult dose: One tablet every six hours.
See enclosure for full prescribing information.

Filmtab — Film-sealed tablets, Abbott
©Abbott

Abbott Laboratories
North Chicago, IL 60064, U.S.A.

2. Medication Ordered: Biaxin 250 mg
   Medication Available: Biaxin 500 mg tablets

Calculation:

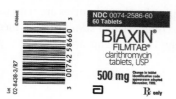

NDC 0074-2586-60
60 Tablets

BIAXIN®
FILMTAB®
clarithromycin
tablets, USP

500 mg

℞ only

6505-01-354-8581
Store tablets at 20° to 25°C (68° to 77°F).
Do not accept if seal over bottle opening
is broken or missing.
Dispense in a USP tight container.
Each tablet contains:
500 mg clarithromycin.
See enclosure for full prescribing
information.
Filmtab – Film-sealed tablets,
Abbott.

Abbott Laboratories
North Chicago, IL 60064, U.S.A.

Abbott Laboratories. Used with permission.

3. Medication Ordered: Furosemide 60 mg
   Medication Available: Furosemide 100 mg/mL

Calculation:

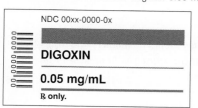

NDC 00xx-0000-0x

FUROSEMIDE

100 mg/mL

℞ only.

4. Medication Ordered: Digoxin 0.125 mg
   Medication Available: Digoxin 0.05 mg/mL

Calculation:

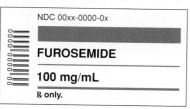

NDC 00xx-0000-0x

DIGOXIN

0.05 mg/mL

℞ only.

5. Medication Ordered: Gantrisin 1.5 mg
   Medication Available: Gantrisin 0.5 mg per tablet

Calculation:

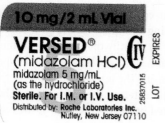

NDC 0004-0009-01   ITEM 73314

Roche

GANTRISIN®
(sulfisoxazole)

0.5 g

Each tablet contains
0.5 g sulfisoxazole.

CAUTION: Federal law prohibits
dispensing without prescription.

100 Tablets

STORE AT 59° TO 86° F (15° TO 30° C).
Dispense in tight, light-resistant
containers as defined in USP/NF.

USUAL DOSAGE: For dosage recommendations and other important
prescribing information, read accompanying insert.
ROCHE LABORATORIES
a division of Hoffmann-La Roche Inc., Nutley, NJ 07110

0004-0009-01

Hoffmann-La Roche Inc. Used with permission.

6. Medication Ordered: Versed 4 mg
   Medication Available: Versed 10 mg/2 mL

Calculation:

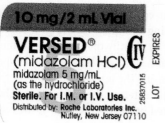

10 mg/2 mL Vial

VERSED®
(midazolam HCl) **C IV**
midazolam 5 mg/mL
(as the hydrochloride)
Sterile. For I.M. or I.V. Use.
Distributed by: Roche Laboratories Inc.
Nutley, New Jersey 07110

EXPIRES

LOT 25837015

Hoffmann-La Roche Inc. Used with permission.

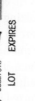

SIX RIGHTS OF MEDICATION ADMINISTRATION

The Six Rights of Medication Administration are a standard of practice that all nurses are required to use each time a medication is administered. Following these "rights" when administering medication ensures that the medication administration is done safely. The six rights are:

- The right medication
- The right dose
- The right route
- The right time
- The right patient
- The right documentation

Some institutions have two additional rights. The patient has a right to refuse or question the medication that is being administered. The other right is that the medication is being administered for the right reason.

The Right Medication

The prescriber orders the medication for the patient. The nurse is responsible for interpreting the prescribed order accurately. If the medication name is not clear or if the medication seems inappropriate for the patient's condition, question the order. Also, read drug labels carefully to ensure that you have the right medication.

(!) **SAFETY ALERT:** *Be very careful when reading medication names from orders and drug labels. Many medications have similar-sounding names, and that can cause you to make a medication error. Check and double check that you have the correct medication.*

The Right Dose

To ensure the right dose of medication, you need to interpret abbreviations accurately. Remember from Chapter 3 the rules about using abbreviations and the use of a leading and trailing zero. If an abbreviation or a dosage in a written order is unclear, call the prescriber for verification. You also need to interpret measurements accurately. This requires:

- Ensuring that the measurement system of the prescribed medication is the same as the measurement system of the available drug.
- Converting unlike measurements of the prescribed medication to an equivalent of that measurement system or unit for the available drug.
- Calculating the medication dosages accurately, using either the formula method or the ratio-proportion method.

The Right Route

For the right route, you need to make sure that the route prescribed for the medication is appropriate for the medication. Additionally, you need to use the correct technique of administration for any route that is ordered. For example, if your patient has an enteric-coated aspirin ordered, do not crush the medication because doing so will destroy the enteric coating and interfere with the action of the drug. When giving intramuscular (IM) injections, make sure to identify the correct anatomic landmarks for injection and select the correct needle size for the injection site selected and the type of solution being administered. When administering a medication using the intravenous (IV) route, make sure that you follow the instructions for preparing and administering the medication. The nurse must make sure that the IV medication is diluted and/or mixed properly and given at the recommended or prescribed rate.

The Right Time

Administering a medication at the prescribed time or right time is important because it will maximize the therapeutic effects of the medication and minimize the potential adverse effects. Medications are administered at specific time intervals to maintain therapeutic blood levels. However, omitting a dose or delaying the administration of a dose of the medication may be necessary when indicated by the patient's condition. Most healthcare institutions have a policy that identifies the usual time interval considered appropriate within which to administer a medication. For example, many institutions state that the medication should be administered within 30 minutes before or after the prescribed time. For a medication that is ordered for 0900, you would administer the medication between 0830 and 0930.

The Right Patient

Identifying the right patient is another critical step in the medication administration process. The National Patient Safety Goals require that you identify the patient using two forms of identification. Acceptable patient identifiers include name, birth date, an assigned hospital identification number, patient telephone number, or other patient-specific identifier. Each healthcare institution will designate which two patient identifiers must be used. Patients in healthcare institutions generally have identification bands. It is permissible to use two identifiers from the identification band. Check the patient's identification band for his or her name and then use the second institutionally-specified patient identifier. As a third identifier, you can ask the patient to state his or her name to help verify that the information on the identification band is correct.

> **(!) SAFETY ALERT:** *Always identify your patient using the two identifiers designated by your institution each time that you administer a medication. This ensures that you have the right patient. This check is even more crucial if there are patients on the unit with the same or similar sounding names. Do not rely on room number as a patient identifier.*

The Right Documentation

The right documentation is the final step in the "right" process to ensure safe medication administration. It involves the prompt documentation of the medication administration on the correct form. Prompt documentation ensures that the patient will not accidentally receive an additional dose of the medication or receive a dose of the medication too early. If an IM injection was given, make sure to document the injection site also.

 CASE STUDY

Now that you have calculated the correct doses of Pepcid and Toradol and prepared them properly, you are ready to administer them to Mr. Dodson. As you administer the medications to Mr. Dodson, follow the "Six Rights of Medication Administration" to ensure safe administration.

Many healthcare institutions are using computerized medication administration systems for documentation. Follow the healthcare institution's policy for documenting medication administration, including the proper method for documenting omitted or late doses of medications. In addition, make sure that your initials and signature on the form are legible.

CASE STUDY

Following the Six Rights of Medication Administration, you safely administer the medications to Mr. Dodson. As he is improving daily, you arrange for the dietician to talk to Mr. Dodson and his wife about a low-cholesterol, no-added-salt diet. The Cardiac Rehabilitation staff has started Mr. Dodson on a regular walking program. He is to be discharged on postoperative day 5.

Critical Thinking/Decision Making Exercise

The nurse received a new medication order for a patient. The order was written:

April 21, 2007   0730
Enalapril (Vasotec) 10 mg   2 tablets p.o. in the A.M.
Dr. Thompson

In reviewing the patient's medication history, the nurse found that the patient normally takes enalapril (Vasotec) 5 mg p.o. daily. The nurse was not sure if the written order meant that the patient should receive 20 mg of Vasotec or if the patient should take 2 tablets of the normally pre-scribed 5 mg dose to equal 10 mg. She placed a call to the physician for clarification of the order. The physician wanted the patient to have only 10 mg of the medication. After rewriting the order for clarification, the nurse prepared to give the patient enalapril (Vasotec) 10 mg.

The new order was added to the Medication Administration Record and 0900 was marked as the time to give the medication. At 0850, the nurse removed enalapril 10 mg from the medication dispensing unit. The nurse entered the patient's room and told the patient that the physician had increased the blood pressure medication. The nurse gave the patient the medication, which the patient took by mouth with a glass of water right away. The nurse left the patient's room and promptly documented the administration of the medication on the Medication Administration Record.

Did the Nurse Practice Safe Medication Administration?

To correctly answer the question, you need to determine if the nurse followed the Six Rights of Medication Administration.

1. *The right medication*—The nurse was able to easily read and interpret the medication that was ordered as enalapril (Vasotec). A comparison was made to the patient's medication history and the nurse noted that the patient takes this medication at home. This step was followed properly because the nurse correctly identified and verified the medication.

2. *The right dose*—The dosage order for the enalapril was confusing to the nurse when compared to the patient's normal dosage of enalapril. The nurse called the physician to clarify the medication order. This step was followed properly because the nurse contacted the physician for clarification of the order so that the correct dose was given to the patient.

3. *The right route*—The physician ordered the medication to be administered p.o. This step was followed properly because the nurse had the patient take the medication by mouth with a glass of water.

4. *The right time*—The medication was ordered to be given to the patient in the A.M. Per institution policy, A.M. medications are to be administered at 0900. The nurse set up the medication at 0850 and administered it right after that. This step was followed properly because the nurse administered the medication at the appropriate time.

5. *The right patient*—The nurse entered the patient's room and informed the patient that the physician had increased the dose of medication. The nurse did not correctly identify the patient by checking the identification band or asking the patient to state his or her name. This step was not followed properly, and the nurse could have given the wrong patient the medication. Always verify that you have the right patient by checking the patient's identification band.

6. *The right documentation*—The nurse promptly documented the administration of the medication on the appropriate form. This step was followed properly because the nurse completed the medication administration process by documenting correctly.

CHAPTER REVIEW PROBLEMS

The answers to the problems can be found at the end of the chapter.

DIRECTIONS: Solve the following medication dosage problems using the formula method.

1. Medication Ordered: Toradol 20 mg p.o.
   Medication Available: Toradol 10 mg per tablet

Calculation:

2. Medication Ordered: Evista 30 mg p.o.
   Medication Available: Evista 60 mg per tablet

Calculation:

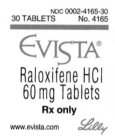 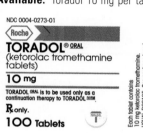

3. Medication Ordered: Strattera 36 mg p.o.
   Medication Available: Strattera 18 mg per capsule

Calculation:

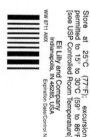 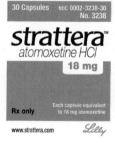 

4. Medication Ordered: Prozac 60 mg p.o.
   Medication Available: Prozac 40 mg per tablet

Calculation:

5. **Medication Ordered:** Morphine sulfate 6 mg IV
   Medication Available: Morphine sulfate 10 mg/ 1mL

Calculation:

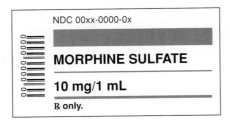

6. **Medication Ordered:** Meperidine 75 mg IM
   Medication Available: Meperidine 100 mg/1 mL

Calculation:

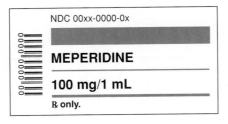

7. **Medication Ordered:** Naprosyn 750 mg
   Medication Available: Naprosyn 250 mg per tablet

Calculation:

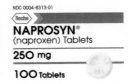

Hoffmann-La Roche Inc. Used with permission.

8. **Medication Ordered:** Romazicon 0.2 mg IV
   Medication Available: Romazicon 0.5 mg/5 mL

Calculation:

ROMAZICON®
(flumazenil)
INJECTION Multiple Use Vial
0.5 mg/5 mL
(0.1 mg/mL) 5 mL Vial
Sterile.
For I.V. Use.
USUAL DOSAGE:
See Package Insert.
STORE AT 59° TO 86° F
(15° TO 30° C).
Roche Laboratories Inc.
Nutley, New Jersey 07110
24992712-0798

EXP.

LOT

Roche Laboratories Inc. Used with permission.

DIRECTIONS: Set up and solve the medication dosage problems using the ratio-proportion method.

1. **Medication Ordered:** Vancomycin HCl 500 mg p.o.
   Medication Available: Vancomycin HCl 125 mg capsule

   Calculation:

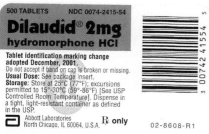

© Copyright Eli Lilly and Company. Used with permission.

2. **Medication Ordered:** Dilaudid 4 mg p.o.
   Medication Available: Dilaudid 2 mg tablet

   Calculation:

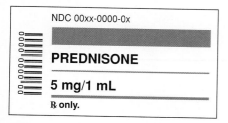

Abbott Laboratories. Used with permission.

3. **Medication Ordered:** Prednisone solution 40 mg
   Medication Available: Prednisone 5 mg/1 mL

   Calculation:

```
NDC 00xx-0000-0x

PREDNISONE

5 mg/1 mL

℞ only.
```

4. **Medication Ordered:** Hytrin 15 mg p.o.
   Medication Available: Hytrin 5 mg capsules

   Calculation:

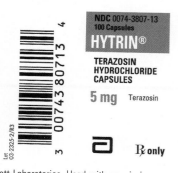

Abbott Laboratories. Used with permission.

5. Medication Ordered: Heparin 3000 units SubQ
   Medication Available: Heparin 10,000 units/1 mL

Calculation:

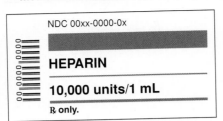

NDC 00xx-0000-0x

HEPARIN

10,000 units/1 mL

℞ only.

---

6. Medication Ordered: CellCept 750 mg p.o.
   Medication Available: CellCept 250 mg per capsule

Calculation:

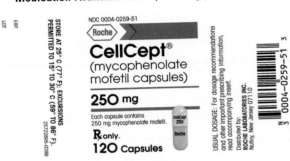

NDC 0004-0259-51

Roche

CellCept®
(mycophenolate mofetil capsules)

250 mg

Each capsule contains 250 mg mycophenolate mofetil.

℞ only.
120 Capsules

STORE AT 25° C (77° F); EXCURSIONS PERMITTED TO 15° TO 30° C (59° TO 86° F).

USUAL DOSAGE: For dosage recommendations and other important prescribing information, read accompanying insert.

Distributed by:
ROCHE LABORATORIES INC.
Nutley, New Jersey 07110

Hoffmann-La Roche Inc. Used with permission.

---

7. Medication Ordered: Valium 20 mg p.o.
   Medication Available: Valium 10 mg per tablet

Calculation:

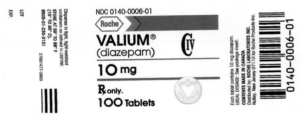

NDC 0140-0006-01

Roche

VALIUM®
(diazepam)   C IV

10 mg

℞ only.
100 Tablets

Hoffmann-La Roche Inc. Used with permission.

---

8. Medication Ordered: Capastat sulfate 0.5 g IM
   Medication Available: Capastat sulfate 1 g/2 mL

Calculation:

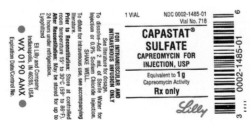

1 VIAL   NDC 0002-1485-01
Vial No. 718

CAPASTAT®
SULFATE
CAPREOMYCIN FOR INJECTION, USP

Equivalent to **1 g**
Capreomycin Activity

Rx only

Lilly

FOR INTRAMUSCULAR AND INTRAVENOUS INFUSION ONLY

Eli Lilly and Company
Indianapolis, IN 46285, USA

© Copyright Eli Lilly and Company. Used with permission.

Answers to Practice Problems

Answers to Practice Problems 6-1

Use the formula below to solve the problems.

$$\frac{D}{H} \times V = A$$

1. **Medication Ordered:** Erythromycin 750 mg
   Medication Available: Erythromycin 250-mg tablet

   $$\frac{750 \text{ mg}}{250 \text{ mg}} \times 1 \text{ tablet}$$

   In this problem because mg appears in both the numerator and denominator, mg is cancelled out and you are left with tablets as the volume of medication in the answer.

   $$\frac{750 \text{ mg}}{250 \text{ mg}} \times 1 \text{ tablet} = 3 \text{ tablets}$$

   Therefore, you would administer 3 tablets.

2. **Medication Ordered:** Biaxin 250 mg
   Medication Available: Biaxin 500 mg tablet

   $$\frac{250 \text{ mg}}{500 \text{ mg}} \times 1 \text{ tablet}$$

   In this problem because mg appears in both the numerator and denominator, mg is cancelled out and you are left with tablet as the volume of medication in the answer.

   $$\frac{250 \text{ mg}}{500 \text{ mg}} \times 1 \text{ tablet} = 0.5 \text{ tablet}$$

   Therefore, you would administer 0.5 tablet.

3. **Medication Ordered:** Furosemide 60 mg
   Medication Available: Furosemide 100 mg/mL

   $$\frac{60 \text{ mg}}{100 \text{ mg}} \times 1 \text{ mL}$$

   In this problem because mg appears in both the numerator and denominator, mg is cancelled out and you are left with mL as the volume of medication in the answer.

   $$\frac{60 \text{ mg}}{100 \text{ mg}} \times 1 \text{ mL} = 0.6 \text{ mL}$$

   Therefore, you would administer 0.6 mL.

4. **Medication Ordered:** Digoxin 0.125 mg
   Medication Available: Digoxin 0.05 mg/mL

   $$\frac{0.125 \text{ mg}}{0.05 \text{ mg}} \times 1 \text{ mL}$$

   In this problem because mg appears in both the numerator and denominator, mg is cancelled out and you are left with mL as the volume of medication in the answer.

   $$\frac{0.125 \text{ mg}}{0.05 \text{ mg}} \times 1 \text{ mL} = 2.5 \text{ mL}$$

   Therefore, you would administer 2.5 mL.

5. **Medication Ordered:** Gantrisin 1.5 g
   Medication Available: Gantrisin 0.5 g tablet

   $$\frac{1.5 \text{ g}}{0.5 \text{ g}} \times 1 \text{ tablet}$$

   In this problem because g appears in both the numerator and denominator, g is cancelled out and you are left with tablet as the volume of medication in the answer.

   $$\frac{1.5 \cancel{\text{g}}}{0.5 \cancel{\text{g}}} \times 1 \text{ tablet} = 3 \text{ tablets}$$

   Therefore, you would administer 3 tablets.

6. **Medication Ordered:** Versed 4 mg
   Medication Available: Versed 10 mg/2mL

   $$\frac{4 \text{ mg}}{10 \text{ mg}} \times 2 \text{ mL}$$

   In this problem because mg appears in both the numerator and denominator, mg is cancelled out and you are left with mL as the volume of medication in the answer.

   $$\frac{4 \cancel{\text{mg}}}{10 \cancel{\text{mg}}} \times 2 \text{ mL} = 0.8 \text{ mL}$$

   Therefore, you would administer 0.8 mL.

Answers to Practice Problems 6-2

Use the formula below to solve the problems.

$$\frac{\text{Dosage on hand (D)}}{\text{Amount on hand (H)}} = \frac{\text{Dosage prescribed (Q)}}{x \text{ Amount desired}}$$

1. **Medication Ordered:** Erythromycin 750 mg
   Medication Available: Erythromycin 250 mg tablet

   Set up:

   $$\frac{250 \text{ mg}}{1 \text{ tablet}} = \frac{750 \text{ mg}}{x}$$

   Cross multiply:

   $$\frac{250 \text{ mg}}{1 \text{ tablet}} \diagdown\diagup \frac{750 \text{ mg}}{x}$$

   $$250 \text{ mg } x = 750 \text{ mg} \times \text{tablet}$$

   Isolate x:

   $$\frac{250 \cancel{\text{mg}} \, x}{250 \cancel{\text{mg}}} = \frac{750 \cancel{\text{mg}} \times \text{tablet}}{250 \cancel{\text{mg}}}$$

   $$x = \frac{750 \text{ tablet}}{250}$$

   $$x = 3 \text{ tablets}$$

2. **Medication Ordered:** Biaxin 250 mg
   Medication Available: Biaxin 500 mg tablet

   Set up:

   $$\frac{500 \text{ mg}}{1 \text{ tablet}} = \frac{250 \text{ mg}}{x}$$

   Cross multiply:

   $$\frac{500 \text{ mg}}{1 \text{ tablet}} \diagdown\diagup \frac{250 \text{ mg}}{x}$$

   $$500 \text{ mg } x = 250 \text{ mg} \times \text{tablet}$$

   Isolate x:

   $$\frac{500 \cancel{\text{mg}} \, x}{500 \cancel{\text{mg}}} = \frac{250 \cancel{\text{mg}} \times \text{tablet}}{500 \cancel{\text{mg}}}$$

   $$x = \frac{250 \text{ tablet}}{500}$$

   $$x = 0.5 \text{ tablet}$$

3. **Medication Ordered:** Furosemide 60 mg
   Medication Available: Furosemide 100 mg/mL
   Set up:

   $$\frac{100 \text{ mg}}{1 \text{ mL}} = \frac{60 \text{ mg}}{x}$$

   Cross multiply:

   $$\frac{100 \text{ mg}}{1 \text{ mL}} \diagdown\!\!\!\!\diagup \frac{60 \text{ mg}}{x}$$

   $$100 \text{ mg } x = 60 \text{ mg} \times \text{mL}$$

   Isolate x:

   $$\frac{100 \text{ mg } x}{100 \text{ mg}} = \frac{60 \text{ mg} \times \text{mL}}{100 \text{ mg}}$$

   $$x = \frac{60 \text{ mL}}{100}$$

   $$x = 0.6 \text{ mL}$$

5. **Medication Ordered:** Gantrisin 1.5 g
   Medication Available: Gantrisin 0.5 g
   tablet
   Set up:

   $$\frac{0.5 \text{ g}}{1 \text{ tablet}} = \frac{1.5 \text{ mg}}{x}$$

   Cross multiply:

   $$\frac{0.5 \text{ g}}{1 \text{ tablet}} \diagdown\!\!\!\!\diagup \frac{1.5 \text{ g}}{x}$$

   $$0.5 \text{ g } x = 1.5 \text{ g} \times \text{tablet}$$

   Isolate x:

   $$\frac{0.5 \text{ g } x}{0.5 \text{ g}} = \frac{1.5 \text{ g} \times \text{tablet}}{0.5 \text{ g}}$$

   $$x = \frac{1.5 \text{ tablet}}{0.5}$$

   $$x = 3 \text{ tablets}$$

4. **Medication Ordered:** Digoxin 0.125 mg
   Medication Available: Digoxin 0.05 mg/mL
   Set up:

   $$\frac{0.05 \text{ mg}}{1 \text{ mL}} = \frac{0.125 \text{ mg}}{x}$$

   Cross multiply:

   $$\frac{0.05 \text{ mg}}{1 \text{ mL}} \diagdown\!\!\!\!\diagup \frac{0.125 \text{ mg}}{x}$$

   $$0.05 \text{ mg } x = 0.125 \text{ mg} \times \text{mL}$$

   Isolate x:

   $$\frac{0.05 \text{ mg } x}{0.05 \text{ mg}} = \frac{0.125 \text{ mg} \times \text{mL}}{0.05 \text{ mg}}$$

   $$x = \frac{0.125 \text{ mL}}{0.05}$$

   $$x = 2.5 \text{ mL}$$

6. **Medication Ordered:** Versed 4 mg
   Medication Available: Versed 10 mg/2mL
   Set up:

   $$\frac{10 \text{ mg}}{2 \text{ mL}} = \frac{4 \text{ mg}}{x}$$

   Cross multiply:

   $$\frac{10 \text{ mg}}{2 \text{ mL}} \diagdown\!\!\!\!\diagup \frac{4 \text{ mg}}{x}$$

   $$10 \text{ mg } x = 8 \text{ mg} \times \text{mL}$$

   Isolate x:

   $$\frac{10 \text{ mg } x}{10 \text{ mg}} = \frac{8 \text{ mg} \times \text{mL}}{10 \text{ mg}}$$

   $$x = \frac{8 \text{ mL}}{10}$$

   $$x = 0.8 \text{ mL}$$

Answers to Chapter Review Problems

Answers to Review Problems 6-1

Remember the formula:

$$\frac{D}{H} \times V = A$$

Where: D = desired or prescribed dosage of the medication
H = dosage of medication available or on hand
V = volume that the medication is available in, such as one tablet or milliliters
A = amount of medication to administer

1. **Medication Ordered:** Toradol 20 mg p.o.
   Medication Available: Toradol 10 mg per tablet

   $$\frac{20 \text{ mg}}{10 \text{ mg}} \times 1 \text{ tablet}$$

   In this problem because mg appears in both the numerator and denominator, mg is cancelled out and you are left with tablet as the volume of medication in the answer.

   $$\frac{20 \cancel{\text{ mg}}}{10 \cancel{\text{ mg}}} \times 1 \text{ tablet} = 2 \text{ tablets}$$

   Therefore, you would administer 2 tablets.

2. **Medication Ordered:** Evista 30 mg p.o.
   Medication Available: Evista 60 mg tablet

   $$\frac{30 \text{ mg}}{60 \text{ mg}} \times 1 \text{ tablet}$$

   In this problem because mg appears in both the numerator and denominator, mg is cancelled out and you are left with tablet as the volume of medication in the answer.

   $$\frac{30 \cancel{\text{ mg}}}{60 \cancel{\text{ mg}}} \times 1 \text{ tablet} = 0.5 \text{ tablet}$$

   Therefore, you would administer 0.5 tablet.

3. **Medication Ordered:** Strattera 36 mg p.o.
   Medication Available: Strattera 18 mg capsule

   $$\frac{36 \text{ mg}}{18 \text{ mg}} \times 1 \text{ capsule}$$

   In this problem because mg appears in both the numerator and denominator, mg is cancelled out and you are left with capsule as the volume of medication in the answer.

   $$\frac{36 \cancel{\text{ mg}}}{18 \cancel{\text{ mg}}} \times 1 \text{ capsule} = 2 \text{ capsules}$$

   Therefore, you would administer 2 capsules.

4. **Medication Ordered:** Prozac 60 mg p.o.
   Medication Available: Prozac 40 mg tablet

   $$\frac{60 \text{ mg}}{40 \text{ mg}} \times 1 \text{ tablet}$$

   In this problem because mg appears in both the numerator and denominator, mg is cancelled out and you are left with tablet as the volume of medication in the answer.

   $$\frac{60 \cancel{\text{ mg}}}{40 \cancel{\text{ mg}}} \times 1 \text{ tablet} = 1.5 \text{ tablet}$$

   Therefore, you would administer 1.5 tablets.

5. **Medication Ordered:** Morphine sulfate 6 mg IV
   Medication Available: Morphine sulfate 10 mg/1mL

   $$\frac{6 \text{ mg}}{10 \text{ mg}} \times 1 \text{ mL}$$

   In this problem because mg appears in both the numerator and denominator, mg is cancelled out and you are left with mL as the volume of medication in the answer.

   $$\frac{6 \cancel{\text{ mg}}}{10 \cancel{\text{ mg}}} \times 1 \text{ mL} = 0.6 \text{ mL}$$

   Therefore, you would administer 0.6 mL intravenously.

6. **Medication Ordered:** Meperidine 75 mg IM
   Medication Available: Meperidine 100 mg/1 mL

   $$\frac{75 \text{ mg}}{100 \text{ mg}} \times 1 \text{ mL}$$

   In this problem because mg appears in both the numerator and denominator, mg is cancelled out and you are left with mL as the volume of medication in the answer.

   $$\frac{75 \cancel{\text{ mg}}}{100 \cancel{\text{ mg}}} \times 1 \text{ mL} = 0.75 \text{ mL}$$

   Therefore, you would administer 0.75 mL by injection.

7. **Medication Ordered:** Naprosyn 750 mg
   Medication Available: Naprosyn 250 mg tablet

   $$\frac{750 \text{ mg}}{250 \text{ mg}} \times 1 \text{ tablet}$$

   In this problem because mg appears in both the numerator and denominator, mg is cancelled out and you are left with tablet as the volume of medication in the answer.

   $$\frac{750 \cancel{\text{ mg}}}{250 \cancel{\text{ mg}}} \times 1 \text{ tablet} = 3 \text{ tablets}$$

   Therefore, you would administer 3 tablets.

8. **Medication Ordered:** Romazicon 0.2 mg IV
   Medication Available: Romazicon 0.5 mg/5 mL

   $$\frac{0.2 \text{ mg}}{0.5 \text{ mg}} \times 5 \text{ mL}$$

   In this problem because mg appears in both the numerator and denominator, mg is cancelled out and you are left with mL as the volume of medication in the answer.

   $$\frac{0.2 \cancel{\text{ mg}}}{0.5 \cancel{\text{ mg}}} \times 5 \text{ mL} = 2 \text{ mL}$$

   Therefore, you would administer 2 mL intravenously.

Answers to Review Problems 6-2

Remember the ratio-proportion equation:

$$\frac{\text{Dosage on hand (D)}}{\text{Amount on hand (H)}} = \frac{\text{Dosage prescribed (Q)}}{x \text{ Amount desired}}$$

1. **Medication Ordered:** Vancomycin HCl 500 mg p.o.
   Medication Available: Vancomycin HCl 125 mg capsule

   Set up:

   $$\frac{125 \text{ mg}}{1 \text{ capsule}} = \frac{500 \text{ mg}}{x}$$

   Cross multiply:

   $$\frac{125 \text{ mg}}{1 \text{ capsule}} \diagdown\diagup \frac{500 \text{ mg}}{x}$$

   $$125 \text{ mg } x = 500 \text{ mg} \times \text{capsule}$$

   Isolate x:

   $$\frac{\cancel{125 \text{ mg}} x}{\cancel{125 \text{ mg}}} = \frac{500 \cancel{\text{ mg}} \times \text{capsule}}{125 \cancel{\text{ mg}}}$$

   $$x = \frac{500 \text{ capsule}}{125}$$

   $$x = 4 \text{ capsules}$$

2. **Medication Ordered:** Dilaudid 4 mg p.o.
   Medication Available: Dilaudid 2 mg tablet

   Set up:

   $$\frac{2 \text{ mg}}{1 \text{ tablet}} = \frac{4 \text{ mg}}{x}$$

   Cross multiply:

   $$\frac{2 \text{ mg}}{1 \text{ tablet}} \diagdown\diagup \frac{4 \text{ mg}}{x}$$

   $$2 \text{mg } x = 4 \text{ mg} \times \text{tablet}$$

   Isolate x:

   $$\frac{\cancel{2 \text{ mg}} x}{\cancel{2 \text{ mg}}} = \frac{4 \cancel{\text{ mg}} \times \text{tablet}}{2 \cancel{\text{ mg}}}$$

   $$x = \frac{4 \text{ tablet}}{2}$$

   $$x = 2 \text{ tablets}$$

3. **Medication Ordered:** Prednisone solution 40 mg
Medication Available: Prednisone 5 mg/1 mL

Set up:

$$\frac{5 \text{ mg}}{1 \text{ mL}} = \frac{40 \text{ mg}}{x}$$

Cross multiply:

$$\frac{5 \text{ mg}}{1 \text{ mL}} \diagdown \frac{40 \text{ mg}}{x}$$

5 mg x = 40 mg × mL

Isolate x:

$$\frac{5 \text{ mg } x}{5 \text{ mg}} = \frac{40 \text{ mg} \times \text{mL}}{5 \text{ mg}}$$

$$x = \frac{40 \text{ mL}}{5}$$

$$x = 8 \text{ mL}$$

4. **Medication Ordered:** Hytrin 15 mg
Medication Available: Hytrin 5 mg capsule

Set up:

$$\frac{5 \text{ mg}}{1 \text{ capsule}} = \frac{15 \text{ mg}}{x}$$

Cross multiply:

$$\frac{5 \text{ mg}}{1 \text{ capsule}} \diagdown \frac{15 \text{ mg}}{x}$$

5 mg x = 15 mg × capsule

Isolate x:

$$\frac{5 \text{ mg } x}{5 \text{ mg}} = \frac{15 \text{ mg} \times \text{capsule}}{5 \text{ mg}}$$

$$x = \frac{15 \text{ capsule}}{5}$$

$$x = 3 \text{ capsules}$$

5. **Medication Ordered:** Heparin 3000 units SubQ
Medication Available: Heparin 10,000 units/1 mL

Set up:

$$\frac{10,000 \text{ units}}{1 \text{ mL}} = \frac{3000 \text{ units}}{x}$$

Cross multiply:

$$\frac{10,000 \text{ units}}{1 \text{ mL}} \diagdown \frac{3000 \text{ units}}{x}$$

10,000 units x = 3000 units × mL

Isolate x:

$$\frac{10,000 \text{ units } x}{10,000 \text{ units}} = \frac{3000 \text{ units} \times \text{mL}}{10,000 \text{ units}}$$

$$x = \frac{3000 \text{ mL}}{10,000}$$

$$x = 0.3 \text{ mL}$$

6. **Medication Ordered:** CellCept 750 mg p.o.
Medication Available: CellCept 250 mg capsule

Set up:

$$\frac{250 \text{ mg}}{1 \text{ capsule}} = \frac{750 \text{ mg}}{x}$$

Cross multiply:

$$\frac{250 \text{ mg}}{1 \text{ capsule}} \diagdown \frac{750 \text{ mg}}{x}$$

250 mg x = 750 mg × capsule

Isolate x:

$$\frac{250 \text{ mg } x}{250 \text{ mg}} = \frac{750 \text{ mg} \times \text{capsule}}{250 \text{ mg}}$$

$$x = \frac{750 \text{ capsules}}{250}$$

$$x = 3 \text{ capsules}$$

7. **Medication Ordered:** Valium 20 mg p.o.
Medication Available: Valium 10 mg tablet

Set up:

$$\frac{10 \text{ mg}}{1 \text{ tablet}} = \frac{20 \text{ mg}}{x}$$

Cross multiply:

$$\frac{10 \text{ mg}}{1 \text{ tablet}} \diagdown \frac{20 \text{ mg}}{x}$$

10 mg x = 20 mg × tablet

Isolate x:

$$\frac{10 \text{ mg } x}{10 \text{ mg}} = \frac{20 \text{ mg} \times \text{tablet}}{10 \text{ mg}}$$

$$x = \frac{20 \text{ tablets}}{10}$$

$$x = 2 \text{ tablets}$$

8. **Medication Ordered:** Capastat sulfate 0.5 g IM
Medication Available: Capastat sulfate 1 g/2 mL

Set up:

$$\frac{1 \text{ g}}{2 \text{ mL}} = \frac{0.5 \text{ g}}{x}$$

Cross multiply:

$$\frac{1 \text{ g}}{2 \text{ mL}} \diagdown \frac{0.5 \text{ g}}{x}$$

1 g x = 1g × mL

Isolate x:

$$\frac{1 \text{ g} x}{1 \text{ g}} = \frac{1 \text{ g} \times \text{mL}}{1 \text{ g}}$$

$$x = \frac{1 \text{ mL}}{1}$$

$$x = 1 \text{ mL}$$

Calculation of Oral Medications

This chapter contains content on:

- **Tablets and Capsules**
- **Liquid Medications**

Learning Objectives

Upon completion of Chapter 7, you will be able to:

- Incorporate the 3-Step Approach to dosage calculation for oral medication dosages.
- Calculate the dosage of capsules and tablets using the formula:

$$\frac{D}{H} \times V = A$$

- Calculate the dosage of capsules and tablets using the ratio-proportion method.
- Calculate the volume of medication required when the medication is in a solution form using the formula and ratio-proportion methods.
- Critically evaluate the calculation process and the accuracy of the answers.

Key Terms

- Capsule
- Elixir
- Emulsion
- Enteric coating
- Suspension
- Sustained release
- Syrup
- Tablet

CASE STUDY

You are the nurse on a busy medical-surgical floor. You are responsible for the nursing care of the four patients:

- Mrs. Billings, a 78-year-old admitted with a respiratory infection, who is receiving antibiotics

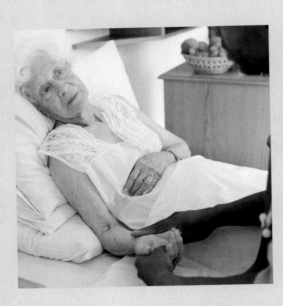

- Mr. Yancy, a 66-year-old with heart failure, who is receiving diuretic therapy and a potassium supplement

- Mrs. Tompkins, a 49-year-old who had an abdominal hysterectomy and is requesting medication for a headache

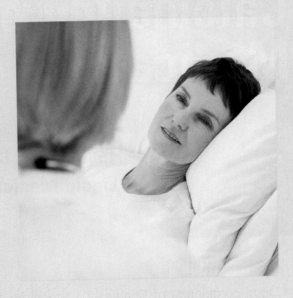

- Ms. Wills, a 34-year-old who is NPO with a nasogastric (NG) tube in place after extensive surgery and now with a urinary tract infection receiving antibiotic therapy via the NG tube

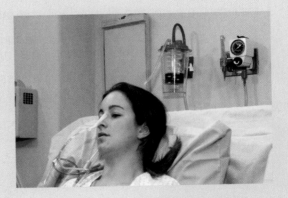

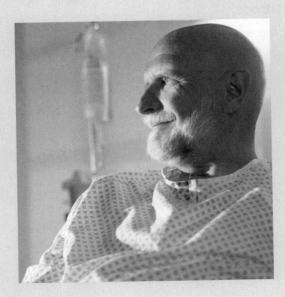

After completing your morning assessments, it is time for you to administer morning medications to the patients. The patients are receiving a variety of oral medications in tablet, capsule, and liquid form. You are responsible for safely calculating, setting up, and administering the medications.

Oral medications come in a variety of forms: tablets, capsules, lozenges, or liquids. Prescribers order these medications to be given by mouth (p.o. or per os). **Tablets** are a solid form of the medication. Some have an **enteric coating**, a wax-like hard coating on the outside of the tablet. This coating prevents the acid environment in the stomach from dissolving the tablet, thereby allowing the tablet to dissolve in a neutral or alkaline environment. **Capsules** are solid medications that have the medication enclosed in a dissolvable shell of hard or soft gelatin. Some solid medications, such as capsules, also come in **sustained release** or timed release form. This form releases a set amount of the medication over an extended period of time.

Liquid medications come in the form of emulsions, syrups, elixirs, or suspensions. An **emulsion** is a combination of two drugs that do not mix well. When shaken, one drug evenly distributes itself through the other drug. **Syrup** contains the medication within a concentrated solution of sugar. An **elixir** is a liquid medication that is generally a combination of the medication, water, and ethanol. A **suspension** is a liquid that contains a finely divided solid medication mixed into a carrier solution.

Oral medications may also be given through nasogastric or gastrostomy tubes. For medications that need to be given through a tube, a liquid form is often available. Medications that do not come in a liquid form will need to be crushed and mixed in water for administration through a tube.

> **! SAFETY ALERT:** *Always check to make sure that a medication can be crushed. Medications that have an enteric coating or come in a sustained or timed-release form cannot be crushed. Crushing these medications can alter the pharmacokinetics of the medication. Contact the prescriber to discuss alternate routes of administration of these medications.*

> **! SAFETY ALERT:** *When crushing medications for administration through a tube, make sure that the particles are fine and fully dissolved in water for easy passage through the tube. Medications with large particles or that are not well dissolved could clog the tube. Make sure to flush the tube well with water after medication administration.*

Frequently pharmaceutical companies supply oral medications for administration in commonly prescribed dosages. This sets a standard so the nurse can recognize the order as either greater or lesser than the usual dose. If the calculation of a medication dosage results in the need to cut a tablet in half, use care to divide the tablet along the scoring created by the manufacturer. If possible, use a pill cutter to divide a tablet in half to help ensure accuracy of the divided tablet.

Prescribers may order oral medications in doses other than the standard or commonly-prescribed dose based on the weight or age of the individual, the status of the patient (for example, critical), the immediacy of the problem, or the type of the medication. Some medications are ordered in smaller doses initially to determine the patient's response. Then subsequent doses are increased to achieve a higher blood level. When a larger-than-usual dose is ordered, it is often to increase the blood level of the medication rapidly. Regardless of the situation, the nurse is responsible for accurately calculating the amount to be administered.

TABLETS AND CAPSULES

Formula Method

When the dosage ordered differs from the dosage available, use the formula method:

$$\frac{D}{H} \times V = A$$

Where: D = desired or ordered dosage
H = dosage on hand
V = volume that the medication is provided in, such as one tablet or milliliters
A = administered medication dose

CASE STUDY

Recall that Mrs. Billings, a 78-year-old who was admitted to the hospital last week with a respiratory infection, requires antibiotics for the treatment of an infection. Today is the first day she will begin taking the antibiotics orally after 4 days of intravenous antibiotic therapy.

The physician has ordered amoxicillin 1 g by mouth this morning. You have available amoxicillin 500 mg in 1 capsule. You recognize that the dosage of the medication that you have available differs from the ordered dosage. Therefore, you decide to use the formula method to calculate the correct dosage of amoxicillin.

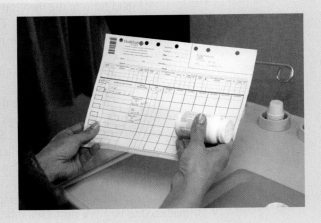

STEP 1: CONVERT

A key step in the process is making sure that the medication dose ordered is in the same dosage system and unit as the medication available. When dosages ordered for medications are in different systems or units than dosage on hand, it is important to convert both the ordered dosage and the dosage on hand to the same system or unit. For Mrs. Billings, both the ordered dosage and dosage on hand need to be in milligrams or grams. To ensure accuracy, it is important to convert grams to milligrams. Based on your understanding of equivalents, you know that there are 1,000 milligrams in 1 gram. You do the conversion by multiplying 1 gram by 1,000.

Multiply: $1 \times 1000 = 1000$

Answer: $1 \text{ g} = 1000 \text{ mg}$

STEP 2: COMPUTE

Determine what data you need and set up the problem correctly. The formula method requires you to know what medication dose is ordered and the dosage available or dosage on hand. This step requires higher-level thinking, not just memorization.

The formula is:
$$\frac{D}{H} \times V = A$$

For this problem: The D (desired or ordered dose) is 1 g, which has been converted to 1000 mg. The H (dosage on hand) is 500 mg. The V (volume medication comes in) is 1 capsule. Therefore, using this method the set-up of the problem would be:

$$\frac{1000 \text{ mg}}{500 \text{ mg}} \times 1 \text{ capsule} = A$$

Reduce the fraction to the lowest common denominator by dividing the numerator and denominator by 500. Cancel out milligrams.

$$\frac{\cancel{1000 \text{ mg}}}{\cancel{500 \text{ mg}}} \frac{2}{1} \times 1 \text{ capsule} = A$$

$$2 \times 1 \text{ capsule} = A$$

$$2 \text{ capsules} = A$$

The correct answer for this problem is 2 capsules.

STEP 3: CRITICALLY THINK

ASK YOURSELF – Does this answer seem logical, correct, and plausible?

This answer is reasonable and plausible in that it meets the safe standard for the number of capsules given at one time. Two capsules is not unusually large or small for a safe dose. It is correct. Think that 1,000 mg is two times as much as 500 mg. Therefore, 2 capsules are correct. To verify this step, have another nurse check your math.

PRACTICE PROBLEMS 7-1. Practice Problems for Tablets and Capsules Using the Formula Method

DIRECTIONS: Solve the following medication dosage problems using the formula method. The answers to the problems can be found at the end of the chapter.

1. **Medication Ordered:** Vancomycin HCl 375 mg p.o. b.i.d.
   Medication Available: Vancomycin HCl 125 mg capsule

   Calculation:

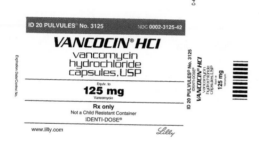

© Eli Lilly and Company. Used with permission.

2. **Medication Ordered:** Dilantin 200 mg p.o. b.i.d.
   Medication Available: Dilantin 100 mg capsule

   Calculation:

Reproduced with permission of Pfizer Inc. All rights reserved.

3. **Medication Ordered:** Metoprolol 25 mg p.o. b.i.d.
   Medication Available: Metoprolol 50 mg tablet

   Calculation:

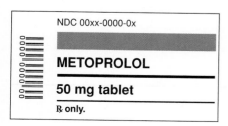

4. **Medication Ordered:** Prednisone 7.5 mg p.o. daily
   Medication Available: Prednisone 2.5 mg tablet

Calculation:

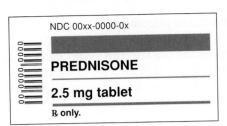

NDC 00xx-0000-0x

PREDNISONE

2.5 mg tablet

℞ only.

---

5. **Medication Ordered:** Potassium 20 mEq p.o. b.i.d.
   Medication Available: Potassium 10 mEq capsule

Calculation:

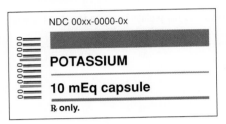

NDC 00xx-0000-0x

POTASSIUM

10 mEq capsule

℞ only.

---

6. **Medication Ordered:** Klonopin 0.5 mg p.o. daily
   Medication Available: Klonopin 1 mg tablet

Calculation:

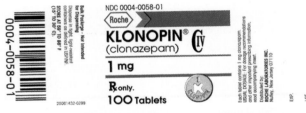

Hoffmann-La Roche Inc. Used with permission.

---

7. **Medication Ordered:** Fortovase 1200 mg p.o. t.i.d.
   Medication Available: Fortovase 200 mg capsule

Calculation:

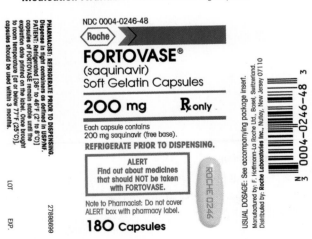

Hoffmann-La Roche Inc. Used with permission.

8. **Medication Ordered:** Aspirin gr 10 p.o. daily
   Medication Available: Aspirin 325 mg tablet

   Calculation:

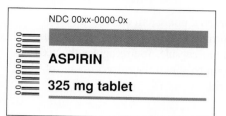

```
NDC 00xx-0000-0x

ASPIRIN

325 mg tablet
```

9. **Medication Ordered:** Depakote DR 500 mg p.o. daily
   Medication Available: Depakote DR 250 mg tablet

   Calculation:

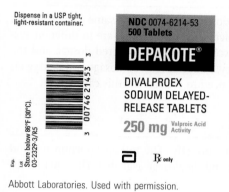

Dispense in a USP tight, light-resistant container.

NDC 0074-6214-53
500 Tablets

DEPAKOTE®

DIVALPROEX
SODIUM DELAYED-
RELEASE TABLETS

250 mg Valproic Acid Activity

℞ only

6505-01-357-8537

Do not accept if band on cap is broken or missing.

Each tablet contains: Divalproex sodium equivalent to valproic acid ....250 mg

Each peach-colored tablet bears the ⊡ and Abbo-Code NR for product identification.

See enclosure for prescribing information.

Pat. No. 4,988,731
©Abbott

Abbott Laboratories
North Chicago, IL60064
U.S.A.

Store below 86°F (30°C).

Abbott Laboratories. Used with permission.

10. **Medication Ordered:** Furosemide 120 mg p.o. q AM
    Medication Available: Furosemide 40 mg tablet

    Calculation:

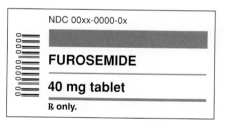

```
NDC 00xx-0000-0x

FUROSEMIDE

40 mg tablet

℞ only.
```

Ratio-Proportion Method

When the medication dosage ordered by the prescriber is different from the dosage of the medication available, the ratio-proportion method can be used to calculate the needed dose of the medication. This method solves for an unknown x in the equation. The equation is:

$$\frac{\text{Dosage on hand}}{\text{Amount on hand}} = \frac{\text{Dosage desired}}{x \text{ Amount desired}}$$

CASE STUDY

Remember Mr. Yancy, a 66-year-old who has been admitted with signs and symptoms of worsening heart failure. His edema is being treated with a diuretic. The physician has also ordered a potassium supplement because of the electrolyte losses with the diuretic.

The physician ordered potassium chloride 30 mEq by mouth every morning. You have available potassium chloride 10 mEq in one capsule. You recognize the need to perform calculation to obtain the correct dosage of the potassium chloride.

STEP 1: CONVERT

This step requires you to make sure that the medication dose ordered is in the same dosage system and unit as the medication available. When dosages ordered for medications are in different systems or units than dosage on hand, it is important to convert both the ordered dosage and the dosage on hand to the same system or unit. For Mr. Yancy, both the ordered dosage and dosage on hand are in the same unit—mEq. Therefore, you do not need to convert for this calculation.

STEP 2: COMPUTE

Determine what data you need and set up the problem correctly. The ratio-proportion method requires you to know what medication dose was ordered and the dosage available. The equation is:

$$\frac{\text{Dosage on hand}}{\text{Amount on hand}} = \frac{\text{Dosage desired}}{x \, \text{Amount desired}}$$

$$\frac{10 \text{ mEq}}{1 \text{ capsule}} = \frac{30 \text{ mEq}}{x}$$

Cross multiply:

$$\frac{10 \text{ mEq}}{1 \text{ capsule}} \bowtie \frac{30 \text{ mEq}}{x}$$

$$10 \text{ mEq } x = 30 \text{ mEq capsule}$$

Isolate x in the equation by dividing both sides of the equation by 10. Cancel out like units.

$$\frac{10 \text{ mEq } x}{10 \text{ mEq}} = \frac{30 \text{ mEq capsule}}{10 \text{ mEq}}$$

$$x = \frac{30 \text{ capsule}}{10}$$

$$x = 3 \text{ capsules}$$

The correct answer for this problem is 3 capsules.

STEP 3: CRITICALLY THINK

ASK YOURSELF – *Does this answer seem logical, correct, and plausible?*

This answer is reasonable and plausible in that it meets the safe standard for the number of capsules given at one time. It is not unusually large or small for a safe dose. Think that 30 mEq is three times as much as 10 mEq. Therefore, 3 capsules are correct. To verify this step, have another nurse check your math.

PRACTICE PROBLEMS 7-2. Practice Problems for Tablets and Capsules Using the Ratio-Proportion Method

DIRECTIONS: Solve the following medication dosage problems using the ratio-proportion method. The answers to the problems can be found at the end of the chapter.

1. **Medication Ordered:** Levothyroxine 0.1 mg p.o. daily
   Medication Available: Levothyroxine 50 mcg tablet

   Calculation:

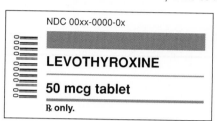

```
NDC 00xx-0000-0x

LEVOTHYROXINE

50 mcg tablet

℞ only.
```

2. **Medication Ordered:** Coumadin 7.5 mg p.o. daily
   Medication Available: Coumadin 5 mg tablet

   Calculation:

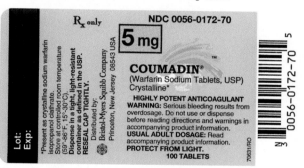

Bristol-Myers Squibb Company. Used with permission.

3. **Medication Ordered:** Atomoxetine 30 mg p.o. daily
   Medication Available: Atomoxetine 10 mg capsule

   Calculation:

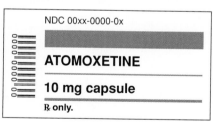

```
NDC 00xx-0000-0x

ATOMOXETINE

10 mg capsule

℞ only.
```

4. **Medication Ordered:** CellCept 500 mg p.o. daily
   Medication Available: CellCept 250 mg capsule

   Calculation:

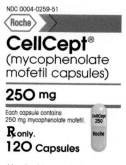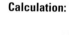

Hoffmann-La Roche Inc. Used with permission.

5. Medication Ordered: Valium 5 mg p.o. in AM
   Medication Available: Valium 10 mg tablet

Calculation:

NDC 0140-0006-01
Roche
VALIUM®
(diazepam) C IV
10 mg
℞ only.
100 Tablets

Hoffmann-La Roche Inc. Used with permission.

6. Medication Ordered: Gantrisin 2.5 g p.o. b.i.d.
   Medication Available: Gantrisin 0.5 g tablet

Calculation:

NDC 0004-0009-01   ITEM 73314
Roche
GANTRISIN®
(sulfisoxazole)
0.5 g
Each tablet contains
0.5 g sulfisoxazole.
CAUTION: Federal law prohibits
dispensing without prescription.
100 Tablets

Hoffmann-La Roche Inc. Used with permission.

7. Medication Ordered: Bumex 1.5 mg p.o. daily
   Medication Available: Bumex 0.5 mg tablet

Calculation:

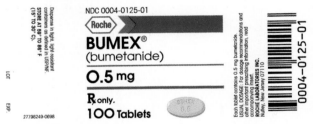

NDC 0004-0125-01
Roche
BUMEX®
(bumetanide)
0.5 mg
℞ only.
100 Tablets

Hoffmann-La Roche Inc. Used with permission.

8. Medication Ordered: Dilaudid 3 mg p.o. q 6h
   Medication Available: Dilaudid 2 mg tablet

Calculation:

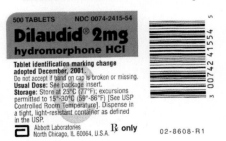

500 TABLETS   NDC 0074-2415-54
Dilaudid® 2mg
hydromorphone HCl
**Tablet identification marking change
adopted December, 2001.**
Do not accept if band on cap is broken or missing.
Usual Dose: See package insert.
Storage: Store at 25°C (77°F); excursions
permitted to 15°-30°C (59°-86°F) [See USP
Controlled Room Temperature]. Dispense in
a tight, light-resistant container as defined
in the USP.
Abbott Laboratories
North Chicago, IL 60064, U.S.A.   ℞ only   02-8608-R1

Abbott Laboratories. Used with permission.

9. **Medication Ordered:** Ibuprofen 600 mg p.o. t.i.d.
   Medication Available: Ibuprofen 200 mg capsule

   Calculation:

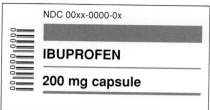

NDC 00xx-0000-0x

IBUPROFEN

200 mg capsule

---

10. **Medication Ordered:** Prozac 40 mg p.o. q a.m.
    Medication Available: Prozac 20 mg tablet

    Calculation:

30 Pulvules® PROZAC®, Fluoxetine Hydrochloride, Equiv. to 20 mg Fluoxetine Keep Tightly Closed Store at 59° to 86°F Control No.

30 Pulvules® PROZAC®, Fluoxetine Hydrochloride, Equiv. to 20 mg Fluoxetine Keep Tightly Closed Store at 59° to 86°F Expiration Date/Control No.

30 NDC 0777-3105-30
PULVULES® No. 3105

℞ Pak
PROZAC®
FLUOXETINE
HYDROCHLORIDE
Equiv. to
20 mg
Fluoxetine

DISTA

Rx only
See accompanying literature for dosage.
Keep Tightly Closed
Store at Controlled Room Temperature 59° to 86°F
(15° to 30°C)
WV 9362 DPX

Eli Lilly and Company
Indianapolis, IN 46285, USA

3 0777-3105-30 8
N

© Eli Lilly and Company. Used with permission.

LIQUID MEDICATIONS

Formula Method

Use the formula method to calculate liquid medications when the dosage ordered differs from the dosage available.

CASE STUDY

Mrs. Tompkins tells you that she has a headache and is requesting medication for the headache. She rates her headache pain as a 7 on the 0 to 10 pain rating scale.

The physician has ordered acetaminophen syrup 600 mg by mouth every 4 to 6 hours as needed. You have available acetaminophen syrup 100 mg/5 mL.

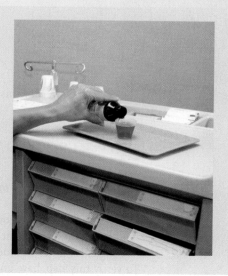

> ⊘ **SAFETY ALERT:** *When giving liquid medications, pay close attention to the amount of solution that the dose per unit contains. Not all medication dosages are in one milliliter.*
> *It is common to find the unit dosage of the medication in a larger volume of liquid. If you use an incorrect volume when performing the calculation, the patient will receive an incorrect dosage of the medication.*
> **Don't make the mistake of thinking that all drug dosages come in 1 mL of volume.**

STEP 1: CONVERT

Remember that the first step in the process is making sure that the medication dose ordered is in the same dosage system and unit as the medication available. When dosages ordered for medications are in different systems or units than dosage on hand it is important to convert both the ordered dosage and the dosage on hand to the same system or unit. For this patient, both the ordered and available medication is in milligrams. No conversion needs to be done in this situation.

STEP 2: COMPUTE

Determining what data you need and setting up the problem correctly is the next step. The formula method requires you to know what medication dose is ordered and the dosage available or dosage on hand. This step requires higher level thinking not just memorization.

The formula is:
$$\frac{D}{H} \times V = A$$

For this problem: The D (desired or ordered dose) is 600 mg. The H (dosage on hand) is 100 mg. The V (volume medication comes in) is 5 mL. Therefore, using this method the set-up of the problem would be:

$$\frac{600 \text{ mg}}{100 \text{ mg}} \times 5 \text{ mL} = A$$

Reduce the fraction to the lowest common denominator by dividing both the numerator and denominator by 100, and cancelling out the units (mg).

$$\frac{\cancel{600 \text{ mg}}}{\cancel{100 \text{ mg}}} \frac{6}{1} \times 5 \text{ mL} = A$$

$$6 \times 5 \text{ mL} = A$$

$$30 \text{ mL} = A$$

The correct answer for this problem is 30 mL.

STEP 3: CRITICALLY THINK

ASK YOURSELF – Does this answer seem logical, correct, and plausible?

This answer is reasonable and plausible in that it meets the safe standard for the amount of liquid medication given at one time. It is not unusually large or small for a safe dose. Think that 600 mg is six times as much as 100 mg. Each 5 mL contains 100 mg. Therefore, 30 mL is correct. To verify this step, have another nurse check your math.

PRACTICE PROBLEMS 7-3. Practice Problems for Liquid Medications Using the Formula Method

DIRECTIONS: Solve the following liquid medication dosage problems using the formula method. The answers to the problems can be found at the end of the chapter.

1. **Medication Ordered:** Lanoxin 0.125 mg p.o. daily
   Medication Available: Lanoxin 0.05 mg/1 mL

   Calculation:

2. **Medication Ordered:** Amoxicillin 0.5 G p.o. q 8h
   Medication Available: Amoxicillin 125 mg/5 mL

   Calculation:

3. **Medication Ordered:** Ibuprofen 400 mg q 6h
   Medication Available: Ibuprofen 100 mg/2.5mL

   Calculation:

4. **Medication Ordered:** Morphine 30 mg p.o. q 6h
   Medication Available: Morphine 10 mg/5 mL

   Calculation:

5. **Medication Ordered:** Zantac 150 mg p.o. b.i.d.
   Medication Available: Zantac 15 mg/1 mL

   Calculation:

6. **Medication Ordered:** Hydrocortisone 20 mg p.o. daily
   Medication Available: Hydrocortisone 10 mg/5 mL

   Calculation:

7. **Medication Ordered:** Aldomet 250 mg p.o. daily
   Medication Available: Aldomet 50 mg/1 mL

   Calculation:

8. **Medication Ordered:** Reglan 10 mg p.o. q 6h
   Medication Available: Reglan 5 mg/5 mL

   Calculation:

9. **Medication Ordered:** Nystatin 600,000 units p.o. t.i.d.
   Medication Available: Nystatin 100,000 units/1 mL

   Calculation:

10. **Medication Ordered:** Zofran 8 mg p.o. t.i.d.
    Medication Available: Zofran 4 mg/5 mL

    Calculation:

Ratio-Proportion Method

When the medication dosage ordered by the prescriber is different from the dosage of the medication available, the ratio-proportion method can be used to calculate the needed dose. This method solves for an unknown x in the equation. The equation is:

$$\frac{\text{Dosage on hand}}{\text{Amount on hand}} = \frac{\text{Dosage desired}}{x \, \text{Amount desired}}$$

CASE STUDY

Think back to Ms. Wills, who developed a urinary tract infection while recovering from extensive surgery. She is receiving ciprofloxacin hydrochloride, an antibiotic used to treat urinary infections. Because she is NPO with a nasogastric tube, she is to receive her medications in liquid form through the nasogastric tube.

The physician ordered ciprofloxacin hydrochloride (Cipro) Suspension 500 mg b.i.d. through the nasogastric tube. You have available ciprofloxacin hydrochloride (Cipro) Suspension 10 g/100 mL. You recognize the need to calculate the correct dosage of ciprofloxacin hydrochloride for your patient.

 SAFETY ALERT: *Remember to always check the volume of the unit dosage in which the medication is supplied. Using the correct volume will prevent dosage errors from occurring.*

STEP 1: CONVERT

You note that the drug dose ordered is in a different dosage unit than the drug available. When the dosage ordered for the medication is in a different system or unit than the dosage on hand, it is important to convert both the ordered dosage and the dosage on hand to the same system or unit. For this patient, the ordered dosage unit and the available dosage unit are different. Therefore, you need to convert. Because the unit of the drug available is in grams, you will want to convert the ordered dosage from milligrams to grams. Remember that 1 g = 1,000 mg. To convert 500 mg to grams, divide 500 by 1,000.

$$500 \div 1000 = 0.5 \text{ g}$$

STEP 2: COMPUTE

Determine what data you need and set up the problem correctly. The ratio-proportion method requires you to know what medication dose is ordered and what the available dosage is. The equation is:

$$\frac{\text{Dosage on hand}}{\text{Amount on hand}} = \frac{\text{Dosage desired}}{x \text{ Amount desired}}$$

$$\frac{10 \text{ g}}{100 \text{ mL}} = \frac{0.5 \text{ g}}{x}$$

Cross multiply:

$$\frac{10 \text{ g}}{100 \text{ mL}} \times \frac{0.5 \text{ g}}{x}$$

$$10 \text{ g } x = 50 \text{ g/mL}$$

Isolate *x* in the equation by dividing both sides of the equation by 10. Cancel out like units.

$$\frac{\cancel{10 \text{ g}}\, x}{\cancel{10 \text{ g}}} = \frac{50 \cancel{\text{ g}}/\text{mL}}{10 \cancel{\text{ g}}}$$

$$x = \frac{50 \text{ mL}}{10}$$

$$x = 5 \text{ mL}$$

The correct answer for this problem is 5 mL.

STEP 3: CRITICALLY THINK

***ASK YOURSELF** – Does this answer seem logical, correct, and plausible?*

This answer is reasonable and plausible in that it meets the safe standard for the amount of liquid medication given at one time. It is not unusually large or small for a safe dose. Think that each 100 mL contains 10 g of ciprofloxacin. Therefore, 5 mL is the correct amount when the dosage is 500 mg. To verify this step, have another nurse check your math.

PRACTICE PROBLEMS 7-4. Practice Problems for Liquid Medications Using Ratio-Proportion Method

DIRECTIONS: Solve the following liquid medication dosage problems using the ratio-proportion method. The answers to the problems can be found at the end of the chapter.

1. **Medication Ordered:** Acetaminophen elixir 240 mg p.o. q.i.d.
   Medication Available: Acetaminophen elixir 80 mg/2.5 mL

   Calculation:

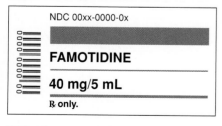

```
NDC 00xx-0000-0x

ACETAMINOPHEN ELIXIR

80 mg/2.5 mL
```

2. **Medication Ordered:** Erythromycin suspension 1 g p.o. q.i.d.
   Medication Available: Erythromycin suspension 250 mg/5 mL

   Calculation:

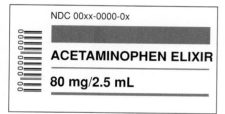

```
NDC 00xx-0000-0x

ERYTHROMYCIN
SUSPENSION

250 mg/5mL

℞ only.
```

3. **Medication Ordered:** Famotidine 20 mg p.o. b.i.d.
   Medication Available: Famotidine 40 mg/5 mL

   Calculation:

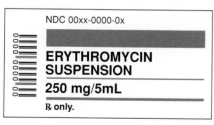

```
NDC 00xx-0000-0x

FAMOTIDINE

40 mg/5 mL

℞ only.
```

4. **Medication Ordered:** Prozac 15 mg p.o. b.i.d.
   Medication Available: Prozac 20 mg/5 mL

Calculation:

NDC 0777-5120-58
120 mL   M-5120

℞

**PROZAC®
LIQUID**
**FLUOXETINE
HYDROCHLORIDE
ORAL SOLUTION**

Equivalent to
20 mg per 5 mL
Base

◻DISTA

Store at Controlled Room Temperature 59° to 86°F
(15° to 30°C)
WV 8601 DPX

Rx only
Keep Tightly Closed

Eli Lilly and Company
Indianapolis, IN 46285, USA
Expiration Date/Control No.

See accompanying literature for dosage.
Dispense in a tight, light-resistant container.
Each 5 mL contains Fluoxetine Hydrochloride
equivalent to 20 mg Fluoxetine base
Contains alcohol 0.23%

3 0777 5120 58 3

© Eli Lilly and Company. All Rights Reserved. Used with permission.
® PROZAC is a registered trademark of Eli Lilly and Company.

---

5. **Medication Ordered:** Dilantin suspension 300 mg b.i.d.
   Medication Available: Dilantin suspension 125 mg/5 mL

Calculation:

NDC 0071-2214-20
8 fl oz (237 mL)   **Rx only**

Dilantin-125®
(Phenytoin
Oral Suspension, USP)

125 mg per 5 mL potency

IMPORTANT—SHAKE WELL
BEFORE EACH USE
NOT FOR PARENTERAL USE

Distributed by
Pfizer **Parke-Davis**
Division of Pfizer Inc, NY, NY 10017

05-5938-00-1

6505-00-890-1110

THIS PRODUCT MUST BE SHAKEN
WELL ESPECIALLY
PRIOR TO INITIAL USE.
Each 5 mL contains phenytoin,
125 mg with a maximum alcohol
content not greater than 0.6 percent.
DOSAGE AND USE
Adults, 1 teaspoonful (5 mL)
three times daily; pediatric patients,
see package insert.
**Advice to Pharmacist and
Patient**—Patient must be advised
to use an accurate measuring
device when using this product.
See package insert for complete
prescribing information.
**Store at Controlled Room
Temperature 20°-25°C
(68°-77°F) [see USP].
Protect from freezing and light.
Keep this and all drugs out
of the reach of children.**

7609

0071-2214-20 8

Exp date and lot

Reproduced with permission of Pfizer Inc. All rights reserved.

---

6. **Medication Ordered:** Hydrocodone syrup 6 mg q 6h
   Medication Available: Hydrocodone syrup 1.5 mg/1 mL

Calculation:

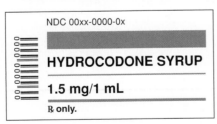

NDC 00xx-0000-0x

HYDROCODONE SYRUP

1.5 mg/1 mL

℞ only.

---

7. **Medication Ordered:** Hydromorphone liquid 2 mg p.o.
   Medication Available: Hydromorphone 5 mg/5 mL

Calculation:

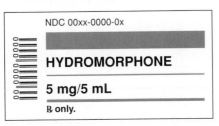

NDC 00xx-0000-0x

HYDROMORPHONE

5 mg/5 mL

℞ only.

8. Medication Ordered: Vistaril Suspension 75 mg p.o. q.i.d.
  Medication Available: Vistaril suspension 25 mg/5 mL

Calculation:

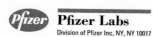

NDC 0069-5440-93

1 Pint (473 mL)

Vistaril®
(hydroxyzine pamoate)

ORAL SUSPENSION
FOR ORAL USE ONLY
IMPORTANT
This closure is not
child-resistant.

25 mg/5 mL*

N 3 0069-5440-93 9

Pfizer **Pfizer Labs**
Division of Pfizer Inc, NY, NY 10017

Vistaril®
(hydroxyzine pamoate)

Store below 77°F (25°C).

Dispense in tight, light-resistant
containers (USP).

USUAL DAILY DOSAGE
Adults: 1 to 4 teaspoonfuls 3-4 times
daily.
Children: 6 years and over–2 to 4
teaspoonfuls daily in divided doses.
Under 6 years–2 teaspoonfuls daily
in divided doses.

READ ACCOMPANYING
PROFESSIONAL INFORMATION.

*Each teaspoonful (5 mL) contains
hydroxyzine pamoate equivalent
to 25 mg hydroxyzine hydrochloride.

SHAKE VIGOROUSLY UNTIL
PRODUCT IS COMPLETELY
RESUSPENDED.

DYE FREE FORMULA

Rx only

MADE IN USA
4387

05-0844-32-5

9. Medication Ordered: Indomethacin suspension 150 mg p.o. q.i.d.
  Medication Available: Indomethacin suspension 25 mg/5 mL

Calculation:

NDC 00xx-0000-0x

**INDOMETHACIN
SUSPENSION**

25 mg/5 mL

℞ only.

10. Medication Ordered: Isoniazid Syrup 300 mg p.o. daily
  Medication Available: Isoniazid 50 mg/5 mL

Calculation:

NDC 00xx-0000-0x

ISONIAZID

50 mg/5 mL

℞ only.

 Critical Thinking/Decision Making Exercise

Making an error in calculating medication dosages leads to inaccuracy and errors in medication administration that could result in serious problems for the patient. *By using these 3 simple steps for medication calculation, medication errors can be avoided.*

What Went Wrong?

The prescriber has ordered levothyroxine 100 mcg for a patient with hypothyroidism.

The medication is available in 0.05 mg tablets. The nurse uses the formula method to do the calculation. Using the formula:

$$\frac{\text{Desired dosage}}{\text{Dosage on hand}} \times \text{Volume of medication}$$

The nurse sets up the calculation:

$$\frac{100 \text{ mcg}}{0.05 \text{ mg}} \times 1 \text{ tablet} = 20 \text{ tablets}$$

> ⚠ **SAFETY ALERT:** *The 20 tablets are a large number of tablets needed to deliver the prescribed dose of the medication. This should alert the nurse to a problem. If this occurs, recheck your problem set-up and recheck your math—an error has occurred. This problem occurred because the nurse did not notice the difference in the drug ordered in the form of micrograms and the drug available as milligrams. It is very important that the nurse read the dosage ordered and the label of the drug available very carefully.*

In not using the 3 steps, the nurse has made a potential medication error and calculated a dose 10 times the ordered dose. This is a critical error. Recognizing that 20 tablets was an excessive dose, the nurse recalculated the medication dosage using the 3 steps.

Correct Way to Calculate the Dosage of This Medication

STEP 1: CONVERT

The nurse committed the first error in this step. The ordered dosage of the medication is in micrograms (mcg) and the dosage of the supplied medication is in milligrams (mg). The nurse needed to recognize the ordered dosage and the dosage on hand needed to be in the same dosage unit. To correctly calculate the ordered dosage, the nurse needed to convert milligrams to micrograms. Remember that 1 mg = 1000 mcg. To convert milligrams to micrograms, multiply the number of milligrams by 1000. In this problem, 0.05 milligrams needed to be multiplied by 1000:

$$0.05 \text{ mg} \times 1000 = 50 \text{ mcg}$$

STEP 2: COMPUTE

The nurse did determine the pieces of data needed to set up the problem using the formula method. However, in not doing the conversion of micrograms to milligrams, an error was made that caused the calculation to be inaccurate. After correctly converting milligrams to micrograms, the nurse should have set up the problem like this:

$$\frac{100 \text{ mcg}}{50 \text{ mcg}} \times 1 \text{ tablet} = A$$

Reduce the fraction to the lowest common denominator by dividing the numerator and denominator by 50. The like units of mcg cancel out.

$$\frac{100 \cancel{\text{ mcg}}}{50 \cancel{\text{ mcg}}} \frac{2}{1} \times 1 \text{ tablet} = A$$

$$2 \times 1 \text{ tablet} = A$$

$$2 \text{ tablets} = A$$

The correct answer is 2 tablets.

STEP 3: CRITICALLY THINK

The nurse then asked herself if this answer was logical, correct, or plausible.

When the nurse calculated the medication dosage to be 20 tablets, this caused the nurse to re-evaluate the answer because it is an excessively large number of tablets that is needed to achieve the ordered dose. In re-evaluating, the nurse went back and made sure to use all 3 steps in the process and that each step was done accurately. The nurse verified the calculated dose for safety by having another nurse independently check the calculation.

(!) SAFETY ALERT: *Request that a second nurse verify the dosage calculation by doing the calculation independently, and then compare the answer with the first nurse. If the calculations are different, both nurses should recalculate and compare answers. Recheck the calculations with each other to see where the problem is occurring.*

This serious medication error was prevented because the nurse used the correct steps for calculating the ordered medication dosage. The nurse's critical evaluation of the first answer identified a problem. Then recalculation of the dosage using all steps provided the nurse with the correct dosage of levothyroxine for this patient.

CHAPTER REVIEW PROBLEMS

The answers to the problems can be found at the end of the chapter.

Review Problems 7-1. Use the formula method to find the correct medication dosage.

1. **Medication Ordered:** Potassium elixir 40 mEq p.o. daily
   Medication Available: Potassium elixir 30 mEq/15 mL

   Calculation:

   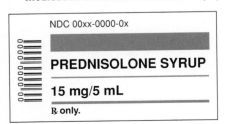

   NDC 00xx-0000-0x

   POTASSIUM ELIXIR

   30 mEq/15 mL

   ℞ only.

2. **Medication Ordered:** Erythromycin 500 mg p.o. t.i.d.
   Medication Available: Erythromycin 250 mg per tablet

   Calculation:

   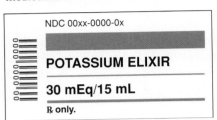

   Dispense in a USP tight container. Keep tightly closed. Store below 86°F (30°C).

   NDC 0074-6326-53
   500 Tablets

   ERYTHROMYCIN Base Filmtab®

   ERYTHROMYCIN TABLETS, USP

   250 mg Erythromycin, USP

   ℞ only

   Do not accept if seal over bottle opening is broken or missing.

   Each tablet contains: Erythromycin, USP ....250 mg

   Usual adult dose: One tablet every six hours. See enclosure for full prescribing information.

   Filmtab — Film-sealed tablets, Abbott

   ©Abbott

   Abbott Laboratories North Chicago, IL 60064, U.S.A.

   Abbott Laboratories. Used with permission.

3. **Medication Ordered:** Hytrin 20 mg p.o. daily
   Medication Available: Hytrin 5 mg capsule

   Calculation:

   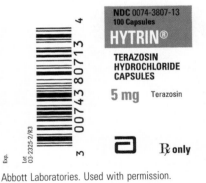

   NDC 0074-3807-13
   100 Capsules

   HYTRIN®

   TERAZOSIN HYDROCHLORIDE CAPSULES

   5 mg   Terazosin

   ℞ only

   Do not accept if seal over bottle opening is broken or missing.

   Dispense in a USP tight, light-resistant container.

   Each capsule contains: terazosin hydrochloride equivalent to terazosin ......5 mg

   Store at controlled room temperature between 20–25°C (68–77°F). See USP. Protect from light and moisture.

   See enclosure for full prescribing information.

   ©Abbott
   Abbott Laboratories North Chicago, IL60064, U.S.A.

   Abbott Laboratories. Used with permission.

4. **Medication Ordered:** Prednisolone 20 mg daily
   Medication Available: Prednisolone Syrup 15 mg/5 mL

   Calculation:

   NDC 00xx-0000-0x

   PREDNISOLONE SYRUP

   15 mg/5 mL

   ℞ only.

5. Medication Ordered: Procainamide 750 mg daily
Medication Available: Procainamide 375 mg capsule

Calculation:

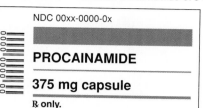

NDC 00xx-0000-0x

PROCAINAMIDE

375 mg capsule

℞ only.

6. Medication Ordered: Prochlorperazine 10 mg p.o. p.r.n. nausea
Medication Available: Prochlorperazine Syrup 5 mg/5 mL

Calculation:

NDC 00xx-0000-0x

PROCHLORPERAZINE SYRUP

5 mg/5 mL

℞ only.

7. Medication Ordered: Bumex 1.5 mg p.o. q a.m.
Medication Available: Bumex 0.5 mg tablet

Calculation:

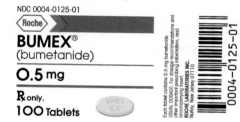

NDC 0004-0125-01

BUMEX®
(bumetanide)

0.5 mg

℞ only.
100 Tablets

0004-0125-01

Hoffman-La Roche, Inc. Used with permission

8. Medication Ordered: Carbamazepine 200 mg p.o. q.i.d.
Medication Available: Carbamazepine suspension 100 mg/5 mL

Calculation:

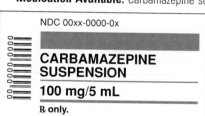

NDC 00xx-0000-0x

CARBAMAZEPINE SUSPENSION

100 mg/5 mL

℞ only.

9. Medication Ordered: Cialis 20 mg p.o. daily
Medication Available: Cialis 10 mg tablet

Calculation:

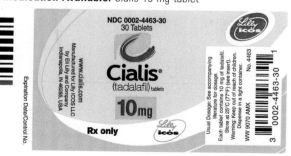

© Eli Lilly and Company. Used with permission.

10. **Medication Ordered:** Ciprofloxacin suspension 750 mg p.o. q 12h

    Medication Available: Ciprofloxacin suspension 500 mg/5 mL

Calculation:

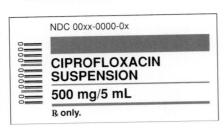

NDC 00xx-0000-0x

CIPROFLOXACIN SUSPENSION

500 mg/5 mL

℞ only.

Review Problems 7-2. Use the ratio-proportion method to find the correct medication dosage.

1. **Medication Ordered:** Cefixime suspension 50 mg p.o. daily

   Medication Available: Cefixime suspension 100 mg/5 mL

Calculation:

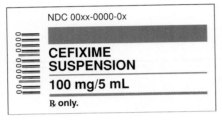

NDC 00xx-0000-0x

CEFIXIME SUSPENSION

100 mg/5 mL

℞ only.

---

2. **Medication Ordered:** Cefzil 500 mg p.o. q 12h

   Medication Available: Cefzil 250 mg tablet

Calculation:

NDC 0087-7720-60   100 Tablets

Cefzil®
(CEFPROZIL)
Tablets

Film-Coated Tablets

EQUIVALENT TO

250 mg
anhydrous cefprozil

U.S. Patent No. 4,520,022

Rx only

Pharmacist: See base label for dispensing directions. Package insert enclosed. Remove before dispensing. See enclosed package insert for indications and dosage schedule. Store at controlled room temperature, 59° F–86° F (15° C–30° C).

Bristol-Myers
Squibb Company
Princeton, New Jersey 08543 USA

1174506
7720600DCL-5   53-004158-05
PULL DOWN TAB TO
OPEN BOOKLET

Lot :
Exp. Date:

Bristol-Myers Squibb Company. Used with permission.

---

3. **Medication Ordered:** Cephradine suspension 1 g p.o. q a.m.

   Medication Available: Cephradine suspension 250 mg/5 mL

Calculation:

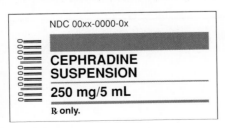

NDC 00xx-0000-0x

CEPHRADINE SUSPENSION

250 mg/5 mL

℞ only.

4. **Medication Ordered:** Chlorothiazide 1.5 g p.o.
   Medication Available: Chlorothiazide 500 mg tablet

   Calculation:

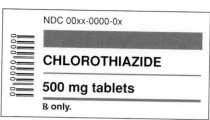

NDC 00xx-0000-0x

CHLOROTHIAZIDE

500 mg tablets

℞ only.

5. **Medication Ordered:** Chlorpromazine Syrup 45 mg p.o. t.i.d.
   Medication Available: Chlorpromazine Syrup 10 mg/5 mL

   Calculation:

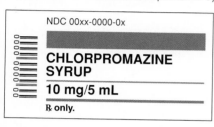

NDC 00xx-0000-0x

**CHLORPROMAZINE
SYRUP**

10 mg/5 mL

℞ only.

6. **Medication Ordered:** Naprosyn 500 mg p.o. t.i.d.
   Medication Available: Naprosyn 250 mg tablet

   Calculation:

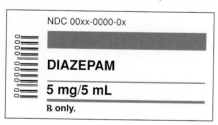

Hoffmann-La Roche Inc. Used with permission.

7. **Medication Ordered:** Diazepam solution 15 mg p.o. b.i.d.
   Medication Available: Diazepam solution 5 mg/mL

   Calculation:

NDC 00xx-0000-0x

DIAZEPAM

5 mg/5 mL

℞ only.

8. **Medication Ordered:** Toradol 15 mg p.o. q 6h
   Medication Available: Toradol 10 mg tablet

   Calculation:

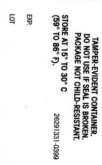

Hoffmann-La Roche Inc. Used with permission.

9. Medication Ordered: Diphenhydramine 50 mg p.o. t.i.d.
    Medication Available: Diphenhydramine 12.5 mg/4 mL

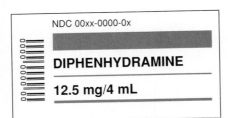

Calculation:

10. Medication Ordered: Synthroid 205.5 mcg daily
     Medication Available: Synthroid 137 mcg tablet

NDC 0074-3727-13
100 TABLETS

SYNTHROID®
(levothyroxine sodium
tablets, USP)

137 mcg (0.137 mg)

Do not accept if seal over bottle
opening is broken or missing.

See full prescribing information for
dosage and administration.

Each tablet contains 137 mcg
(0.137 mg) levothyroxine sodium.

Dispense in a tight, light-resistant
container as described in USP.

Store at 25°C (77°F); excursions
permitted to 15°-30°C (59°-
86°F). [See USP Controlled Room
Temperature]. Protect from light
and moisture.

©Abbott

Abbott Laboratories
North Chicago, IL 60064,
U.S.A.

℞ only   02-8669-R2

Abbott Laboratories. Used with permission.

Calculation:

Answers to Practice Problems

Practice Problem Answers 7-1

1. $\dfrac{375}{125} \times 1 = \dfrac{\cancel{375}}{\cancel{125}} \dfrac{3}{1} \times 1 = 3 \times 1 \text{ capsule} = 3 \text{ capsules}$

2. $\dfrac{200}{100} \times 1 = \dfrac{\cancel{200}}{\cancel{100}} \dfrac{2}{1} \times 1 = 2 \times 1 \text{ capsule} = 2 \text{ capsules}$

3. $\dfrac{25}{50} \times 1 = \dfrac{\cancel{25}}{\cancel{50}} \dfrac{1}{2} \times 1 = \dfrac{1}{2} \times 1 \text{ tablet} = \dfrac{1}{2} \text{ tablet}$

4. $\dfrac{7.5}{2.5} \times 1 = \dfrac{\cancel{7.5}}{\cancel{2.5}} \dfrac{3}{1} \times 1 = 3 \times 1 \text{ tablet} = 3 \text{ tablets}$

5. $\dfrac{20}{10} \times 1 = \dfrac{\cancel{20}}{\cancel{10}} \dfrac{2}{1} \times 1 = 2 \times 1 \text{ capsule} = 2 \text{ capsules}$

6. $\dfrac{0.5}{1} \times 1 = 0.5 \times 1 \text{ tablet} = \dfrac{1}{2} \text{ tablet}$

7. $\dfrac{1200}{200} \times 1 = \dfrac{\cancel{1200}}{\cancel{200}} \dfrac{6}{1} \times 1 = 6 \times 1 \text{ capsule} = 6 \text{ capsules}$

8. gr 1 = 60 mg $10 \times 60 = 600 \text{ mg}$

    $\dfrac{600}{325} \times 1 = 1.85, \text{ round to 2 tablets}$

9. $\dfrac{500}{250} \times 1 = \dfrac{\cancel{500}}{\cancel{250}} \dfrac{2}{1} \times 1 = 2 \times 1 \text{ tablet} = 2 \text{ tablets}$

10. $\dfrac{120}{40} \times 1 = \dfrac{\cancel{120}}{\cancel{40}} \dfrac{3}{1} \times 1 = 3 \times 1 \text{ tablet} = 3 \text{ tablets}$

Practice Problem Answers 7-2

1. Convert: 1000 mcg = 1 mg

    $$\dfrac{1 \text{ mg}}{1000 \text{ mcg}} = \dfrac{0.1 \text{ mg}}{x}$$

    $1 \text{ mg } x = 1000 \text{ mcg} \times 0.1 \text{ mg}$

    $$\dfrac{\cancel{1 \text{ mg}} \, x}{\cancel{1 \text{ mg}}} = \dfrac{1000 \text{ mcg} \times 0.1 \, \cancel{\text{mg}}}{1 \, \cancel{\text{mg}}}$$

    $x = 1000 \text{ mcg} \times 0.1 = 100 \text{ mcg}$

    Set up: $\dfrac{50 \text{ mcg}}{1 \text{ tablet}} = \dfrac{100 \text{ mcg}}{x}$

    Cross multiply the set-up equation to get: $50x = 100$

    Isolate x in the equation by dividing by 50. $\dfrac{\cancel{50}x}{\cancel{50}} = \dfrac{100}{50}$ $x = \dfrac{2}{1}$

    $x = 2 \text{ tablets}$

2. $\dfrac{5}{1} = \dfrac{7.5}{x}$

Cross multiply the set-up equation to get: $5x = 7.5$

Isolate x in the equation by dividing by 5. $\dfrac{\cancel{5}x}{\cancel{5}} = \dfrac{7.5}{5}$ $\quad x = \dfrac{1.5}{1}$

$x = 1.5$ tablets

3. $\dfrac{10}{1} = \dfrac{30}{x}$

Cross multiply the set-up equation to get: $10x = 30$

Isolate x in the equation by dividing by 10: $\dfrac{\cancel{10}x}{\cancel{10}} = \dfrac{30}{10}$

$x = 3$ capsules

4. $\dfrac{250}{1} = \dfrac{500}{x}$

Cross multiply the set-up equation to get: $250x = 500$

Isolate x in the equation by dividing by 250. $\dfrac{\cancel{250}x}{\cancel{250}} = \dfrac{500}{250}$

$x = 2$ capsules

5. $\dfrac{10}{1} = \dfrac{5}{x}$

Cross multiply the set-up equation to get: $10x = 5$

Isolate x in the equation by dividing by 10. $\dfrac{\cancel{10}x}{\cancel{10}} = \dfrac{5}{10}$

$x = 0.5$ tablet

6. $\dfrac{0.5}{1} = \dfrac{2.5}{x}$

Cross multiply the set-up equation to get: $0.5x = 2.5$

Isolate x in the equation by dividing by 0.5. $\dfrac{\cancel{0.5}x}{\cancel{0.5}} = \dfrac{2.5}{0.5}$

$x = 5$ tablets

7. $\dfrac{0.5}{1} = \dfrac{1.5}{x}$

Cross multiply the set-up equation to get: $0.5x = 1.5$

Isolate x in the equation by dividing by 0.5. $\dfrac{\cancel{0.5}x}{\cancel{0.5}} = \dfrac{1.5}{0.5}$

$x = 3$ tablets

8. $\dfrac{2}{1} = \dfrac{3}{x}$

Cross multiply the set-up equation to get: $2x = 3$

Isolate x in the equation by dividing by 2. $\dfrac{\cancel{2}x}{\cancel{2}} = \dfrac{3}{2}$

$x = 1.5$ tablets

9. $\dfrac{200}{1} = \dfrac{600}{x}$

Cross multiply the set-up equation to get: $200x = 600$

Isolate x in the equation by dividing by 200. $\dfrac{200x}{200} = \dfrac{600}{200}$

$x = 3$ capsules

10. $\dfrac{20}{1} = \dfrac{40}{x}$

Cross multiply the set-up equation to get: $20x = 40$

Isolate x in the equation by dividing by 20. $\dfrac{20x}{20} = \dfrac{40}{20}$

$x = 2$ tablets

Practice Problem Answers 7-3

1. $\dfrac{0.125}{0.05} \times 1 = \dfrac{\cancel{0.125}\;2.5}{\cancel{0.05}\;1} \times 1 = 2.5$ mL

2. Convert 1000 mg = 1 g

$\dfrac{1\,g}{1000\,mg} = \dfrac{0.5\,g}{x}$ $x = 500$ mg

$\dfrac{500}{125} \times 5 = \dfrac{\cancel{500}\;4}{\cancel{125}\;1} \times 5 = 20$ mL

3. $\dfrac{400}{100} \times 2.5 = \dfrac{\cancel{400}\;4}{\cancel{100}\;1} \times 2.5 = 10$ mL

4. $\dfrac{30}{10} \times 5 = \dfrac{\cancel{30}\;3}{\cancel{10}\;1} \times 5 = 15$ mL

5. $\dfrac{150}{15} \times 1 = \dfrac{\cancel{150}\;10}{\cancel{15}\;1} \times 1 = 10$ mL

6. $\dfrac{20}{10} \times 5 = \dfrac{\cancel{20}\;2}{\cancel{10}\;1} \times 5 = 10$ mL

7. $\dfrac{250}{50} \times 1 = \dfrac{\cancel{250}\;5}{\cancel{50}\;1} \times 1 = 5$ mL

8. $\dfrac{10}{5} \times 5 = \dfrac{\cancel{10}\;2}{\cancel{5}\;1} \times 5 = 10$ mL

9. $\dfrac{600,000}{100,000} \times 1 = \dfrac{\cancel{600,000}\;6}{\cancel{100,000}\;1} \times 1 = 6$ mL

10. $\dfrac{8}{4} \times 5 = \dfrac{\cancel{8}\;2}{\cancel{4}\;1} \times 5 = 10$ mL

Practice Problem Answers 7-4

1. $\dfrac{80}{2.5} = \dfrac{240}{x}$

   Cross multiply the set-up equation to get: $80x = 600$

   Isolate x in the equation by dividing by 80. $\dfrac{\cancel{80}x}{\cancel{80}} = \dfrac{600}{80}$

   $x = 7.5$ mL

2. Convert 1 g $= 1,000$ mg

   $\dfrac{250}{5} = \dfrac{1000}{x}$

   Cross multiply the set-up equation to get: $250x = 5,000$

   Isolate x in the equation by dividing by 250. $\dfrac{\cancel{250}x}{\cancel{250}} = \dfrac{5,000}{250}$

   $x = 20$ mL

3. $\dfrac{40}{5} = \dfrac{20}{x}$

   Cross multiply the set-up equation to get: $40x = 100$

   Isolate x in the equation by dividing by 40. $\dfrac{\cancel{40}x}{\cancel{40}} = \dfrac{100}{40}$

   $x = 2.5$ mL

4. $\dfrac{20}{5} = \dfrac{15}{x}$

   Cross multiply the set-up equation to get: $20x = 75$

   Isolate x in the equation by dividing by 20. $\dfrac{\cancel{20}x}{\cancel{20}} = \dfrac{75}{20}$

   $x = 3.75$ mL

5. $\dfrac{125}{5} = \dfrac{300}{x}$

   Cross multiply the set-up equation to get: $125x = 1,500$

   Isolate x in the equation by dividing by 125. $\dfrac{\cancel{125}x}{\cancel{125}} = \dfrac{1,500}{125}$

   $x = 12$ mL

6. $\dfrac{1.5}{1} = \dfrac{6}{x}$

   Cross multiply the set-up equation to get: $1.5x = 6$

   Isolate x in the equation by dividing by 1.5. $\dfrac{\cancel{1.5}x}{\cancel{1.5}} = \dfrac{6}{1.5}$

   $x = 4$ mL

7. $\dfrac{5}{5} = \dfrac{2}{x}$

   Cross multiply the set-up equation to get: $5x = 10$

   Isolate x in the equation by dividing by 5. $\dfrac{\cancel{5}x}{\cancel{5}} = \dfrac{10}{5}$

   $x = 2$ mL

8. $\dfrac{25}{5} = \dfrac{75}{x}$

   Cross multiply the set-up equation to get: $25x = 375$

   Isolate x in the equation by dividing by 25. $\dfrac{\cancel{25}x}{\cancel{25}} = \dfrac{375}{25}$

   $x = 15$ mL

9. $\dfrac{25}{5} = \dfrac{150}{x}$

   Cross multiply the set-up equation to get: $25x = 750$

   Isolate x in the equation by dividing by 25. $\dfrac{\cancel{25}x}{\cancel{25}} = \dfrac{750}{25}$

   $x = 30$ mL

10. $\dfrac{50}{5} = \dfrac{300}{x}$

   Cross multiply the set-up equation to get: $50x = 1500$

   Isolate x in the equation by dividing by 50. $\dfrac{\cancel{50}x}{\cancel{50}} = \dfrac{1500}{50}$

   $x = 30$ mL

Answers to Chapter Review Problems

Chapter Review Problem Answers 7-1

Remember the formula: $\dfrac{D}{H} \times V = A$

1. $\dfrac{40}{30} \times 15 = \dfrac{\cancel{40}}{\cancel{30}} \ \dfrac{4}{3} \times 15 = \dfrac{60}{3} = 20$ mL

2. $\dfrac{500}{250} \times 1 = \dfrac{\cancel{500}}{\cancel{250}} \ \dfrac{2}{1} \times 1 = 2$ tablets

3. $\dfrac{20}{5} \times 1 = \dfrac{\cancel{20}}{\cancel{5}} \ \dfrac{4}{1} \times 1 = 4$ capsules

4. $\dfrac{20}{15} \times 5 = \dfrac{\cancel{20}}{\cancel{15}} \ \dfrac{4}{3} \times 5 = \dfrac{20}{3} = 6.67$ mL

5. $\dfrac{750}{375} \times 1 = \dfrac{\cancel{750}}{\cancel{375}} \dfrac{2}{1} \times 1 = 2$ capsules

6. $\dfrac{10}{5} \times 5 = \dfrac{\cancel{10}}{\cancel{5}} \dfrac{2}{1} \times 5 = 10$ mL

7. $\dfrac{1.5}{0.5} \times 1 = \dfrac{\cancel{1.5}}{\cancel{0.5}} \dfrac{3}{1} \times 1 = 3$ tablets

8. $\dfrac{200}{100} \times 5 = \dfrac{\cancel{200}}{\cancel{100}} \dfrac{2}{1} \times 5 = 10$ mL

9. $\dfrac{20}{10} \times 1 = \dfrac{\cancel{20}}{\cancel{10}} \dfrac{2}{1} \times 1 = 2$ tablets

10. $\dfrac{750}{500} \times 5 = \dfrac{\cancel{750}}{\cancel{500}} \dfrac{1.5}{1} \times 5 = 7.5$ mL

Chapter Review Problem Answers 7-2

Remember this equation: $\dfrac{\text{Dosage on hand}}{\text{Amount on hand}} = \dfrac{\text{Dosage desired}}{x\,\text{Amount desired}}$

1. $\dfrac{100}{5} = \dfrac{50}{x}$

   Cross multiply the set-up equation to get: $100x = 250$

   Isolate x in the equation by dividing by 100. $\dfrac{100x}{100} = \dfrac{250}{100}$

   $x = 2.5$ mL

2. $\dfrac{250}{1} = \dfrac{500}{x}$

   Cross multiply the set-up equation to get: $250x = 500$

   Isolate x in the equation by dividing by 250. $\dfrac{250x}{250} = \dfrac{500}{250}$

   $x = 2$ tablets

3. Need to convert 1 g to 1000 mg

   $\dfrac{250}{5} = \dfrac{1{,}000}{x}$

   Cross multiply the set-up equation to get: $250x = 5000$

   Isolate x in the equation by dividing by 250. $\dfrac{250x}{250} = \dfrac{5000}{250}$

   $x = 20$ mL

4. Need to convert 1.5g to 1500 mg

   $\dfrac{500}{1} = \dfrac{1500}{x}$

   Cross multiply the set-up equation to get: $500x = 1500$

   Isolate x in the equation by dividing by 500. $\dfrac{500x}{500} = \dfrac{1500}{500}$

   $x = 3$ tablets

5. $\dfrac{10}{5} = \dfrac{45}{x}$

Cross multiply the set-up equation to get: $10x = 225$

Isolate x in the equation by dividing by 10. $\dfrac{\cancel{10}x}{\cancel{10}} = \dfrac{225}{10}$

$x = 22.5$ mL

6. $\dfrac{250}{1} = \dfrac{500}{x}$

Cross multiply the set-up equation to get: $250x = 500$

Isolate x in the equation by dividing by 250. $\dfrac{\cancel{250}x}{\cancel{250}} = \dfrac{500}{250}$

$x = 2$ tablets

7. $\dfrac{5}{1} = \dfrac{15}{x}$

Cross multiply the set-up equation to get: $5x = 15$

Isolate x in the equation by dividing by 5. $\dfrac{\cancel{5}x}{\cancel{5}} = \dfrac{15}{5}$

$x = 3$ mL

8. $\dfrac{10}{1} = \dfrac{15}{x}$

Cross multiply the set-up equation to get: $10x = 15$

Isolate x in the equation by dividing by 10. $\dfrac{\cancel{10}x}{\cancel{10}} = \dfrac{15}{10}$

$x = 1.5$ tablets

9. $\dfrac{12.5}{4} = \dfrac{50}{x}$

Cross multiply the set-up equation to get: $12.5x = 200$

Isolate x in the equation by dividing by 12.5. $\dfrac{\cancel{12.5}x}{\cancel{12.5}} = \dfrac{200}{12.5}$

$x = 16$ mL

10. $\dfrac{137}{1} = \dfrac{205.5}{x}$

Cross multiply the set-up equation to get: $137x = 205.5$

Isolate x in the equation by dividing by 137. $\dfrac{\cancel{137}x}{\cancel{137}} = \dfrac{205.5}{137}$

$x = 1.5$ tablets

Calculation of Parenteral Medications

This chapter contains content on:

- **Injection Equipment**
- **Parenteral Routes**
- **Calculation of Dosages in the Same System of Measurement**
- **Calculations with Different Units of Measurement**
- **Calculations in Different Systems**
- **Calculations for Drugs Combined in One Syringe**
- **Preparing Parenteral Medications From Drugs Supplied as Powders**

Learning Objectives

Upon completion of Chapter 8, you will be able to:

- Select the correct syringe for the amount of medication calculated.
- Calculate the correct dose of medication for parenteral administration.
- Convert to the same system for accuracy in calculations.

Key Terms

- Parenteral route
- Subcutaneous (SubQ) route
- Intradermal (ID) route
- Intramuscular (IM) route
- Z-Track technique

CASE STUDY

As a nurse working on the orthopedic unit, you are caring for Sandy Henson, age 34, who was admitted to the unit after being involved in an automobile accident. Sandy experienced a fracture of two ribs on her right side and a fractured femur. She underwent an open reduction of the femur today. Her postoperative plan of care identifies pain as a priority. The physician has ordered morphine sulfate 8 mg IM every 3 to 4 hours prn for pain.

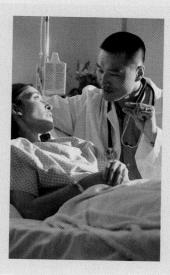

Medications may be administered by the **parenteral route,** which means by injection of the medication into body tissues. Parenteral medication administration is preferred when the oral route for drug administration is unavailable or inappropriate, or when there is a need for a more rapid rate of absorption and distribution.

Parenteral medications are usually provided as a sterile solution or liquid that can be readily absorbed and distributed without irritating the tissues. These solutions are supplied in ampules, multiple- or single-dose vials, and in prefilled syringes (see Figure 8-1).

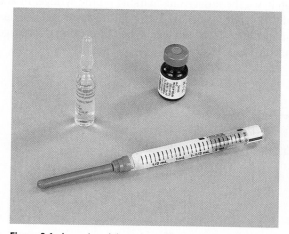

Figure 8-1. Ampule, vial, and prefilled syringe cartridge. (Photo © B. Proud.)

INJECTION EQUIPMENT

The parenteral medications are administered via a syringe to which a needle is attached (see Figure 8-2). Syringes come in a variety of sizes. In most situations, a 3-mL syringe is used. However, when the calculated dose is small, it is usually safer and more accurate to use a 1-mL syringe. The 1-mL syringe is also called a tuberculin syringe. When administering insulin, U-100 insulin-specific syringes are used. (For more information, see Chapter 3.)

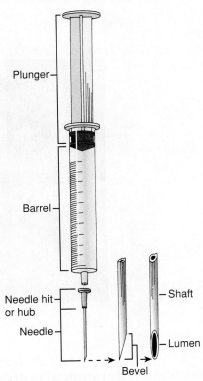

Figure 8-2. Parts of a syringe. (From Taylor, C., Lillis, C., & LeMone, P. [2005.] *Fundamentals of Nursing.* 5th ed. Philadelphia: Lippincott Williams & Wilkins.)

Regardless of the type of syringe being used, precision with the dose is essential. Therefore, you must be expert at reading the markings, or calibrations, on the syringes. View the syringe at eye level to accurately see the dosage line marking on the syringe. In addition, always use the top of the black ring of the plunger as the measuring line to ensure precise dosage measurements. Some syringes have a rounded top on the plunger. When measuring the dosage, use the top of the black ring, not the rounded tip (see Figure 8-3).

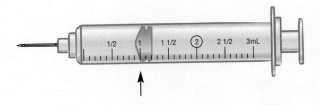

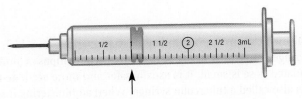

Figure 8-3. Measurement of 1 mL.

PARENTERAL ROUTES

Parenteral routes include the following: intradermal, subcutaneous, intramuscular, and intravenous. Intravenous administration is discussed in Chapter 9. Regardless of the route used, dosage calculation remains the same. Due to the more rapid absorption rate of medications, accuracy in calculation is absolutely crucial.

> **SAFETY ALERT:** *Prior to administering a parenteral medication, always check the patient's medication history to determine if there is a drug allergy, especially with anti-infective agents and narcotics. Remember that parenteral medications are more rapidly absorbed.*

Intradermal Route

The **intradermal (ID) route** involves injection of the medication into the dermis, the layer of tissue located directly beneath the outer layer of skin. The medication is injected at a 15-degree angle with the bevel of the needle facing up. Typically a 25- to 27-gauge needle is used. The needle size should be $\frac{1}{4}$ to $\frac{5}{8}$ inches long. The dosage usually is small, ranging between 0.1 to 0.5 mL. This route is most commonly used for allergy testing and administering a tuberculin skin test.

Subcutaneous Route

The **subcutaneous (SubQ) route** involves the injection of medication into tissue below the skin and above the muscle, usually at an angle of 45 to 90 degrees. Often, a fine-gauge needle, such as a 25- to 27-gauge, is preferred. Generally, a $\frac{5}{16}$- to 1-inch needle is appropriate for subcutaneous injections. This route is used for administering heparin and insulin. The amount injected is typically 1 mL or less.

Intramuscular Route

The **intramuscular (IM) route** involves the injection of medication directly into the muscle, which is located below the subcutaneous tissue. The needle is usually 20- to 25-gauge, 1 to $1\frac{1}{2}$ inches in length, and is inserted at a 90-degree angle. The average dose is 1.0 mL, but can range from 0.5 mL to 4.0 mL. When using the intramuscular route, aspirate for blood prior to giving the injection to prevent inadvertent injection into a blood vessel.

> **SAFETY ALERT:** *The maximum single injection amount to be administered to an adult ranges from 3 to 4 mL.*

The **Z-track technique** is an intramuscular injection technique that is used to prevent the medication from leaking out following the injection. This technique involves pulling the skin to the side, then inserting the needle at a 90-degree angle, aspirating for blood, injecting the medication, removing the needle, and then releasing the patient's skin. Letting go of the skin seals the solution beneath the tissues and prevents leakage (see Figure 8-4).

CALCULATION OF DOSAGES IN THE SAME SYSTEM OF MEASUREMENT

 CASE STUDY

Sandy has been back from surgery for an hour. When you do your assessment, she rates the pain in her leg as an 8 on a 0 to 10 scale. You prepare to give her a dosage of morphine. The morphine is available in injectable form at 10 mg/mL. You need to calculate the amount to administer.

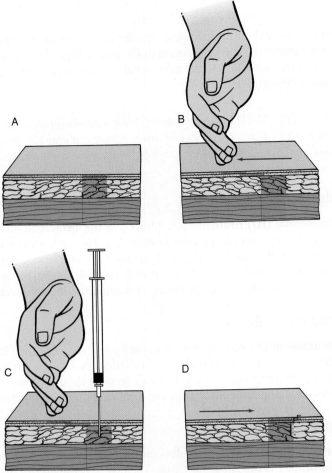

Figure 8-4. Z-track technique. **A.** Normal skin position. **B.** Pulling skin to the side. **C.** Injecting the medication. **D.** Releasing the skin after syringe removal. (From Taylor, C., Lillis, C., & LeMone, P. [2005.] *Fundamentals of Nursing.* 5th ed. Philadelphia: Lippincott Williams & Wilkins.)

Formula Method

When you have the same system and unit of measurement for the dosage ordered and the dosage on hand, use the formula method to do the calculation.

Sandy's order for pain medication reads 8 mg of morphine. You have 10 mg/mL of morphine available. You recognize it is necessary to perform a calculation to obtain the correct dosage of morphine.

When the dosage ordered differs from the dosage available, use the formula method:

$$\frac{D}{H} \times V = A$$

Where: D = desired or prescribed dosage of the medication

H = dosage of medication available or on hand

V = volume that the medication is available in, such as one tablet or milliliters

A = amount of medication to administer

STEP 1: CONVERT

The first step requires you to make sure that the medication dose ordered is in the same dosage system and unit as the medication available. When dosages ordered for medications are in different systems or units than the dosage on hand, it is important to convert both the ordered dosage and the dosage on hand to the same system or unit. For Sandy, both the ordered dosage and dosage on hand are in the same unit—mg. Therefore, you do not need to convert for this calculation.

STEP 2: COMPUTE

Determine what data you need and set up the problem correctly. The formula method required you to know what medication dose is ordered and the dosage available or dosage on hand. This step requires higher-level thinking, not just memorization.

The formula is:

$$\frac{D}{H} \times V = A$$

For this problem, D (desired or ordered dose) is 8 mg, H (dosage on hand) is 10 mg, and V (volume medication comes in) is 1 mL. Therefore, using the formula method, the problem would be set up as follows:

$$\frac{8 \text{ mg}}{10 \text{ mg}} \times 1 \text{ mL} = A$$

Cancel out milligrams. Solve the equation.

$$\frac{8 \text{ mg}}{10 \text{ mg}} \times 1 \text{ mL} = A$$

$$\frac{8}{10} \times 1 \text{ mL} = A$$

$$0.8 \text{ mL} = A$$

The correct answer for this problem is 0.8 mL.

STEP 3: CRITICALLY THINK

ASK YOURSELF – Does this answer seem logical, correct, and plausible?

This answer is reasonable and plausible in that it meets the safe standard for the amount of morphine to be given at one time. It is not an unusually large or small amount for a safe dose. It is correct. Think that 0.8 mL is slightly less than 1 mL. Therefore, 0.8 mL is correct. To verify the accuracy of this step, have another nurse check your math.

PRACTICE PROBLEMS 8-1. Practice Problems for Calculating Dosages in the Same Measurement System, Using the Formula Method

DIRECTIONS: Solve the following medication dosage problems using the formula method. The answers to the problems can be found at the end of the chapter.

1. **Medication Ordered:** Diazepam 10 mg IM daily
   Medication Available: Diazepam 5 mg/mL

   Calculation:

2. **Medication Ordered:** Dexamethasone 2 mg IV daily
   Medication Available: Dexamethasone 4 mg/mL

   Calculation:

3. **Medication Ordered:** Bumetanide 0.75 mg IM daily
   Medication Available: Bumetanide 0.5 mg/mL

   Calculation:

4. **Medication Ordered:** Atropine 0.3 mg IM
   Medication Available: Atropine 0.5 mg/mL

   Calculation:

5. **Medication Ordered:** Methylprednisolone 60 mg IM daily
   Medication Available: Methylprednisolone 80 mg/mL

   Calculation:

6. **Medication Ordered:** Propranolol 0.5 mg IV now
   Medication Available: Propranolol 1 mg/mL

   Calculation:

7. **Medication Ordered:** Solu-Cortef 20 mg IM
   Medication Available: Solu-Cortef 50 mg/mL

   Calculation:

CASE STUDY

Remember Sandy, the 34-year-old woman who had an open reduction for a fractured femur following an automobile accident. The physician has also ordered ampicillin 250 mg IM to prevent infection. The pharmacy supplies a vial containing ampicillin 1000 mg/5 mL.

- The physician ordered ampicillin 250 mg IM twice a day
- You have available ampicillin 1000 mg/5 mL

You recognize the need to perform calculation to obtain the correct dosage of ampicillin.

Ratio-Proportion Method

When the medication dose ordered by the prescriber is different from the dosage of the medication available, the ratio-proportion method can be used to calculate the needed dose of the medication. This method solves for an unknown x in the equation. The equation is:

$$\frac{\text{Dosage on hand}}{\text{Amount on hand}} = \frac{\text{Dosage desired}}{x\,\text{Amount desired}}$$

STEP 1: CONVERT

This step requires you to make sure that the medication dose ordered is in the same dosage system and unit as the medication available. When medication dosages ordered are in different systems or units than the dosage on hand, it is important to convert both the ordered dosage and the dosage on hand to the same system or unit. For Sandy, both the ordered dosage and dosage on hand are in the same unit—mg. Therefore, you do not need to convert for this calculation.

STEP 2: COMPUTE

Determine what data you need and set up the problem correctly. The ratio-proportion method requires you to know what medication dose is ordered and the dosage available. The equation is:

$$\frac{\text{Dosage on hand}}{\text{Amount on hand}} = \frac{\text{Dosage desired}}{x\,\text{Amount desired}}$$

$$\frac{1000\ \text{mg}}{5\ \text{mL}} = \frac{250\ \text{mg}}{x}$$

Cross multiply:

$$\frac{1{,}000 \text{ mg}}{5 \text{ mL}} \diagdown \diagup \frac{250 \text{ mg}}{x}$$

1000 mg x = 1250 mg × mL

Isolate x in the equation by dividing both sides of the equation by 1000. Cancel out like units.

$$\frac{\cancel{1000 \text{ mg}} \, x}{\cancel{1000 \text{ mg}}} = \frac{1250 \cancel{\text{ mg}} \times \text{mL}}{1000 \cancel{\text{ mg}}}$$

$$x = \frac{1250 \text{ mL}}{1000}$$

$$x = 1.25 \text{ mL}$$

The correct answer for this problem is 1.25 mL.

 SAFETY ALERT: *When preparing medications, pay close attention to the amount of solution that contains the dose per unit. Not all medication dosages are in one milliliter. It is common to find the unit dosage of the medication in a larger volume. If you use an incorrect amount when performing the calculation, the patient will receive an incorrect dosage of the medication.* **Don't make the mistake of thinking that all drug dosages come in 1 mL.**

STEP 3: CRITICALLY THINK

ASK YOURSELF – *Does this answer seem logical, correct, and plausible?*

This answer is reasonable and plausible in that it meets the safe standard for the amount to be given at one time. It is not an unusually large or small amount for a safe dose. It is correct. Think that 250 mg is smaller than 1000 mg and is being used to prevent an infection. Therefore, 1.25 mL is correct. To verify this step, have another nurse check your math.

SAFETY ALERT: *When withdrawing a medication from a single-dose vial, always discard any unused portion. When using a multi-dose vial, label the vial with the date and time it was opened, and store according to the directions on the vial or according to the agency policy. Store the opened vial only the length of time as indicated on the vial.*

CASE STUDY

You check on Sandy 2 hours later and she tells you that the morphine did not relieve her pain. She continues to rate her pain as a 9 on a 0 to 10 scale. You contact the physician and he orders a one-time dose of Dilaudid 3 mg intramuscularly. The Dilaudid is available in 2 mg/mL. You recognize the need to perform a calculation to obtain the correct dosage of the Dilaudid.

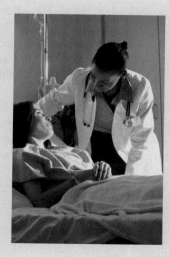

Use the ratio-proportion method again, and follow the three steps.

STEP 1: CONVERT

This step requires you to make sure that the medication dose ordered is in the same dosage system and unit as the medication available. When dosages ordered for medications are in different systems or units than the dosage on hand, it is important to convert both the ordered dosage and the dosage on hand to the same system or unit. For Sandy, both the ordered dosage and dosage on hand are in the same unit—mg. Therefore, you do not need to convert for this calculation.

STEP 2: COMPUTE

Determine what data you need and set up the problem correctly. The ratio-proportion method requires you to know what medication dose is ordered and the dosage available. The equation is:

$$\frac{\text{Dosage on hand}}{\text{Amount on hand}} = \frac{\text{Dosage desired}}{x\,\text{Amount desired}}$$

To calculate this problem using the ratio-proportion method, set up the problem like this:

$$\frac{2\text{ mg}}{1\text{ mL}} = \frac{3\text{ mg}}{x}$$

Cross multiply:

$$\frac{2\text{ mg}}{1\text{ mL}} \diagdown\diagup \frac{3\text{ mg}}{x}$$

$$2\text{ mg } x = 3\text{ mg} \times 1\text{ mL}$$

Isolate the x by dividing both sides by 2. Milligrams (mg) in the numerator and denominator cancel each other out, and you are left with mL as the volume of medication in the answer.

$$\frac{2\text{ mg } x}{2\text{ mg}} = \frac{3\text{ mg} \times \text{mL}}{2\text{ mg}}$$

Solve for x.

$$x = \frac{3\text{ mL}}{2} = 1.5\text{ mL}$$

Therefore, the answer to the problem is 1.5 mL. You prepare 1.5 mL in the syringe to be given to Sandy.

STEP 3: CRITICALLY THINK

ASK YOURSELF – Does this answer seem logical, correct, and plausible?

This answer is reasonable and plausible in that it meets the safe standard for the amount to be given at one time. It is not unusually large or small for a safe dose. It is correct. Think that 3 mg is 2 mg larger than the available dose. Therefore, 1.5 mL is correct. To verify this step, have another nurse check your math.

PRACTICE PROBLEMS 8-2. Practice Problems for Calculating Dosages in the Same Measurement System, Using the Ratio-Proportion Method

DIRECTIONS: Solve the following medication dosage problems using the ratio-proportion method. The answers to the problems can be found at the end of the chapter.

1. **Medication Ordered:** Vistaril 50 mg 1M
   Medication Available: Vistaril 100 mg/2 mL

   Calculation:

2. **Medication Ordered:** Robinul 0.1 mg
   Medication Available: Robinul 0.2 mg/mL

   Calculation:

3. **Medication Ordered:** Chloroquine 250 mg
   Medication Available: Chloroquine 50 mg/mL

   Calculation:

4. **Medication Ordered:** Lanoxin 0.125 mL
   Medication Available: Lanoxin 0.25 mg/mL

   Calculation:

5. **Medication Ordered:** Garamycin 60 mg
   Medication Available: Garamycin 40 mg/mL

   Calculation:

6. **Medication Ordered:** Clindamycin 250 mg
   Medication Available: Clindamycin 150 mg/mL

   Calculation:

7. **Medication Ordered:** Furosemide 60 mg
   Medication Available: Furosemide 10 mg/mL

   Calculation:

8. **Medication Ordered:** Rifampin 500 mg
   Medication Available: Rifampin 600 mg/mL

   Calculation:

CALCULATIONS WITH DIFFERENT UNITS OF MEASUREMENT

Sometimes, medications are ordered in one unit of measurement, but the medication is supplied in another unit of measurement. However, the units are in the same system of measurement—for example, the metric system.

Formula Method

First determine that the units of measurement are different but in the same system. Always convert to equivalent units. Then use the formula method.

For example: The physician orders Synthroid 0.2 mg intramuscular daily. The medication is supplied as 1000 mcg/mL. Use the formula method to determine the dose:

$$\frac{D}{H} \times V = A$$

Where: D = desired or prescribed dosage of the medication

H = dosage of medication available or on hand

V = volume that the medication is available in, such as one tablet or milliliters

A = amount of medication to administer

STEP 1: CONVERT

This step requires you to make sure that the medication dose ordered is in the same dosage system and unit as the medication available. When dosages ordered for medications are in different systems or units than dosage on hand, it is important to convert both the ordered dosage and the dosage on hand to the same system or unit. Remember that 1 mg = 1000 mcg. For this example, convert the 0.2 mg to mcg by multiplying 0.2 by 1000. The results are

$$0.2 \times 1000 = 200 \text{ mcg.}$$

Now the ordered dosage and dosage on hand are in the same unit—mcg.

STEP 2: COMPUTE

Determine what data you need and set up the problem correctly. The formula method required you to know what medication dose is ordered and the dosage available or dosage on hand.

The formula is:

$$\frac{D}{H} \times V = A$$

Using the formula method, set up the problem:

$$\frac{200 \text{ mcg}}{1000 \text{ mcg}} \times 1 \text{ mL}$$

Since mcg appears in both the numerator and denominator, mcg is cancelled out and you are left with mL as the volume of medication in the answer.

$$\frac{200 \cancel{\text{mcg}}}{1000 \cancel{\text{mcg}}} \times 1 \text{ mL} = 0.2 \text{ mL}$$

Therefore, you would administer 0.2 mL of Synthroid.

STEP 3: CRITICALLY THINK

ASK YOURSELF – *Does this answer seem logical, correct, and plausible?*

This answer is reasonable and plausible in that it meets the safe standard for the amount of Synthroid to be given at one time. It is not an unusually small amount for a safe dose. It is correct. Think that 0.2 mL is smaller than 1 mL. Therefore, 0.2 mL is correct. To verify the accuracy of this step, have another nurse check your math. Since it is correct, you would administer 0.2 mL of Synthroid.

PRACTICE PROBLEMS 8-3. Practice Problems for Calculating Dosages With Different Units of Measurement, Using the Formula Method

DIRECTIONS: Solve the following medication dosage problems using the formula method. The answers to the problems can be found at the end of the chapter.

1. **Medication Ordered:** Aztreonam 1.5g 1M
   Medication Available: Aztreonam 1000 mg/mL

   Calculation:

2. **Medication Ordered:** Fentanyl 0.1 mg
   Medication Available: Fentanyl 50 mcg/mL

   Calculation:

3. **Medication Ordered:** Cefepime hydrochloride 1g
   Medication Available: Cefepime hydrochloride 500 mg/mL

   Calculation:

4. **Medication Ordered:** Vitamin B_{12}, 1000 mcg
   Medication Available: Vitamin B_{12}, 5 mg/mL

   Calculation:

5. **Medication Ordered:** Ampicillin 250 mg
   Medication Available: Ampicillin 2 g/mL

   Calculation:

Ratio-Proportion Method

When the prescriber orders medication in one unit of measurement but the medication is supplied in another unit of measurement, you must convert the medications to the same measurement system. Then the ratio-proportion method can be used to calculate the needed dose. This method solves for an unknown x in the equation. The equation is:

$$\frac{\text{Dosage on hand}}{\text{Amount on hand}} = \frac{\text{Dosage desired}}{x \, \text{Amount desired}}$$

Consider this example. The physician orders ampicillin 500 mg IV. The pharmacy supplies a vial of ampicillin, 2 g/50 mL. You recognize the need to calculate the correct dosage of ampicillin for your patient.

STEP 1: CONVERT

You note that the drug dose ordered is in a different dosage unit than the drug available. When the dosage ordered for the medication is in a different system or unit than the dosage on hand, it is important to convert both the ordered dosage and the dosage on hand to the same system or unit. For this patient, the ordered dosage unit and the available dosage unit are different. Therefore, you need to convert. Because the unit of the drug available is in grams, convert the ordered dosage from milligrams to grams. Remember that 1 g = 1000 mg. To convert 500 mg to grams, divide 500 by 1000.

$$500 \div 1000 = 0.5 \text{ g}$$

STEP 2: COMPUTE

Determine what data you need and set up the problem correctly. The ratio-proportion method requires you to know what medication dose is ordered and what the available dosage is. The equation is:

$$\frac{\text{Dosage on hand}}{\text{Amount on hand}} = \frac{\text{Dosage desired}}{x \, \text{Amount desired}}$$

$$\frac{2 \text{ g}}{50 \text{ mL}} = \frac{0.5 \text{ g}}{x}$$

Cross multiply:

$$\frac{2 \text{ g}}{50 \text{ mL}} \diagdown\!\!\!\!\diagup \frac{0.5 \text{ g}}{x}$$

$$2 \text{ g } x = 25 \text{ g} \times \text{mL}$$

Isolate x in the equation by dividing both sides of the equation by 2. Like units cancel out.

$$\frac{2 \text{ g } x}{2 \text{ g}} = \frac{25 \text{ g} \times \text{mL}}{2 \text{ g}}$$

$$x = \frac{25 \text{ mL}}{2}$$

$$x = 12.5 \text{ mL}$$

The correct answer for this problem is 12.5 mL.

STEP 3: CRITICALLY THINK

ASK YOURSELF – Does this answer seem logical, correct, and plausible?

This answer is reasonable and plausible in that it meets the safe standard for the amount of IV medication to be given. It is not unusually large or small for a safe dose. It is correct. Think that each 50 mL contains 2 g of ampicillin. Therefore, 12.5 mL is the correct amount when the dosage is 500 mg. To verify this step, have another nurse check your math.

PRACTICE PROBLEMS 8-4. Practice Problems for Calculating Dosages With Different Units of Measurement, Using the Ratio-Proportion Method

DIRECTIONS: Solve the following medication dosage problems using the ratio-proportion method. The answers to the problems can be found at the end of the chapter.

1. **Medication Ordered:** Quinidine 0.2 g
   Medication Available: Quinidine 80 mg/mL

   Calculation:

2. **Medication Ordered:** Vancomycin 1.5 g
   Medication Available: Vancomycin 500 mg/mL

   Calculation:

3. **Medication Ordered:** Methylprednisolone 0.25 g
   Medication Available: Methylprednisolone 1000 mg/mL

   Calculation:

4. **Medication Ordered:** Fentanyl 0.2 mg
   Medication Available: Fentanyl 50 mcg/mL

   Calculation:

5. **Medication Ordered:** Rocephin 250 mg
   Medication Available: Rocephin 1 g/mL

   Calculation:

CALCULATIONS IN DIFFERENT SYSTEMS

At times, a drug may be ordered in a unit of measurement in one system, for example the apothecary system. However, the drug may be supplied in a unit of measurement in another system, such as the metric system. When this occurs, you will need to convert the ordered drug to the same system as that for the supplied drug.

Formula Method

A physician has ordered codeine, gr ss of codeine IM every 4 hours prn. Codeine 60 mg/mL is available. Use the formula method to calculate the correct dose.

In the formula method:

$$\frac{D}{H} \times V = A$$

Where: D = desired or prescribed dosage of the medication

H = dosage of medication available or on hand

V = volume that the medication is available in, such as one tablet or milliliters

A = amount of medication to administer

STEP 1: CONVERT

This step requires you to make sure that the medication dose ordered is in the same dosage system and unit as the medication available. When dosages ordered for medications are in different systems or units than dosage on hand, it is important to convert both the ordered dosage and the dosage on hand to the same system or unit. For example, both the ordered dosage and dosage on hand for codeine need to be in mg. Therefore, you need to convert for this calculation.

First, convert to the same system. Be certain to use the system in which the drug is available. Then, work your answer as a fraction or ratio format and use the formula method.

$$\text{Remember that} \qquad gr\ 1 = 60\ mg.$$

$$\text{Use the formula} \quad gr\ 1{:}60\ mg :: gr\ \frac{1}{2}{:}\ x\ mg$$

$$gr\ 1 \times x = gr\ \frac{1}{2} \times 60\ mg$$

$$1x = \frac{1}{2} \times 60\ mg$$

$$x = 30\ mg$$

STEP 2: COMPUTE

Determine what data you need and set up the problem correctly. The formula method required you to know what medication dose is ordered and the dosage available or dosage on hand. This step requires higher-level thinking, not just memorization.

The formula is:
$$\frac{D}{H} \times V = A$$

For this problem, the D (desired or ordered dose) is 30 mg, the H (dosage on hand) is 60 mg, and the V (volume medication comes in) is 1 mL. Set up the problem as follows:

$$\frac{30\ mg}{60\ mg} \times 1\ mL = A$$

Since mg appears in both the numerator and denominator, mg is cancelled out and you are left with mL as the volume of medication in the answer.

$$\frac{30\ \cancel{mg}}{60\ \cancel{mg}} \times 1\ mL = A$$

$$\frac{30}{60} \times 1\ mL = A$$

$$0.5\ mL = A$$

The correct answer for this problem is 0.5 mL.

STEP 3: CRITICALLY THINK

ASK YOURSELF – Does this answer seem logical, correct, and plausible?

This answer is reasonable and plausible in that it meets the safe standard for the amount of codeine to be given at one time. It is not an unusually small amount for a safe dose. It is correct. Think that 0.5 mL is smaller than 1 mL. Therefore, 0.5 mL is correct. So you would prepare 0.5 mL in the syringe for administration. To verify the accuracy of this step, have another nurse check your math.

(!) **SAFETY ALERT:** *Always critically analyze the answers to your calculations. Ask yourself this question: Is the answer much larger than the available dose? For example, if the available dose is 25 mg/mL, is it likely that the calculated answer would be much greater than 1 mL? The answer is no when you see that the dose is much larger than the available dosage. Always verify with an approved drug reference or with the pharmacist.*

PRACTICE PROBLEMS 8-5. Practice Problems for Calculating Dosages in Different Systems, Using the Formula Method

DIRECTIONS: Solve the following medication dosage problems using the formula method. The answers to the problems can be found at the end of the chapter.

1. **Medication Ordered:** Phenobarbital gr $1\frac{1}{2}$

   Medication Available: Phenobarbital 60 mg/mL

   Calculation:

2. **Medication Ordered:** Scopolamine gr $\frac{1}{150}$

   Medication Available: Scopolamine 0.5 mg

   Calculation:

3. **Medication Ordered:** AquaMEPHYTON gr $\frac{1}{6}$

   Medication Available: AquaMEPHYTON 2 mg/mL

   Calculation:

4. **Medication Ordered:** Thiamine hydrochloride gr 3
   Medication Available: Thiamine hydrochloride 200 mg/mL

   Calculation:

5. **Medication Ordered:** Codeine gr $\frac{1}{4}$

   Medication Available: Codeine 60 mg/mL

   Calculation:

Ratio-Proportion Method

When the medication is ordered by the prescriber in a unit of measurement different from the dosage of the medication available, the ratio-proportion method can be used to calculate the needed dose. The ordered medication needs to be converted to the same system as the available medication. The ratio-proportion method solves for an unknown x in the equation. The equation is:

$$\frac{\text{Dosage on hand}}{\text{Amount on hand}} = \frac{\text{Dosage desired}}{x \, \text{Amount desired}}$$

A physician orders diphenhydramine (Benadryl) gr $\frac{1}{2}$ for a patient because she has developed a rash. The pharmacy supplies Benadryl 50 mg/mL. You recognize the need to calculate the correct dosage in the same measurement system of Benadryl for your patient.

STEP 1: CONVERT

You note that the drug dose ordered is in a different dosage unit than the drug available. When the dosage ordered for the medication is in a different system or unit than the dosage on hand, it is important to convert both the ordered dosage and the dosage on hand to the same system or unit.

For this patient, the ordered dosage unit and the available dosage unit are different. Therefore, you need to convert. Because the unit of the drug available is in grams, you will want to convert the ordered dosage from grains to milligrams. Remember that gr 1 = 60 mg. So, gr $\frac{1}{2}$ would equal 30 mg.

STEP 2: COMPUTE

Determine what data you need and set up the problem correctly. The ratio-proportion method requires you to know what medication dose is ordered and what the available dosage is. The equation is:

$$\frac{\text{Dosage on hand}}{\text{Amount on hand}} = \frac{\text{Dosage desired}}{x \, \text{Amount desired}}$$

$$\frac{50 \text{ mg}}{1 \text{ mL}} = \frac{30 \text{ mg}}{x}$$

Cross multiply:

$$\frac{50 \text{ mg}}{1 \text{ mL}} \diagdown\!\!\!\!\diagup \frac{30 \text{ mg}}{x}$$

$$50 \text{ mg}x = 30 \text{ mg} \times \text{mL}$$

Isolate x in the equation by dividing both sides of the equation by 50. Like units cancel out.

$$\frac{\cancel{50 \text{ mg}} \, x}{\cancel{50 \text{ mg}}} = \frac{30 \cancel{\text{ mg}} \times \text{mL}}{50 \cancel{\text{ mg}}}$$

$$x = \frac{30 \text{ mL}}{50}$$

$$x = 0.6 \text{ mL}$$

The correct answer for this problem is 0.6 mL.

STEP 3: CRITICALLY THINK

ASK YOURSELF – Does this answer seem logical, correct, and plausible?

This answer is reasonable and plausible in that it meets the safe standard for the amount of medication given at one time. It is not unusually large or small for a safe dose. It is correct. Think that 1 mL contains 50 mg of Benadryl. Therefore, 30 mg is smaller than the 50 mg available dose. So it is logical that the calculated dose is 0.6 mL and it is the correct amount. To verify this step, have another nurse check your math.

PRACTICE PROBLEMS 8-6. Practice Problems for Calculating Dosages in Different Systems, Using the Ratio-Proportion Method

DIRECTIONS: Solve the following medication dosage problems using the ratio-proportion method. The answers to the problems can be found at the end of the chapter.

1. **Medication Ordered:** Phenobarbital gr $1\frac{1}{2}$

   Medication Available: Phenobarbital 130 mg/mL

   Calculation:

2. **Medication Ordered:** Atropine gr $\frac{1}{200}$

   Medication Available: Atropine 0.4 mg/mL

   Calculation:

3. **Medication Ordered:** Morphine gr $\frac{1}{4}$

   Medication Available: Morphine 10 mg/mL

   Calculation:

4. **Medication Ordered:** Benadryl gr 1

   Medication Available: Benadryl 50 mg/mL

   Calculation:

5. **Medication Ordered:** Aztreonam gr 10

   Medication Available: Aztreonam 1000 mg/mL

   Calculation:

CALCULATIONS FOR DRUGS COMBINED IN ONE SYRINGE

Sometimes, two drugs may need to be combined in a syringe and administered as one injection. When preparing two parenteral medications for one injection, it is safer to prepare each in a separate syringe and then combine the two into one. Doing so helps to prevent a calculation error by drawing up more volume of one of the medications.

Formula Method

Consider this example: A physician orders atropine sulfate 0.3 mg IM and morphine sulfate 8 mg IM 30 minutes prior to surgery. Atropine is supplied as 0.4 mg/mL. The morphine sulfate is supplied as 10 mg/mL in a prefilled syringe.

Using the formula method:

$$\frac{D}{H} \times V = A$$

Where: D = desired or prescribed dosage of the medication

H = dosage of medication available or on hand

V = volume that the medication is available in, such as one tablet or milliliters

A = amount of medication to administer

First you will have to calculate the dosage for atropine and then the dosage for morphine.

STEP 1: CONVERT

This step requires you to make sure that the medication dose ordered is in the same dosage system and unit as the medication available. When dosages ordered for medications are in different systems or units than the dosage on hand, it is important to convert both the ordered dosage and the dosage on hand to the same system or unit. For example, both the ordered dosage and dosage on hand for each drug are in the same unit—mg. Therefore, you do not need to convert for this calculation.

STEP 2: COMPUTE

Determine what data you need and set up the problem correctly. The formula method required you to know what medication dose is ordered and the dosage available or dosage on hand. This step requires higher-level thinking, not just memorization.

The formula is:

$$\frac{D}{H} \times V = A$$

To calculate the atropine dosage: the D (desired or ordered dose) is 0.3 mg. The H (dosage on hand) is 0.4 mg. The V (volume medication comes in) is 1 mL. Therefore, using this method the set-up of the problem would be:

$$\frac{0.3 \text{ mg}}{0.4 \text{ mg}} \times 1 \text{ mL} = A$$

Since mg appears in both the numerator and denominator, mg is cancelled out and you are left with mL as the volume of medication in the answer.

$$\frac{0.3 \cancel{\text{ mg}}}{0.4 \cancel{\text{ mg}}} \times 1 \text{ mL} = A$$

$$\frac{0.3}{0.4} \times 1 \text{ mL} = A$$

$$0.75 \text{ mL} = A$$

The correct answer for the atropine dose is 0.75 mL.

Next, use the formula method to calculate the morphine dosage. The morphine sulfate is supplied as 10 mg/mL in a prefilled syringe. To calculate the morphine dosage: The D (desired or ordered dose) is 8 mg. The H (dosage on hand) is 10 mg. The V (volume medication comes in) is 1 mL. Therefore, using this method the set-up of the problem would be:

$$\frac{8 \text{ mg}}{10 \text{ mg}} \times 1 \text{ mL} = A$$

Since mg appears in both the numerator and denominator, mg is cancelled out and you are left with mL as the volume of medication in the answer.

$$\frac{8 \cancel{\text{ mg}}}{10 \cancel{\text{ mg}}} \times 1 \text{ mL} = A$$

$$\frac{8}{10} \times 1 \text{ mL} = A$$

$$0.8 \text{ mL} = A$$

The correct answer for this problem is 0.8 mL. Therefore, you would need 0.75 mL of atropine and 0.8 mL of morphine.

STEP 3: CRITICALLY THINK

ASK YOURSELF – Does this answer seem logical, correct, and plausible?

This answer is reasonable and plausible in that it meets the safe standard for the amount of atropine to be given at one time. It is not an unusually small amount for a safe dose. It is correct. Think that 0.75 mL is slightly smaller than 1 mL. Therefore, 0.75 mL is correct.

For the morphine dosage, this answer is reasonable and plausible in that it meets the safe standard for the amount of morphine to be given at one time. It is not an unusually small amount for a safe dose. It is correct. Think that 0.8 mL is slightly smaller than 1 mL. Therefore, 0.8 mL is correct. To verify the accuracy of this step, have another nurse check your math.

Since the morphine was available in a prefilled syringe it is important to waste 0.2 mL so the remainder is equal to the calculation of 0.8 mL. Next, add the atropine dose of 0.75 mL to the syringe. Therefore, when properly combined, the total volume in the syringe will be 1.55 mL—0.75 mL of atropine and 0.8 mL of morphine.

> (!) **SAFETY ALERT:** *Be certain to follow agency policy when wasting a medication that is a controlled substance. Also be very careful when wasting medication so that you have the exact dose remaining as determined by the calculation.*

Ratio-Proportion Method

The ratio-proportion method may be used when drugs may need to be combined and administered as one injection. Remember when preparing two parenteral medications for one injection, it is safer to prepare each in a separate syringe and then combine the two into one. Doing so helps to prevent a calculation error by drawing up more volume of one of the medications.

For example, an order reads Vistaril 25 mg IM and meperidine 75 mg IM 30 minutes prior to surgery. Vistaril is supplied as 50 mg/mL. The meperidine is supplied as 100 mg/mL in a 3-mL prefilled syringe.

STEP 1: CONVERT

This step requires you to make sure that the medication dose ordered is in the same dosage system and unit as the medication available. The dosages ordered for both medications are in the same systems or units as the dosage on hand—mg. Therefore, you do not need to convert for this calculation.

STEP 2: COMPUTE

Determine what data you need and set up the problem correctly. The ratio-proportion method requires you to know what medication dose is ordered and the dosage available. The ratio-proportion is as follows:

$$\frac{\text{Dosage on hand}}{\text{Amount on hand}} = \frac{\text{Dosage desired}}{x\,\text{Amount desired}}$$

Set up the ratio-proportion for the Vistaril:

$$\frac{50\text{ mg}}{1\text{ mL}} = \frac{25\text{ mg}}{x}$$

Cross multiply:

$$\frac{50 \text{ mg}}{1 \text{ mL}} \diagdown \diagup \frac{25 \text{ mg}}{x}$$

$$50 \text{ mg } x = 25 \text{ mg} \times 1 \text{ mL}$$

Isolate x in the equation by dividing both sides of the equation by 50. Cancel out like units.

$$\frac{50 \text{ mg } x}{50 \text{ mg}} = \frac{25 \text{ mg} \times \text{mL}}{50 \text{ mg}}$$

$$x = \frac{25 \text{ mL}}{50}$$

$$x = 0.5 \text{mL}$$

The correct answer for this problem is 0.5 mL.

To calculate the meperidine dose, set up the problem as follows:

$$\frac{100 \text{ mg}}{1 \text{ mL}} = \frac{75 \text{ mg}}{x}$$

Cross multiply:

$$\frac{100 \text{ mg}}{1 \text{ mL}} \diagdown \diagup \frac{75 \text{ mg}}{x}$$

$$100 \text{ mg } x = 75 \text{ mg} \times 1 \text{ mL}$$

Isolate the x by dividing both sides by 100. Milligrams (mg) in the numerator and denominator cancel each other out and you are left with mL as the volume of medication in the answer.

$$\frac{100 \text{ mg } x}{100 \text{ mg}} = \frac{75 \text{ mg} \times \text{mL}}{100 \text{ mg}}$$

Solve for x. $x = 0.75$ mL

Therefore, you need 0.75 mL of meperidine.

STEP 3: CRITICALLY THINK

ASK YOURSELF – Does this answer seem logical, correct, and plausible?

Both answers are reasonable and plausible in that each meets the safe standard for the amount of meperidine and Vistaril to be given at one time. It is not an unusually small amount for a safe dose. Is it correct? For meperidine, think that 0.75 mL is slightly smaller than 1 mL. Therefore, 0.75 mL is correct. For the Vistaril, think that 0.5 mL is smaller than 1 mL. Therefore, 0.5 mL is correct.

Then, think about the total volume to be administered. Since the meperidine is available in a prefilled syringe, you must waste 0.25 mL so the remainder is equal to 0.75 mL.

Next, add the Vistaril dose of 0.5 mL to the meperidine syringe. Therefore the prepared dose will now equal 0.75 mL of meperidine plus 0.5 mL of Vistaril for a total volume of 1.25 mL. This amount is within the safe range for one injection. To verify the accuracy of these steps, have another nurse check your math.

(!) SAFETY ALERT: *Before combining parenteral medications in the same syringe, it is imperative that you consult a reliable reference to verify compatibility. If a reference is not available, then contact the pharmacist.*

PREPARING PARENTERAL MEDICATIONS FROM DRUGS SUPPLIED AS POWDERS

Some medications are available in a powder or dry form and must be dissolved or reconstituted with a solution or diluent before the drug may be administered. The package insert or the drug label will state the diluent to be used and the exact amount to be added. When adding a solution or diluent to the powder, you will notice that the directions will state the volume and dose after the solution has been added. Remember the powder takes up space. For example, the directions may read to add 1.5 mL of normal saline to a vial and when added to the powder, the solution contains a total of 2 mL. In addition follow the label or package insert about proper storage and the length of time the drug may be kept before it must be discarded.

> (!) **SAFETY ALERT:** *Remember that sterile solutions are always used for reconstitution. Always label the vial with the date, time, the solution added, the dose per mL, and the signature of the nurse doing the reconstitution.*

Formula Method

A patient is to receive ampicillin 300 mg intravenously every 6 hours. The label on the vial of ampicillin reads: add 3.5 mL of diluent. According to the manufacturer's label, after reconstitution the vial contains 250 mg/mL.

Use the formula method to calculate the dose:

$$\frac{D}{H} \times V = A$$

Where: D = desired or prescribed dosage of the medication

H = dosage of medication available or on hand

V = volume that the medication is available in, such as one tablet or milliliters

A = amount of medication to administer

STEP 1: CONVERT

This step requires you to make sure that the medication dose ordered is in the same dosage system and unit as the medication available. When dosages ordered for medications are in different systems or units than the dosage on hand, it is important to convert both the ordered dosage and the dosage on hand to the same system or unit. Both the ordered dosage and dosage on hand are in the same unit—mg. Therefore, you do not need to convert for this calculation.

STEP 2: COMPUTE

Determine what data you need and set up the problem correctly. The formula method required you to know what medication dose is ordered and the dosage available or dosage on hand. This step requires higher-level thinking, not just memorization.

The formula is: $$\frac{D}{H} \times V = A$$

For this problem: The D (desired or ordered dose) is 300 mg. The H (dosage on hand) is 250 mg. The V (volume medication comes in) is 1 mL. Therefore, using this method the set-up of the problem would be:

$$\frac{300 \text{ mg}}{250 \text{ mg}} \times 1 \text{ mL} = A$$

Since mg appears in both the numerator and denominator, mg is cancelled out and you are left with mL as the volume of medication in the answer.

$$\frac{300 \, \cancel{mg}}{250 \, \cancel{mg}} \times 1 \, mL = A$$

$$\frac{300}{250} \times 1 \, mL = A$$

$$1.2 \, mL = A$$

The correct answer for this problem is 1.2 mL.

STEP 3: CRITICALLY THINK

ASK YOURSELF – *Does this answer seem logical, correct, and plausible?*

This answer is reasonable and plausible in that it meets the safe standard for the amount of ampicillin to be given at one time. It is not an unusually large amount for a safe dose. It is correct. Think that 1.2 mL is slightly larger than 1 mL. Therefore, 1.2 mL is correct. To verify the accuracy of this step, have another nurse check your math.

PRACTICE PROBLEMS 8-7. Practice Problems for Calculating Dosages of Parenteral Medications From Drugs Supplied as Powders, Using the Formula Method

DIRECTIONS: Solve the following medication dosage problems using the formula method. The answers to the problems can be found at the end of the chapter.

1. Synthroid 150 mcg intravenous is ordered daily. After reconstitution the vial contains a total of 5 mL and there is 100 mcg/mL.
   Give _____ mL.

2. Cefazolin sodium 250 mg IV every 8 hours. Reconstitute with 2.5 mL sterile normal saline. After reconstitution the vial contains 225 mg/mL.
   Give _____ mL.

3. Ampicillin 250 mg IM every 12 hours is ordered. After reconstitution there is 125 mg/mL. Give _____ mL.

4. Cefazolin sodium 125 mg IV every 12 hours is ordered. After reconstitution the vial contains 225 mg/mL. Give _____ mL.

Ratio-Proportion Method

When the medication is ordered by the prescriber is supplied in powder form, you add a diluent according to the directions on the label. Remember that the label will also provide the volume of medication in the vial after reconstitution as well as the dose per mL. The ratio-proportion method can be used to calculate the needed dose. The ratio-proportion method solves for an unknown x in the equation. The equation is:

$$\frac{\text{Dosage on hand}}{\text{Amount on hand}} = \frac{\text{Dosage desired}}{x \, \text{Amount desired}}$$

The physician ordered Rocephin 250 mg IM. You have available Rocephin 1 g in powder form. The directions state to add 9.6 mL to the vial to arrive at a solution that will contain 100 mg/mL.

STEP 1: CONVERT

You note that the drug dose ordered after it has been reconstituted is in the same dosage unit as the drug available. In this example there is no need to convert as both the ordered dose and available dose are in mg.

STEP 2: COMPUTE

Determine what data you need and set up the problem correctly. The ratio-proportion method requires you to know what medication dose is ordered and what the available dosage is. To calculate this problem using the ratio-proportion method, set up the problem to calculate for the Rocephin dose of 250 mg when on hand there is 100 mg/mL:

$$\frac{100 \text{ mg}}{1 \text{ mL}} = \frac{250 \text{ mg}}{x}$$

Cross multiply:

$$\frac{100 \text{ mg}}{1 \text{ mL}} \times \frac{250 \text{ mg}}{x}$$

$$100 \text{ mg } x = 250 \text{ mg} \times 1 \text{ mL}$$

Isolate the x by dividing both sides by 100; mg in the numerator and denominator cancel each other out and you are left with mL as the volume of medication in the answer.

$$\frac{100 \text{ mg } x}{100 \text{ mg}} = \frac{250 \text{ mg} \times \text{mL}}{100 \text{ mg}}$$

Solve for x.

$$x = 2.5 \text{ mL}$$

Therefore, the answer to the problem is to administer 2.5 mL of Rocephin.

STEP 3: CRITICALLY THINK

ASK YOURSELF – Does this answer seem logical, correct, and plausible?

This answer is reasonable and plausible in that it meets the safe standard for the amount of medication given at one time. It is not unusually large or small for a safe dose. It is correct. Think that the 2.5 mL contains 250 mg of Rocephin. Since 250 mg is larger than the 100 mg available dose, it is logical that the calculated dose is 2.5 mL, and it is the correct amount. To verify this step, have another nurse check your math.

PRACTICE PROBLEMS 8-8. Practice Problems for Calculating Dosages of Parenteral Medications From Drugs Supplied as Powders, Using the Ratio-Proportion Method

DIRECTIONS: Solve the following medication dosage problems using the ratio-proportion method. The answers to the problems can be found at the end of the chapter.

1. Ampicillin 350 mg IM is ordered daily. After reconstitution with 3.5 mL of sterile water, the vial contains a total of 500 mg/mL.
   Give _____ mL.

2. Claforan 500 mg IV every 12 hours. Reconstitute with 2.4 mL sterile water. After reconstitution the vial contains 230 mg/mL.
   Give _____ mL.

3. Rocephin 500 mg IM every 12 hours is ordered. After reconstitution there are 250 mg/mL. Give _____ mL.

4. Cefotetan 1 g IV every 12 hours. After reconstitution the vial contains 400 mg/mL. Give _____ mL.

5. Ceftazidime 1 gram IV every 8 hours. After reconstitution the vial contains 100 mg/mL. Give _____ mL.

Critical Thinking/Decision Making Exercise

The physician orders terbutaline 0.125 mg IM for your patient this morning for her respiratory distress. The drug is supplied in a vial labeled 1 mg/mL. As you prepare the equipment, you plan to use a 3-mL syringe and you begin to calculate the dose.

Set up the problem using the formula method:

$$\frac{D}{H} \times V = A$$

$$\frac{0.125 \text{ mg}}{1 \text{ mg}} \times 1 \text{ mL} = A$$

$$0.125 \text{ mL} = A \text{ Round to } 0.13 \text{ mL}$$

So you realize that you should rethink your preparation.

Problem

What problem do you have? What is the rationale for your decision? After performing the calculation, you realize that you need to use a 1-mL syringe because of the small dose.

Solution

Instead of using a 3-mL syringe, you use a 1-mL syringe and withdraw the solution to the 0.13 mL marking. Follow the rules for rounding, which state that when the number is at or above 5, you round to the next unit. Since the unit is hundredths, you would round to 0.13 mL.

If you used the 3-mL syringe, you would have likely made a medication error. The markings of the 3-mL syringe are in intervals of tenths of a mL. Therefore, measuring 0.13 mL would be extremely difficult, making the dose inaccurate.

CHAPTER REVIEW PROBLEMS

Answers to the problems can be found at the end of the chapter.

Review Problems 8-1. Calculate the amount of medication for parenteral injections.

1. Amoxicillin 250 mg is prescribed. The drug dose on hand is 1 g amoxicillin in 2 mL. Give _0.5_ mL.

2. Furosemide 60 mg IV is prescribed. The available drug dose is furosemide 40 mg/mL. You would administer _____ mL.

3. Digoxin 0.75 mg as an initial dose is ordered. Available is 0.5 mg/2 mL. You will administer _____ mL.

4. Ceftriaxone sodium 0.3 g IV is ordered. Available is ceftriaxone sodium 1000 mg/mL. Give _____ mL.

5. Dilaudid 1.5 mg subcutaneous is prescribed. On hand is Dilaudid 2 mg/mL. Administer _____ mL.

6. Metoclopramide 20 mg is ordered IV for relief of nausea. Available is metoclopramide 10 mg/mL. The calculated dose is _____ mL.

7. Diazepam 4 mg is ordered. The drug on hand is diazepam 5 mg/mL. You calculate the correct dose as _.8_ mL.

Answers to Practice Problems

Practice Problem Answers 8-1

1. Diazepam

The problem is set up:

$$\frac{10\ mg}{5\ mg} \times 1\ mL$$

$$\frac{10\ \cancel{mg}}{5\ \cancel{mg}} \times 1\ mL = 2\ mL.$$

Give 2 mL of diazepam.

2. Dexamethasone

The problem is set up:

$$\frac{2\ mg}{4\ mg} \times 1\ mL$$

$$\frac{2\ \cancel{mg}}{4\ \cancel{mg}} \times 1\ mL = 0.5\ mL.$$

Give 0.5 mL of dexamethasone.

3. Bumetanide

The problem is set up:

$$\frac{0.75\ mg}{0.5\ mg} \times 1\ mL$$

$$\frac{0.75\ \cancel{mg}}{0.5\ \cancel{mg}} \times 1\ mL = 1.5\ mL$$

Give 1.5 mL of bumetanide.

4. Atropine

The problem is set up:

$$\frac{0.3\ mg}{0.5\ mg} \times 1\ mL$$

$$\frac{0.3\ \cancel{mg}}{0.5\ \cancel{mg}} \times 1\ mL = 0.6\ mL.$$

Give 0.6 mL of atropine.

5. Methylprednisolone

The problem is set up:

$$\frac{60\ mg}{80\ mg} \times 1\ mL$$

$$\frac{60\ \cancel{mg}}{80\ \cancel{mg}} \times 1\ mL = 0.75\ mL$$

Give 0.75 mL of methylprednisolone.

6. Propranolol

The problem is set up:

$$\frac{0.5\ mg}{1\ mg} \times 1\ mL$$

$$\frac{0.5\ \cancel{mg}}{1\ \cancel{mg}} \times 1\ mL = 0.5\ mL$$

Give 0.5 mL of propranolol.

7. Solu-Cortef

The problem is set up:

$$\frac{20\ mg}{50\ mg} \times 1\ mL$$

$$\frac{20\ \cancel{mg}}{50\ \cancel{mg}} \times 1\ mL = 0.4\ mL$$

Give 0.4 mL of Solu-Cortef.

Practice Problem Answers 8-2

1. Vistaril

   Set up the problem:

   $$\frac{100 \text{ mg}}{2 \text{ mL}} = \frac{50 \text{ mg}}{x}$$

   Cross multiply the set-up equation to get: 100 mg x = 100 mg $\times$ mL

   Isolate x in the equation by dividing by 100 mg.

   $$\frac{100 \text{ mg } x}{100 \text{ mg}} = \frac{100 \text{ mg} \times \text{mL}}{100 \text{ mg}}$$

   x = 1 mL

2. Robinul

   $$\frac{0.2 \text{ mg}}{1 \text{ mL}} = \frac{0.1 \text{ mg}}{x}$$

   Cross multiply the set-up equation to get: 0.1 mg $\times$ mL = 0.2 mg x

   Isolate x in the equation by dividing by 0.2 mg.

   $$\frac{0.1 \text{ mg} \times \text{mL}}{0.2 \text{ mg}} = \frac{0.2 \text{ mg } x}{0.2 \text{ mg}}$$

   x = 0.5 mL

3. Chloroquine

   $$\frac{50 \text{ mg}}{1 \text{ mL}} = \frac{250 \text{ mg}}{x}$$

   Cross multiply the set-up equation to get: 250 mg $\times$ mL = 50 mg x.

   Isolate x in the equation by dividing by 50 mg:

   $$\frac{250 \text{ mg} \times \text{mL}}{50 \text{ mg}} = \frac{50 \text{ mg } x}{50 \text{ mg}}$$

   x = 5 mL

4. Lanoxin

   $$\frac{0.25 \text{ mg}}{1 \text{ mL}} = \frac{0.125 \text{ mg}}{x}$$

   Cross multiply the set-up equation to get: 0.25 mg x = 0.125 mg $\times$ mL

   Isolate x in the equation by dividing by 0.25 mg:

   $$\frac{0.25 \text{ mg } x}{0.25 \text{ mg}} = \frac{0.125 \text{ mg} \times \text{mL}}{0.25 \text{ mg}}$$

   x = 0.5 mL

5. Garamycin

   $$\frac{40 \text{ mg}}{1 \text{ mL}} = \frac{60 \text{ mg}}{x}$$

   Cross multiply the set-up equation to get: 60 mg $\times$ mL = 40 mg x

   Isolate x in the equation by dividing by 40 mg:

   $$\frac{40 \text{ mg } x}{40 \text{ mg}} = \frac{60 \text{ mg} \times \text{mL}}{40 \text{ mg}}$$

   x = 1.5 mL

6. Clindamycin

$$\frac{150 \text{ mg}}{1 \text{ mL}} = \frac{250 \text{ mg}}{x}$$

Cross multiply the set-up equation to get: 250 mg × mL = 150 mg x

Isolate x in the equation by dividing by 150 mg:

$$\frac{\cancel{150 \text{ mg}} \, x}{\cancel{150 \text{ mg}}} = \frac{250 \cancel{\text{ mg}} \times \text{mL}}{150 \cancel{\text{ mg}}}$$

$x = 1.66$ mL, round to 1.7 mL

7. Furosemide

$$\frac{10 \text{ mg}}{1 \text{ mL}} = \frac{60 \text{ mg}}{x}$$

Cross multiply the set-up equation to get: 60 mg × mL = 10 mg x

Isolate x in the equation by dividing by 10 mg.

$$\frac{\cancel{10 \text{ mg}} \, x}{\cancel{10 \text{ mg}}} = \frac{60 \cancel{\text{ mg}} \times \text{mL}}{10 \cancel{\text{ mg}}}$$

$x = 6$ mL

8. Rifampin

$$\frac{600 \text{ mg}}{1 \text{ mL}} = \frac{500 \text{ mg}}{x}$$

Cross multiply the set-up equation to get: 600 mg $x = 500$ mg × mL

Isolate x in the equation by dividing by 600 mg:

$$\frac{\cancel{600 \text{ mg}} \, x}{\cancel{600 \text{ mg}}} = \frac{500 \cancel{\text{ mg}} \times \text{mL}}{600 \cancel{\text{ mg}}}$$

$x = 0.83$ mL, round to 0.8 mL

Practice Problem Answers 8-3

1. Aztreonam

Convert g to mg. Remember 1 g = 1000 mg.

$1.5 \times 1000 = 1500$ mg

$$\frac{1500 \cancel{\text{ mg}}}{1000 \cancel{\text{ mg}}} \times 1 \text{ mL} = 1.5 \text{ mL}$$

The answer is 1.5 mL.

2. Fentanyl

Convert the 0.1 mg to mcg by moving the decimal three places to the right, giving 100 mcg.

The problem is set up:

$$\frac{100 \text{ mcg}}{50 \text{ mcg}} \times 1 \text{ mL}$$

$$\frac{100 \cancel{\text{ mcg}}}{50 \cancel{\text{ mcg}}} \times 1 \text{ mL} = 2 \text{ mL}$$

3. Cefepime hydrochloride

Convert the g to mg. Remember 1 g = 1000 mg.

$1 \times 1000 = 1000$ mg

The problem is set up:

$$\frac{1000 \text{ mg}}{500 \text{ mg}} \times 1 \text{ mL} = 2 \text{ mL}$$

The answer is 2 mL.

4. Vitamin B_{12}

Convert the 1000 mcg to mg by moving the decimal three places to the left, giving 1 mg.

The problem is set up:

$$\frac{1 \text{ mg}}{5 \text{ mg}} \times 1 \text{ mL} = 0.2 \text{ mL}$$

5. Ampicillin

Convert the 2 g to mg by moving the decimal three places to the right, giving 2000 mg.

The problem is set up:

$$\frac{250 \text{ mg}}{2000 \text{ mg}} \times 1 \text{ mL} = 0.125 \text{ mL}$$

Practice Problem Answers 8-4

1. Quinidine

Remember 1000 mg = 1 g. Convert 0.2 g to mg by moving the decimal 3 places to the right; 0.2 g becomes 200 mg.

$$\frac{80 \text{ mg}}{1 \text{ mL}} = \frac{200 \text{ mg}}{x}$$

Cross multiply the set-up equation to get: 80 mg x = 200 mg $\times$ 1 mL

Isolate x in the equation by dividing by 80 mg:

$$\frac{80 \text{ mg } x}{80 \text{ mg}} = \frac{200 \text{ mg} \times \text{mL}}{80 \text{ mg}}$$

x = 2.5 mL

2. Vancomycin

Remember 1000 mg = 1 g. Convert 1.5 g to mg by moving the decimal 3 places to the right; 1.5 g becomes 1500 mg.

$$\frac{500 \text{ mg}}{1 \text{ mL}} = \frac{1500 \text{ mg}}{x}$$

Cross multiply the set-up equation to get: 500 mg x = 1500 mg $\times$ mL

Isolate x in the equation by dividing by 500 mg:

$$\frac{500 \text{ mg } x}{500 \text{ mg}} = \frac{1500 \text{ mg} \times \text{mL}}{500 \text{ mg}}$$

x = 3 mL

3. Methylprednisolone

   Remember there are 1000 mg in a gram. Convert 0.25 g to mg by moving the decimal 3 places to the right; 0.25 g becomes 250 mg.

   $$\frac{1000 \text{ mg}}{1 \text{ mL}} = \frac{250 \text{ mg}}{x}$$

   Cross multiply the set-up equation to get: 250 mg × mL = 1000 mg x

   Isolate x in the equation by dividing by 1000 mg:

   $$\frac{250 \text{ mg} \times \text{mL}}{1000 \text{ mg}} = \frac{1000 \text{ mg } x}{1000 \text{ mg}} = 0.25 \text{ mL}$$

   $x = 0.25$ mL

4. Fentanyl

   Remember there are 1000 mcg in a milligram. Convert the 0.2 mg to mcg by moving the decimal three places to the right; 0.2 mg becomes 200 mcg.

   The problem is set up:

   $$\frac{50 \text{ mcg}}{1 \text{ mL}} = \frac{200 \text{ mcg}}{x}$$

   Cross multiply the set-up equation to get: 50 mcg x = 200 mcg × mL

   Isolate x in the equation by dividing by 50 mcg.

   $$\frac{50 \text{ mcg } x}{50 \text{ mcg}} = \frac{200 \text{ mcg} \times \text{mL}}{50 \text{ mcg}}$$

   $x = 4$ mL

5. Rocephin

   Remember there are 1000 mg in a gram. Convert 1 g to mg by moving the decimal three places to the right; 1 g becomes 1000 mg.

   $$\frac{1000 \text{ mg}}{1 \text{ mL}} = \frac{250 \text{ mg}}{x}$$

   Cross multiply the set-up equation to get: 1000 mg x = 250 mg × mL

   Isolate x in the equation by dividing by 1000 mg:

   $$\frac{1000 \text{ mg } x}{1000 \text{ mg}} = \frac{250 \text{ mg} \times \text{mL}}{1000 \text{ mg}}$$

   $x = 0.25$ mL

Practice Problem Answers 8-5

1. Phenobarbital

   Remember 60 mg = gr 1. Convert gr $1\frac{1}{2}$ to mg.

   $$\frac{60 \text{ mg}}{\text{gr } 1} \times \text{gr } 1.5 = 90 \text{ mg}$$

   The problem is set up:

   $$\frac{90 \text{ mg}}{60 \text{ mg}} \times 1 \text{ mL}$$

   $$\frac{90 \text{ mg}}{60 \text{ mg}} \times 1 \text{ mL} = 1.5 \text{ mL}$$

2. Scopolamine

   Convert grains to mg; remember, 60 mg = gr 1.

   $$\frac{gr\ 1}{150} \times \frac{60\ mg}{gr\ 1} = 0.4\ mg$$

   The problem is set up:

   $$\frac{0.4\ mg}{0.5\ mg} \times 1\ mL$$

   $$\frac{0.4\ \cancel{mg}}{0.5\ \cancel{mg}} \times 1\ mL = 0.8\ mL$$

3. AquaMEPHYTON

   First convert grains to mg.

   $$\frac{gr\ 1}{6} \times \frac{60\ mg}{gr\ 1} = 10\ mg$$

   The problem is set up:

   $$\frac{10\ mg}{2\ mg} \times 1\ mL$$

   $$\frac{10\ \cancel{mg}}{2\ \cancel{mg}} \times 1\ mL = 5\ mL$$

4. Thiamine

   Convert grains to milligrams: $gr\ 3 \times \frac{60\ mg}{gr\ 1} = 180\ mg$

   The problem is set up:

   $$\frac{180\ mg}{200\ mg} \times 1\ mL$$

   $$\frac{180\ \cancel{mg}}{200\ \cancel{mg}} \times 1\ mL = 0.9\ mL$$

5. Codeine

   Convert grains to mg: $\frac{gr\ 1}{4} \times \frac{60\ mg}{gr\ 1} = 15\ mg$

   The problem is set up:

   $$\frac{15\ mg}{60\ mg} \times 1\ mL$$

   $$\frac{15\ \cancel{mg}}{60\ \cancel{mg}} \times 1\ mL = 0.25\ mL$$

Practice Problem Answers 8-6

1. Phenobarbital

   Remember 60 mg = gr 1. Convert grain $1\frac{1}{2}$ to mg by multiplying by 60, then gr $1\frac{1}{2}$ becomes 90 mg.

   $$\frac{130\ mg}{1\ mL} = \frac{90\ mg}{x}$$

   Cross multiply the set-up equation: 130 mg x = 90 mg × mL

Isolate x in the equation by dividing by 130 mg

$$\frac{\cancel{130\ mg}\ x}{\cancel{130\ mg}} = \frac{90\ \cancel{mg} \times mL}{130\ \cancel{mg}}$$

$x = 0.69$ mL, round to 0.7 mL

2. Atropine

Remember 60 mg = gr 1. Convert gr $\frac{1}{200}$ to mg by multiplying by 60; gr $\frac{1}{200}$ becomes 0.3 mg.

$$\frac{gr\ 1}{200} \times \frac{60\ mg}{gr\ 1} = 0.3\ mg$$

$$\frac{0.4\ mg}{1\ mL} = \frac{0.3\ mg}{x}$$

Cross multiply the set-up equation to get: 0.4 mg $x = 0.3$ mg $\times$ mL

Isolate x in the equation by dividing by 0.4 mg:

$$\frac{\cancel{0.4\ mg}\ x}{\cancel{0.4\ mg}} = \frac{0.3\ \cancel{mg} \times mL}{0.4\ \cancel{mg}}$$

$x = 0.75$ mL

3. Morphine

Remember 60 mg = gr 1. Convert gr $\frac{1}{4}$ to mg by multiplying by 60; gr $\frac{1}{4}$ becomes 15 mg.

$$\frac{10\ mg}{1\ mL} = \frac{15\ mg}{x}$$

Cross multiply the set-up equation to get: 10 mg $x = 15$ mg $\times$ mL

Isolate x in the equation by dividing by 10 mg:

$$\frac{\cancel{10\ mg}\ x}{\cancel{10\ mg}} = \frac{15\ \cancel{mg} \times mL}{10\ \cancel{mg}}$$

$x = 1.5$ mL

4. Benadryl

Remember 60 mg = gr 1. Convert gr 1 by multiplying by 60; gr 1 becomes 60 mg.

$$\frac{50\ mg}{1\ mL} = \frac{60\ mg}{x}$$

Cross multiply the set-up equation to get: 50 mg $x = 60$ mg $\times$ mL

Isolate x in the equation by dividing by 50 mg:

$$\frac{\cancel{50\ mg}\ x}{\cancel{50\ mg}} = \frac{60\ \cancel{mg} \times mL}{50\ \cancel{mg}}$$

$x = 1.2$ mL

5. Aztreonam

Remember 60 mg = gr 1. Convert gr 10 to mg by multiplying by 60; gr 10 becomes 600 mg.

$$\frac{1000\ mg}{1\ mL} = \frac{600\ mg}{x}$$

Cross multiply the set-up equation to get: 1000 mg $x = 600$ mg $\times$ mL

Isolate x in the equation by dividing by 1000 mg:

$$\frac{\cancel{1000\ mg}\ x}{\cancel{1000\ mg}} = \frac{600\ \cancel{mg} \times mL}{1000\ \cancel{mg}}$$

$x = 0.6$ mL

Practice Problem Answers 8-7

1. Synthroid

The problem is set up:

$$\frac{150 \text{ mcg}}{100 \text{ mcg}} \times 1 \text{ mL}$$

$$\frac{150 \text{ mcg}}{100 \text{ mcg}} \times 1 \text{ mL} = 1.5 \text{ mL}$$

Give 1.5 mL of Synthroid.

2. Cefazolin

The problem is set up:

$$\frac{250 \text{ mg}}{225 \text{ mg}} \times 1 \text{ mL}$$

$$\frac{250 \text{ mg}}{225 \text{ mg}} \times 1 \text{ mL} = 1.1 \text{ mL}$$

Give 1.1 mL of Cefazolin.

3. Ampicillin

The problem is set up:

$$\frac{250 \text{ mg}}{125 \text{ mg}} \times 1 \text{ mL}$$

$$\frac{250 \text{ mg}}{125 \text{ mg}} \times 1 \text{ mL} = 2 \text{ mL}$$

Give 2 mL of ampicillin.

4. Cefazolin

The problem is set up:

$$\frac{125 \text{ mg}}{225 \text{ mg}} \times 1 \text{ mL}$$

$$\frac{125 \text{ mg}}{225 \text{ mg}} \times 1 \text{ mL} = 0.55 \text{ mL, round to } 0.6 \text{ mL}$$

Give 0.6 mL of Cefazolin.

Practice Problem Answers 8-8

1. Ampicillin

$$\frac{500 \text{ mg}}{1 \text{ mL}} = \frac{350 \text{ mg}}{x}$$

Cross multiply the set-up equation to get: 500 mg x = 350 mg × mL

Isolate x in the equation by dividing by 500 mg:

$$\frac{500 \text{ mg } x}{500 \text{ mg}} = \frac{350 \text{ mg} \times \text{mL}}{500 \text{ mg}}$$

$x = 0.7$ mL

2. Claforan

$$\frac{230 \text{ mg}}{1 \text{ mL}} = \frac{500 \text{ mg}}{x}$$

Cross multiply the set-up equation to get: 230 mg x = 500 mg × mL

Isolate x in the equation by dividing by 230 mg:

$$\frac{230 \text{ mg } x}{230 \text{ mg}} = \frac{500 \text{ mg} \times \text{mL}}{230 \text{ mg}}$$

$x = 2.17$ mL, round to 2.2 mL.

3. Rocephin

$$\frac{250 \text{ mg}}{1 \text{ mL}} = \frac{500 \text{ mg}}{x}$$

Cross multiply the set-up equation to get: 250 mg x = 500 mg × mL

Isolate x in the equation by dividing by 250 mg:

$$\frac{250 \text{ mg } x}{250 \text{ mg}} = \frac{500 \text{ mg} \times \text{mL}}{250 \text{ mg}}$$

$x = 2$ mL

4. Cefotetan

$$\frac{400 \text{ mg}}{1 \text{ mL}} = \frac{1000 \text{ mg}}{x}$$

Cross multiply the set-up equation to get: $400 \text{ mg } x = 1000 \text{ mg} \times \text{mL}$

Isolate x in the equation by dividing by 400 mg:

$$\frac{400 \text{ mg } x}{400 \text{ mg}} = \frac{1000 \text{ mg} \times \text{mL}}{400 \text{ mg}}$$

$x = 2.5 \text{ mL}$

5. Ceftazidime

$$\frac{100 \text{ mg}}{1 \text{ mL}} = \frac{1000 \text{ mg}}{x}$$

Cross multiply the set-up equation to get: $100 \text{ mg } x = 1000 \text{ mg} \times \text{mL}$

Isolate x in the equation by dividing by 100 mg:

$$\frac{100 \text{ mg } x}{100 \text{ mg}} = \frac{1000 \text{ mg} \times \text{mL}}{100 \text{ mg}}$$

$x = 10 \text{ mL}$

Chapter Review Problem Answers

1. Amoxicillin

   Convert g to mg. 1000 mg = 1 g

   Set up the problem:

   $$\frac{250 \text{ mg}}{1000 \text{ mg}} \times 2 \text{ mL} = 0.5 \text{ mL}$$

2. Furosemide

   Set up the problem:

   $$\frac{60 \text{ mg}}{40 \text{ mg}} \times 1 \text{ mL} = 1.5 \text{ mL}$$

3. Digoxin

   Set up the problem:

   $$\frac{0.75 \text{ mg}}{0.5 \text{ mg}} \times 2 \text{ mL} = 3 \text{ mL}$$

4. Ceftriaxone

   Set up the problem:

   $$\frac{300 \text{ mg}}{1000 \text{ mg}} \times 1 \text{ mL} = 0.3 \text{ mL}$$

5. Dilaudid

   Set up the problem:

   $$\frac{1.5 \text{ mg}}{2 \text{ mg}} \times 1 \text{ mL} = 0.75 \text{ mL}$$

6. Metoclopramide

   Set up the problem:

   $$\frac{20 \text{ mg}}{10 \text{ mg}} \times 1 \text{ mL} = 2 \text{ mL}$$

7. Diazepam

   Set up the problem:

   $$\frac{4 \text{ mg}}{5 \text{ mg}} \times 1 \text{ mL} = 0.8 \text{ mL}$$

Calculation of Intravenous Rates

This chapter contains content on:

- **Intravenous Fluid Administration Equipment**
- **Calculation of Amount of Solute per Intravenous Solution**
- **Calculation of Intravenous Flow Rates in mL/hour**
- **Calculation of Intravenous Flow Rates in gtt/min**

Learning Objectives

Upon completion of Chapter 9, you will be able to:

- Select the correct IV solution and equipment based on the physician's order.
- Identify the drop calibration factor on IV tubing package.
- Calculate the amount of solute in intravenous solutions.
- Calculate mL/hour flow rate for intravenous solutions.
- Calculate gtt/min flow rate of intravenous solution using the formula and "quick" methods.

Key Terms

- Drop factor
- Intravenous
- Macro-drip tubing
- Micro-drip tubing
- Osmolarity
- Primary tubing
- Secondary tubing

CASE STUDY

Mr. Sampson, age 54, is admitted to the nursing unit with a diagnosis of acute pancreatitis secondary to biliary disease. He has been complaining of severe abdominal pain for the last two days. His laboratory work shows elevated serum amylase and lipase levels that are consistent with the diagnosis of acute pancreatitis. The physician made Mr. Sampson NPO and ordered a peripheral IV started. The order for the intravenous infusion reads: Infuse 1000 mL of 5% dextrose in 0.45% normal saline with 20 mEq of potassium chloride over 8 hours.

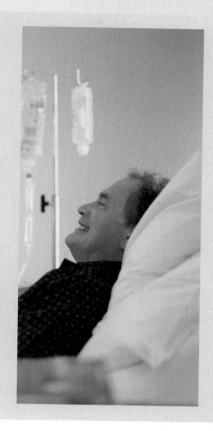

Medications, electrolyte solutions, and other fluids are frequently ordered and administered to a patient directly into a vein. This method is called **intravenous (IV)** administration. Fluid and electrolyte solutions are given intravenously to restore or maintain fluid and electrolyte balance. For example, the patient may require intravenous fluids if they are NPO (nothing by mouth) for an extended period of time, or have experienced fluid loss through bleeding, vomiting, or diarrhea. Intravenous administration allows the infusion of a specified amount of solution for rapid absorption by the patient. You can also administer a large volume of fluid over a short period of time when the patient is hypovolemic (volume depleted).

Blood and blood products are also administered intravenously. In addition, a patient's nutritional needs may also be met by administering concentrated glucose, amino acid, and electrolyte solutions.

Medications are administered intravenously for a variety of reasons. Patients may be NPO or unable to swallow medications. Some drugs, such as certain antibiotics, are supplied only in solution for intravenous use. If the patient status is critical, and rapid absorption and distribution of emergency medications is needed, then the intravenous route is the route of choice. Medications administered intravenously have a faster absorption and distribution rate.

Intravenous solutions are administered via an intravenous catheter inserted peripherally or centrally (see Figure 9-1). Peripherally inserted catheters typically are placed in veins located in the extremities, such as the arm or leg. In infants, scalp veins may be used for peripheral insertion. Peripherally inserted catheters are used to administer smaller volumes of fluids or for short-term therapy. Blood products may be administered through larger peripheral veins.

Centrally inserted catheters are placed in large veins in the chest, such as the subclavian vein, or the neck, such as the jugular vein. Central lines are used when large volumes of fluids need to be administered rapidly, the patient is receiving parenteral nutritional therapy, or the patient is expected to require long-term IV therapy.

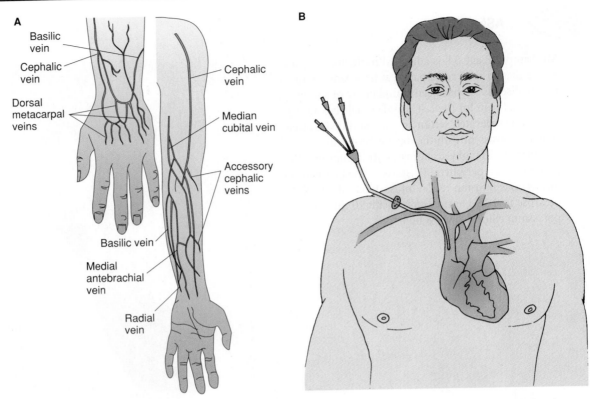

Figure 9-1. Intravenous insertion sites. **A.** Peripheral. **B.** Central. (From Taylor, C., Lillis, C., and LeMone, P. [2005]. *Fundamentals of Nursing,* 5th ed. Philadelphia: Lippincott Williams & Wilkins.)

INTRAVENOUS FLUID ADMINISTRATION EQUIPMENT

Intravenous Solutions

Intravenous solutions are administered to patients to restore or maintain fluid and electrolyte balance. The specific type of intravenous solution is ordered by the prescriber based on patient needs. The nurse is responsible for ensuring that the correct solution is infusing at the correct rate, and for monitoring the patient for tolerance and response to the area. Always monitor the patient to determine if he or she is able to tolerate the infusion at the prescribed rate. Also assess for any evidence of too much or too little fluid administration.

Intravenous solutions can be either colloids or crystalloids. Colloid solutions contain proteins or starch molecules. Examples of colloid intravenous solutions are blood products, albumin, hetastarch, and parenteral nutrition solutions.

Crystalloid solutions are clear electrolyte solutions that have the potential to be distributed throughout the extracellular compartment. The common components found in crystalloid solutions are: water, dextrose, sodium chloride or saline (NaCl), and electrolytes. Examples of crystalloid solutions are lactated Ringer's and dextrose in water or saline solutions (see Figure 9-2).

Both colloid and crystalloid solutions are used for fluid replacement in patients who are hypovolemic. Crystalloid solutions are readily available, easy to administer, and less expensive than colloid solutions. The disadvantage of crystalloids is that it takes 3 to 4 times greater volume than colloid solutions to replace the fluid deficit. The physician will consider the patient's underlying clinical problems when selecting the intravenous solution.

OSMOLARITY

Osmolarity is another characteristic considered when intravenous solutions are ordered. **Osmolarity** is the number of particles, or amount of substance, in a liter of solution. Osmolarity is reported as milliosmoles per liter (mOsm/L).

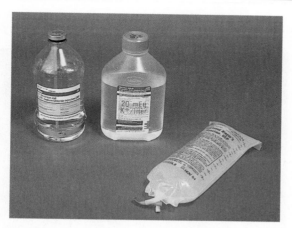

Figure 9-2. Examples of IV solutions.

SOLUTION STRENGTH

Solution strength is written as a percent (%). This percent indicates the specific number of grams per 100 mL of the specified component. For example, 5% dextrose in water means that there are 5 grams of dextrose in each 100 mL of solution.

SOLUTION CONCENTRATION

Intravenous solutions are categorized based on their osmolarity, as isotonic, hypotonic, or hypertonic concentrations. Isotonic solutions are ordered to increase circulating volume when the patient is experiencing hypovolemia. These solutions have an osmolarity that is equal to the osmotic pressure found in cells, ranging from 250 to 275 mOsm/L. Examples of isotonic solutions include 5% dextrose in water (D5W), 0.9% NaCl (normal saline or physiologic saline), and lactated Ringer's solution.

Hypotonic solutions are ordered when the patient needs cellular hydration and can be used to lower serum osmolarity. These solutions have an osmotic pressure that is lower than the cell. Thus the osmolarity of hypotonic solutions is less than 250 mOsm/L. Examples of hypotonic solutions include: 0.225% NaCl (1/4 strength saline) and 0.45% NaCl (1/2 strength saline).

Hypertonic solutions are used to raise serum osmolarity or pull fluid from the cell or interstitial tissues into the vascular space. These solutions have a higher osmotic pressure than the cell. Thus the osmolarity of hypertonic solutions is 375 mOsm/L or higher. Examples of hypertonic solutions include: 5% dextrose in 0.45% NaCl, 10% dextrose in water (D10W), and 5% dextrose in 0.9% NaCl.

ADDITIONAL COMPONENTS

Intravenous solutions can have electrolytes added to them. Potassium chloride (KCl) is the most common electrolyte added to standard solutions. Potassium chloride is ordered in milliequivalents (mEq). Common dosages of potassium chloride in intravenous solutions are 20 mEq or 40 mEq.

PACKAGING

Intravenous solutions are normally packaged in flexible or rigid plastic containers. These plastic containers typically collapse under atmospheric pressure as the solution infuses into the patient. Infusion bags most often contain 500 or 1000 mL of solution. Smaller plastic bags with 50, 100, or 250 mL also are available. These smaller-sized containers are most often used to mix medications such as antibiotics when the medication is to be administered over a period of time. Because some medications adhere to plastic, intravenous solutions are also available in glass bottles.

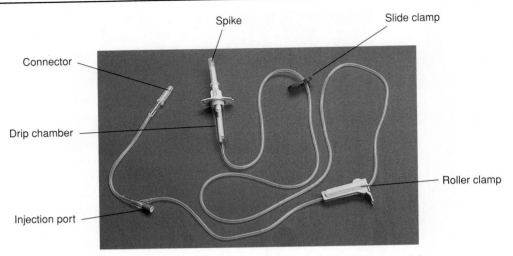

Figure 9-3. IV administration set. (Courtesy of Abbott Laboratories, North Chicago, IL.)

Intravenous Tubing

Intravenous solutions are administered using intravenous tubing, also called an IV administration set (see Figure 9-3). The tubing is inserted into the bag or bottle containing the solution through a small tube or spike. The tubing has a drip chamber near the end of the tubing that is closest to the bag or bottle. The flow rate is calculated by counting the drops per minute that fall into the drip chamber. The rate of flow is controlled by a roller clamp, which helps to regulate the speed at which the drops enter the drip chamber.

The number of drops per milliliter that is delivered by the intravenous tubing is called the **drop factor**. This information can be found on the package of the tubing. The drip chamber is continuous with the tubing that is connected to the patient via the intravenous catheter. The diameter of the tubing attached to the drip chamber controls the size of the drop. Tubing is calibrated, based on the diameter of tubing, to deliver a preset number of drops per milliliter. The larger the diameter of the tubing, the more drops per milliliter that are delivered. Along the tubing are one or more injection ports.

TYPES OF TUBING

Tubing may be categorized based on the number of drops delivered per milliliter of fluid as macro-drip and micro-drip tubing (see Figure 9-4). **Macro-drip tubing** is tubing that delivers 10, 15, or 20 drops per milliliter. Primary tubing is one type of macro-drip tubing. **Micro-drip tubing** is intravenous tubing with a small diameter that delivers 60 drops per mL. This type of tubing is used with pediatric patients, elderly patients, or in other situations where it is important to deliver small amounts of solution or when a more precise measurement of intravenous solution is needed.

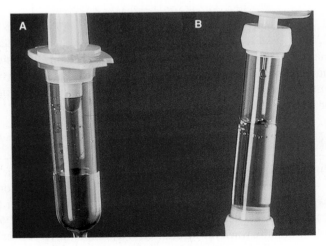

Figure 9-4. IV Tubing. **A.** Macro-drip. **B.** Micro-drip.

Tubing also may be categorized based on its purpose. **Primary tubing** is used for intravenous solution administration or when larger amounts of fluid are delivered. **Secondary tubing** is used to administer intravenous medications. It is attached to an injection port on the primary tubing. This is called piggybacking the secondary tubing into the primary tubing. When administering the two solutions together, hang the secondary intravenous solution bag higher than the primary bag to ensure that the secondary medication infuses first.

Administration of blood requires tubing made specifically for this purpose. Blood tubing is shaped like a "Y". Two ports are located above a built-in filter (porous enough to allow the blood cells to pass through) on the tubing. One port is spiked into the blood product and the other port is spiked into the IV bag containing normal saline solution, the solution required for blood administration (see Figure 9-5). Blood tubing is a type of macro-drip tubing.

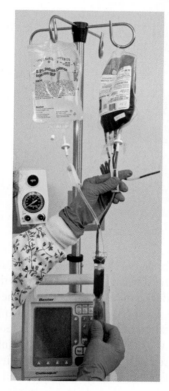

Figure 9-5. Blood administration.

Both primary and blood tubing may be supplied as tubing designed for gravity infusion, controlled using a manual roller-type clamp, or as tubing designed for use with an electronic infusion device.

> ⓘ **SAFETY ALERT:** *Never administer any intravenous solution, with the exception of 0.9% NaCl or intravenous medications, via the intravenous tubing used for administering blood while blood administration is occurring. Administration of solutions other than 0.9% NaCl or intravenous medications with the blood can adversely affect the blood product and harm the patient.*

Electronic Infusion Devices

Electronic infusion devices can be used to control intravenous flow rates. The infusion devices infuse solution at the prescribed amount of fluid per hour. These devices are used to administer IV solutions in situations where patient safety is critical, such as administration of chemotherapy, parenteral nutrition solutions, or potent medications such as heparin, insulin, antiarrhythmics, or inotropic medications. They are used regularly on general floors within the hospital, critical care areas, pediatrics, and surgery based on the patient's age, condition, and prescribed therapy.

Electronic infusion devices vary from simple to complex depending upon the manufacturer. Some devices are single channel units in which only one IV solution can be programmed to infuse at a time. There are also multichannel units that allow you to infuse up to three or four different IV solutions, each on a separate channel, through a single device. Figure 9-6 shows an example of an electronic device. Generally each device requires specialized tubing supplied by the manufacturer. Newer devices can calculate infusion rates.

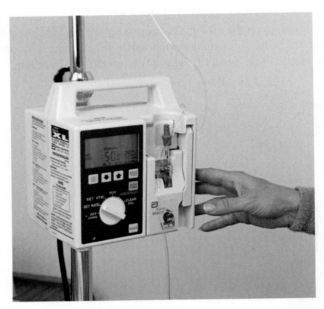

Figure 9-6. Electronic infusion device.

Infusion devices are equipped with alarms that signal problems with the infusion. Devices also are equipped with an internal rechargeable battery backup so that the device can operate during patient care situations requiring the device to be unplugged from the electrical current, such as when the patient is ambulating or being transported to another department or unit.

The Joint Commission on Accreditation of Healthcare Organization's 2005 National Patient Safety Goals established a goal to improve patient safety when using infusion pumps. Healthcare organizations are required to ensure free-flow protection on all infusion devices and patient-controlled analgesia (PCA) pumps. Free-flow protection means that the tubing has a built in mechanism like a slide clamp that is mobilized when the tubing is removed from the pump. The free-flow mechanism prevents flow of fluid into the patient when the pump is stopped or the tubing is taken out of the infusion pump.

TYPES OF DEVICES

There are four types of electronic infusion devices: controllers, positive-pressure infusion pumps, syringe pumps, and patient-controlled analgesia (PCA) pumps.

- Controller-type devices deliver fluid at a preset hourly flow rate. This type of pump uses an electronically controlled clamp that pinches the IV tubing to control fluid flow. A drop sensor is attached to the IV tubing drip chamber that counts drops to monitor the flow rate.
- Positive-pressure infusion pumps control the flow of IV solution via the application of pressure in the IV system. The pressure keeps the IV solution flowing at the preset mL/hour rate.
- Syringe pumps deliver a preset amount of fluid in a preset time period directly from a syringe. The pump can also be programmed to deliver the IV solution in mL/hour. It is generally used in pediatric and critical care settings to infuse medications or small volumes of fluid.
- Patient-controlled analgesia (PCA) pumps deliver a preset amount of analgesic medication, providing the patient control over their own pain management. The machine is programmed to

allow the patient to receive a preset dosage of medication in a specified time period. The machine can be programmed to deliver medication continuously, or intermittently by pressing a button. The PCA pump has a "lock out" period that prevents a patient from receiving additional medication during a specific time period. The pump keeps a record of the amount of medication that a patient receives during a specified time period.

> **(!) SAFETY ALERT:** *Monitor the patient and the electronic infusion device per institution policy. Safe functioning of the infusion device, and patient response to the fluids or medications being administered are essential.*

CALCULATION OF AMOUNT OF SOLUTE PER INTRAVENOUS SOLUTION

Solution strength of an intravenous solution is expressed as a percent that identifies the number of grams of a specified component contained in 100 mL of solution. For example, a solution of 5% dextrose means there are 5 g of dextrose in each 100 mL of solution. This percent, together with knowledge of the total milliliters per solution, can be used to calculate the amount of the specified component in the intravenous solution.

Use the ratio-proportion method to calculate the solutes in an intravenous solution. The ratio-proportion is set up as follows:

$$\frac{\#\,g}{100\,mL} = \frac{x\,g}{total\,mL\,solution}$$

Remember the number of grams (# g) per 100 mL is the percentage expressed in the solution. The total mL solution is the total number of milliliters of the intravenous solution in which the solute is dissolved.

Consider this example: An order for intravenous solution reads: 500 mL of 10% dextrose in water. You need to determine the amount of dextrose being delivered.

Use the formula:
$$\frac{\#\,g}{100\,mL} = \frac{x\,g}{total\,mL\,solution}$$

Set up the problem: Remember that 10% dextrose is equal to 10 g dextrose per 100 mL.

$$\frac{10\,g}{100\,mL} = \frac{x\,g}{500\,mL}$$

Cross multiply:
$$\frac{10\,g}{100\,mL} \diagdown\diagup \frac{x\,g}{500\,mL}$$

$$100x\,mL = 5000\,g/mL$$

Isolate x in the equation by dividing both sides by 100. Cancel out mL.

$$\frac{100\,x\,\cancel{mL}}{100\,\cancel{mL}} = \frac{5000\,g/\cancel{mL}}{100\,\cancel{mL}}$$

$$x = \frac{5000\,g}{100}$$

$$x = 50\,g$$

The answer is 50 g of dextrose in 500 mL of 10% dextrose in water.

Another order for intravenous solution reads: 1000 mL of 0.45% NaCl.

Set up the problem: Remember 0.45% NaCl is equal to 0.45 g NaCl per 100 mL.

$$\frac{0.45 \text{ g}}{100 \text{ mL}} = \frac{x \text{ g}}{1000 \text{ mL}}$$

Cross multiply:

$$\frac{0.45 \text{ g}}{100 \text{ mL}} \diagdown\diagup \frac{x \text{ g}}{1000 \text{ mL}}$$

$$100x \text{ mL} = 450 \text{ g/mL}$$

Isolate x in the equation by dividing both sides by 100. Cancel out mL.

$$\frac{100x \text{ mL}}{100 \text{ mL}} = \frac{450 \text{ g/mL}}{100 \text{ mL}}$$

$$x = \frac{450 \text{ g}}{100}$$

$$x = 4.5 \text{ g}$$

The answer is 4.5 g of NaCl in 1000 mL of solution.

CASE STUDY

Remember Mr. Sampson, the patient with acute pancreatitis. His order for the intravenous infusion reads: Infuse 1000 mL of 5% dextrose in 0.45% normal saline with 20 mEq of potassium chloride over 8 hours. This solution contains two components: dextrose and NaCl. You will need to calculate the amount for each component in this solution.

Set up the problem: Remember 0.45% normal saline is equal to 0.45 g NaCl per 100 mL.

$$\frac{0.45 \text{ g}}{100 \text{ mL}} = \frac{x \text{ g}}{1000 \text{ mL}}$$

Cross multiply:

$$\frac{0.45 \text{ g}}{100 \text{ mL}} \diagdown\diagup \frac{x \text{ g}}{1000 \text{ mL}}$$

$$100x \text{ mL} = 450 \text{ g mL}$$

Isolate x in the equation by dividing both sides by 100. Cancel out mL.

$$\frac{100x \text{ mL}}{100 \text{ mL}} = \frac{450 \text{ g/mL}}{100 \text{ mL}}$$

$$x = \frac{450 \text{ g}}{100}$$

$$x = 4.5 \text{ g}$$

Set up the problem: Remember 5% dextrose is equal to 5 g dextrose per 100 mL.

$$\frac{5 \text{ g}}{100 \text{ mL}} = \frac{x \text{ g}}{1000 \text{ mL}}$$

Cross multiply:

$$\frac{5 \text{ g}}{100 \text{ mL}} \diagdown\diagup \frac{x \text{ g}}{1000 \text{ mL}}$$

$$100x \text{ mL} = 5000 \text{ g/mL}$$

Isolate x in the equation by dividing both sides by 100. Cancel out mL.

$$\frac{100 \, x \text{ mL}}{100 \text{ mL}} = \frac{5000 \text{ g/mL}}{100 \text{ mL}}$$

$$x = \frac{5000 \text{ g}}{100}$$

$$x = 50 \text{ g}$$

The answer: In a solution of 1000 mL of 5% dextrose in 0.9% NaCl, there are 50 g of dextrose and 4.5 g of NaCl.

PRACTICE PROBLEMS 9-1. Practice Problems for Calculating the Amount of Solute in Solution

DIRECTIONS: Calculate the amount of dextrose and/or NaCl in the ordered IV solutions. The answers to the problems can be found at the end of the chapter.

1. 250 mL of 0.9% NaCl

2. 1000 mL 10% dextrose in 0.45% NaCl

3. 500 mL of 5% dextrose in water

4. 500 mL of 0.45% NaCl

5. 2 L of 5% dextrose in 0.45% NaCl

6. 4 L of 5% dextrose in 0.9% NaCl

CALCULATION OF INTRAVENOUS FLOW RATES IN mL/hour

The prescriber orders intravenous fluids and flow rates to typically infuse in milliliters per hour. As the nurse, you are responsible for correctly administering the intravenous solution using the prescribed flow rate.

Formula Method

For example, some prescribers will order the solution to infuse at 150 mL/hour. In this case, set the prescribed mL/hour rate on the electronic infusion device or use that information to calculate gtt/min to manually adjust the IV rate. Other prescribers will order 2000 mL/24 hours or 1000 mL/10 hours. With this type of order, calculate the mL/hour to correctly set the infusion rate on an electronic infusion device or manually regulate the infusion rate.

The formula for calculating mL/hour for intravenous infusions is:

$$\frac{\text{mL of solution ordered}}{\text{Total hours ordered}} = \text{mL/hour}$$

The answer that you obtain should be rounded to the nearest whole number.

Use the 3-step approach—*convert, compute, and critically think*—that you learned in Chapter 6. For example, the patient's order reads: 1000 mL to infuse over 10 hours.

STEP 1: CONVERT

The first step requires ensuring that all the prescribed solution is ordered in the correct units of measurement that are found in the formula. The formula requires that the solution ordered is in mL and the time for infusion is in hours ordered. If the prescriber would order the intravenous solution in liters rather than milliliters, you would need to convert the liters to milliliters so that the unit of measurement for the solution is the same as the unit of measurement for the formula. In this example, no conversion is needed because the solution ordered is 1000 mL and the time for infusion is 10 hours.

STEP 2: COMPUTE

This step requires you to determine the data you need to solve the dose problem, to set up the problem correctly, and to calculate an answer. Using the above formula, set up the problem as follows:

$$\frac{1000 \text{ mL}}{10 \text{ hours}} = \text{mL/hour}$$

Reduce the fraction to the lowest common denominator by dividing the numerator and denominator by 10.

$$\frac{\cancel{1000}}{\cancel{10}} = \frac{100}{1} = \text{mL/hour}$$

The answer to the above problem is 100 mL/hour.

STEP 3: CRITICALLY THINK

ASK YOURSELF – *Does this answer seem logical, correct, and plausible?*

The answer is logical, correct and plausible. In rechecking your math, you know that $10 \times 100 = 1000$. This double check verifies your calculation in Step 2 is correct.

CASE STUDY

After inserting a 20-gauge intravenous catheter into Mr. Sampson's left forearm, you set up the intravenous solution using primary intravenous tubing and connect the tubing to Mr. Sampson's IV catheter. The solution is to run in by gravity. The order reads 1000 mL over an 8 hour period. You need to calculate the mL per hour infusion rate. Applying the formula previously presented, calculate the intravenous flow rate as follows:

$$\frac{1000 \text{ mL}}{8 \text{ hours}} = 125 \text{ mL/hour}$$

Ratio-Proportion Method

In some cases, prescribers may order intravenous antibiotics or small amounts of solution to be infused in minutes rather than hours. However, when using an electronic infusion device to administer these solutions, you must set the infusion rate in mL/hours. Consider this example: An order reads to infuse ceftazidime 1 g in 100 mL normal saline over 30 minutes.

STEP 1: CONVERT

For the example, the solution infusion order rate is in minutes and the formula requires that you have total hours ordered. In such a case, use the ratio-proportion method to find the correct infusion rate by converting minutes into hours. The ratio-proportion formula is:

$$\frac{\text{mL solution ordered}}{\text{Total minutes ordered}} = \frac{x \text{ mL/hour}}{60 \text{ min}}$$

In the above formula, remember that 60 minutes = 1 hour.

STEP 2: COMPUTE

To calculate the infusion rate of the ordered medication, set up the problem inserting the correct values into the proportion.

$$\frac{100\ mL}{30\ min} = \frac{x\ mL/hour}{60\ min}$$

Cross multiply:

$$\frac{100\ mL}{30\ min} \diagdown\diagup \frac{x\ mL/hour}{60\ min}$$

$$6000 = 30x$$

Isolate x in the equation by dividing both sides of the equation by 30.

$$\frac{6000}{30} = \frac{30\,x}{30}$$

$$\frac{6000}{30} = x$$

$$200 = x$$

The answer to the problem is 200 mL/hour. This is the rate you would set on the electronic infusion device or adjust the controller to deliver by gravity flow.

STEP 3: CRITICALLY THINK

ASK YOURSELF – *Does this answer seem logical, correct, and plausible?*

The answer is logical, correct, and plausible. Think about the fact that the infusion is to be set at mL/hour. There are 60 minutes in one hour and the infusion is ordered to run over 30 minutes. Sixty is two times greater than 30, so 100 mL times two is 200 mL/hour.

PRACTICE PROBLEMS 9-2. Practice Problems for Calculating Intravenous Flow Rates in mL/hour

DIRECTIONS: Calculate the flow rate for the ordered IV solutions. The answers to the problems can be found at the end of the chapter.

1. 500 mL of normal saline to infuse in 4 hours

2. 1000 mL of lactated Ringer's to infuse in 6 hours

3. 250 mL of antibiotic to infuse in 3 hours

4. 3 L of normal saline to infuse in 24 hours

5. 2 L of 5% dextrose in 0.45% normal saline to infuse in 24 hours

6. 150 mL of antibiotic to infuse in 45 minutes

CALCULATION OF INTRAVENOUS FLOW RATES IN gtt/min

Intravenous solutions can be administered by gravity flow using the manual roller clamp on the intravenous tubing to adjust flow rate. To correctly adjust the rate, first calculate the mL/hour as described above. The second step is to calculate the drops per minute, or gtt/min. Drops per minute are the number of drops falling per minute in the drip chamber. Use the manual roller clamp on the tubing to control the gtt/min.

Recall that each type of IV tubing delivers a specific number of drops (gtt) per mL (drop factor). Check the tubing package to identify the drop factor for the tubing.

Two methods can be used to calculate gtt/min. These methods are: the formula method, and the "quick" method.

Formula Method

The formula for calculating gtt/min is:

$$\frac{\text{mL of IV solution}}{\text{Time in minutes}} \times \text{drop factor (gtt/mL)} = \text{gtt/min}$$

In this formula, mL of IV solution is the milliliters per hour of solution ordered by the prescriber. Time in minutes is the number of minutes ordered by the prescriber. If the prescriber orders the total volume of solution to be administered over a total number of hours, first you need to calculate mL/hour. Once you have calculated the mL/hour, you need to convert hours to minutes. Drop factor is the calibration of drops/mL of the tubing being used to administer the solution. Remember to locate the drop factor on the tubing package. If the answer you get is a decimal, round to the nearest whole number.

For example, the prescriber orders: 1000 mL of normal saline to infuse at 125 mL/hour. The tubing you are using has a drop factor of 15 gtt/mL. Set up the problem using the formula:

$$\frac{125 \text{ mL}}{60 \text{ min}} \times 15 \text{ gtt/mL} = \text{gtt/min}$$

$$\frac{125 \text{ mL}}{60 \text{ min}} \times \frac{15 \text{ gtt}}{1 \text{ mL}} = \text{gtt/min}$$

$$\frac{125 \text{ m\!L}}{\underset{4}{60} \text{ min}} \times \frac{\overset{1}{\cancel{15}} \text{ gtt}}{1 \text{ m\!L}} = \text{gtt/min}$$

$$\frac{125 \text{ gtt}}{4 \text{ min}} = 31.25 \text{ gtt/min, which is rounded to 31 gtt/min}$$

You would regulate this solution to infuse at 31 gtt/min.

Consider this example. The prescriber orders: 100 mL antibiotic to infuse over 30 minutes. The drop factor for the tubing is 10 gtt/mL. Set up the problem using the formula:

$$\frac{100 \text{ mL}}{30 \text{ min}} \times 10 \text{ gtt/mL} = \text{gtt/min}$$

$$\frac{100 \text{ mL}}{30 \text{ min}} \times \frac{10 \text{ gtt}}{1 \text{ mL}} = \text{gtt/min}$$

$$\frac{100 \text{ m\!L}}{\underset{3}{30} \text{ min}} \times \frac{\overset{1}{\cancel{10}} \text{ gtt}}{1 \text{ m\!L}} = \text{gtt/min}$$

$$\frac{100 \text{ gtt}}{3 \text{ min}} = 33.33, \text{ which is rounded to 33 gtt/min}$$

You would set the antibiotic to infuse at 33 gtt/min.

Another prescriber orders IV solution to infuse at 100 mL/hour. The available tubing is micro-drip tubing with a drop factor of 60 gtt/mL. Set up the problem using the formula:

$$\frac{100 \text{ mL}}{60 \text{ min}} \times 60 \text{ gtt/mL} = \text{gtt/min}$$

$$\frac{100 \text{ mL}}{60 \text{ min}} \times \frac{60 \text{ gtt}}{1 \text{ mL}} = \text{gtt/min}$$

$$\frac{100 \text{ mL}}{\underset{1}{60 \text{ min}}} \times \frac{\overset{1}{60 \text{ gtt}}}{1 \text{ mL}} = \text{gtt/min}$$

$$\frac{100 \text{ gtt}}{1 \text{ min}} = 100 \text{ gtt/min}$$

This example illustrates that when using micro-drip tubing with a drop factor of 60 gtt/mL, the gtt/min rate is equal to the mL/hour infusion rate.

CASE STUDY

You previously calculated Mr. Sampson's intravenous flow rate to be 125 mL/hour. The intravenous solution is to flow by gravity. To ensure that Mr. Sampson receives 125 mL/hour as ordered, you need to calculate the drops per minute that need to be infused. Using the formula just described and remembering that primary intravenous tubing is calibrated to deliver 10 drops per mL, calculate the gtt/min as follows:

$$\frac{125 \text{ mL}}{60 \text{ min}} \times 10 \text{ gtt/mL} = \text{gtt/min}$$

$$\frac{125 \text{ mL}}{60 \text{ min}} \times \frac{10 \text{ gtt}}{1 \text{ mL}} = \text{gtt/min}$$

$$\frac{125 \text{ mL}}{\underset{6}{60 \text{ min}}} \times \frac{\overset{1}{10 \text{ gtt}}}{1 \text{ mL}} = \text{gtt/min}$$

$$\frac{125 \text{ mL}}{6 \text{ min}} = 20.83, \text{ round to } 21 \text{ gtt/min}$$

You would adjust the drip rate on Mr. Sampson's IV to 21 gtt/min to administer 125 mL/hour.

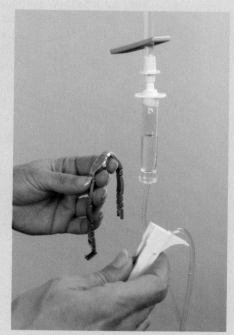

Photo by Rick Brady.

PRACTICE PROBLEMS 9-3. Practice Problems for Calculating Intravenous Flow Rates in gtt/min

DIRECTIONS: Calculate the flow rate in gtt/min for the ordered IV solutions. The answers to the problems can be found at the end of the chapter.

1. 0.9% normal saline to infuse at 150 mL/hour. Tubing has drop factor of 15 gtt/mL

2. Unit of blood to infuse at 100 mL/hour. Tubing has drop factor of 10 gtt/mL

3. 5% dextrose in water to infuse at 75 mL/hour. Tubing has drop factor of 20 gtt/mL

4. 250 mL antibiotic to infuse at 125 mL/hour. Tubing has drop factor of 60 gtt/mL

5. 1000 mL lactated Ringer's to infuse over 12 hours. Tubing has drop factor of 10 gtt/mL

6. 500 mL of 0.45% normal saline to infuse at 50 mL/hour. Tubing has drop factor of 15 gtt/mL

"Quick Method"

The "quick method" is another way to calculate flow rates in gtt/min. Each type of tubing has a constant that can be calculated. This constant is the number obtained in the formula method when canceling out the drop factor on one side of the formula to be equal to 1 and then dividing 60 minutes by the drop factor. For example, in a problem where the drop factor is 20, you would calculate the constant as $\frac{60}{20} = 3$. Table 9-1 shows the constant calculated based on the drop factor for the tubing.

Table 9-1. Quick Method Constants

Drop Factor of Tubing	Constant Calculation
10 gtt/mL	$\frac{60}{10} = 6$
15 gtt/mL	$\frac{60}{15} = 4$
20 gtt/mL	$\frac{60}{20} = 3$
60 gtt/mL	$\frac{60}{60} = 1$

Once you obtain the constant, then you divide the mL/hour by the constant. The "quick method" formula to calculate gtt/min flow rate looks like this:

$$\frac{mL/hour}{Constant} = gtt/min$$

CASE STUDY

Mr. Sampson's intravenous solution, 1000 mL, was ordered to infuse over 8 hours. You want to use the "Quick Method" to calculate the gtt/min needed to regulate Mr. Sampson's IV. First, you identify that the tubing you are using delivers 15 gtt/mL. Then, you need to calculate the mL/hour for the IV. To do this, divide the total mL by the total hours: 1000 mL ÷ 8 hours = 125 mL/hour. Remember the constant for tubing with a drop factor of 15 gtt/mL is 4 (60 ÷ 15 = 4). You then set up and solve your problem using the "quick method": 125 mL/hour ÷ 4 = 31.25 which is rounded to 31 gtt/min.

When using micro-drip tubing that delivers 60 gtt/mL, the gtt/min is equal to mL/hour because the constant is 1. Remember from your math that a number divided by 1 is equal to the number. Review the following example:

IV solution to infuse at 100 mL/hour using micro-drip tubing with a drop factor of 60 gtt/mL. Using the "quick method":

$$\frac{mL/hour}{Constant} = \frac{100\ mL/hour}{1} = 100\ gtt/min$$

Another prescriber orders lactated Ringer's to infuse at 150 mL/hour. Primary IV tubing with a drop factor of 10 gtt/min is used. Solve the problem:

$$\frac{mL/hour}{Constant} = \frac{150\ mL/hour}{6} = 25\ gtt/min$$

If the intravenous solution is ordered in total mL over a total hour period, first calculate mL/hour. Then use the "quick method" to calculate gtt/min.

Consider this example: 0.9% normal saline 500 mL to infuse over 2 hours using primary tubing with a drop factor of 15 gtt/mL.

First calculate the mL/hour:
$$\frac{500\ mL}{2\ hours} = 250\ mL/hour$$

Having calculated mL/hour, then use the "quick method":

$$\frac{mL/hour}{Constant} = \frac{250\ mL/hour}{4} = 62.5\ gtt/min,\ \text{which is rounded to 63 gtt/min.}$$

PRACTICE PROBLEMS 9-4. Practice Problems for Calculating Intravenous Flow Rates in gtt/min

DIRECTIONS: Calculate the flow rate in gtt/min for the ordered IV solutions. The answers to the problems can be found at the end of the chapter.

1. 3000 mL to infuse over 24 hours using tubing with a drop factor of 10 gtt/mL

2. Lactated Ringer's to infuse at 75 mL/hour using tubing with a drop factor of 15 gtt/mL

3. 1000 mL 0.45% normal saline to infuse over 8 hours using tubing with a drop factor of 60 gtt/mL

4. Antibiotic solution to infuse at 50 mL/hour using tubing with a drop factor of 20 gtt/mL

5. IV solution to infuse at 200 mL/hour using tubing with a drop factor of 15 gtt/mL

6. 250 mL 5% dextrose in water to infuse at 80 mL/hour using tubing with a drop factor of 10 gtt/mL

Critical Thinking/Decision Making Exercise

You are caring for Mr. Williams following his surgery for repair of an abdominal aortic aneurysm. You check his postoperative orders and see that he is ordered to have an IV of 1000 mL 5% dextrose in 0.45% NaCl to infuse over 10 hours to start after his IV from surgery is completed. The tubing you will use with this IV has a drop factor of 15 gtt/min. He also will be getting four doses of an intravenous antibiotic in the next 24 hours. You note that his IV from surgery is lactated Ringer's to infuse at 100 mL/hour. It is infusing through blood tubing, which has a drop factor of 20 gtt/mL. When you check the rate, you find that it is infusing at a rate of 55 gtt/min.

What Action Should You Take At This Time?

At this time, you want to calculate the flow rate for the current IV that is to infuse at 100 mL/hour. Compare your calculated flow rate with the actual flow rate that you assessed. Based on your observations, you find that his current IV is infusing too rapidly. You need to slow his current IV to the correct rate. Use the 3-Step Approach to find the correct flow rate.

STEP 1: CONVERT

This step requires that the prescribed solution ordered is in the correct units of measurement as found in the formula. Remember the formula requires you to use mL/hour. In this problem, the lactated Ringer's solution from surgery was ordered to be infused at 100 mL/hour. No conversion is needed at this time because the unit measurement required for the "quick method" is mL/hour, the same as the unit in which the IV was ordered.

STEP 2: COMPUTE

This step requires you to determine the data needed to solve the calculation correctly. Using the "quick method" set up the problem: 100 mL/hour ÷ 3 (remember that the tubing you are using has a drop factor of 20 gtt/mL so the constant is 3) = 33.33 or 33 gtt/min.

STEP 3: CRITICALLY THINK

ASK YOURSELF – *Does this answer seem logical, correct, and plausible?*

Double check your math and multiply 33.33 × 3 = 100. You find the answer is logical, correct, and plausible.

Once you have slowed the IV to the correct gtt/min rate of 33, you monitor the infusion of the solution until it is time to change the solution.

What Is Your Next Step?

Next, you set up the new IV solution of 5% dextrose in 0.45% NaCl with primary tubing having a drop factor of 15 gtt/mL. You select primary tubing because the patient is to receive IV antibiotics and this type of tubing has a high port, which is used as the secondary medication infusion port. Once you have the IV set up, change the lactated Ringer's IV to the solution that is ordered postoperatively. Once this is completed, make sure to recalculate the flow rate and regulate the IV solution at the newly calculated rate.

CHAPTER REVIEW PROBLEMS

The answers to the problems can be found at the end of the chapter.

Review Problems 9-1. Calculate the mL/hour flow rate for each of the ordered intravenous solutions.

1. 500 mL 0.9% normal saline to infuse over 3 hours
2. 2 L lactated Ringer's to infuse over 24 hours
3. 1000 mL 5% dextrose in water to infuse over 6 hours
4. 4 L 0.45% NaCl to infuse over 36 hours
5. 250 mL medication to infuse over 2 hours

6. 1.5 L 0.9% NaCl to infuse over 10 hours
7. 750 mL 5% dextrose in 0.225% NaCl to infuse over 5 hours
8. 100 mL antibiotic to infuse over 30 minutes
9. 250 mL normal saline to infuse over 3 hours
10. 2.5 L lactated Ringer's to infuse over 48 hours

Review Problems 9-2. Calculate the amount of dextrose and/or NaCl in the ordered IV solutions.

1. 750 mL of 0.9% NaCl
2. 1000 mL of 5% dextrose in 0.225% NaCl
3. 1000 mL of 5% dextrose in water
4. 1000 mL of 0.45% NaCl
5. 2 L of 10% dextrose in 0.9% NaCl

6. 3 L of 5% dextrose in 0.45% NaCl
7. 4 L of 5% dextrose in water
8. 1.5 L of 0.33% NaCl
9. 2 L of 50% dextrose in 0.9% NaCl
10. 100 mL of 5% dextrose in 0.45% NaCl

Review Problems 9-3. Calculate the gtt/min for each of the ordered intravenous solutions using the ratio-proportion method. The drop factor is given for each problem.

1. 100 mL antibiotic to infuse at 50 mL/hour with tubing that has a drop factor of 10 gtt/mL
2. 2 L of lactated Ringer's over 24 hours with tubing that has a drop factor of 15 gtt/mL
3. 1000 mL of 0.9% NaCl over 6 hours with tubing that has a drop factor of 60 gtt/mL
4. 500 mL 0.45% NaCl over 10 hours with tubing that has a drop factor of 20 gtt/mL
5. 250 mL 5% dextrose in water over 4 hours with tubing with a drop factor of 60 gtt/min

6. 3 L of 5% dextrose in 0.225% NaCl to run at 125 mL/hour with tubing with a drop factor of 10 gtt/mL
7. 1000 mL lactated Ringer's at 83 mL/hour with tubing with a drop factor of 15 gtt/mL
8. 500 mL antibiotic solution to run at 100 mL/hour with tubing with a drop factor of 20 gtt/mL
9. 750 mL of intravenous solution to run at 250 mL/hour with tubing with a drop factor of 15 gtt/mL
10. 1500 mL 0.45% NaCl with 20 mEq KCl to infuse at 150 mL/hour with tubing with a drop factor of 10 gtt/mL

Review Problems 9-4. Calculate the gtt/min for each ordered intravenous solution using the "quick method." The drop factor is given for each problem.

1. 250 mL of antibiotic solution to infuse over 2 hours with tubing with a drop factor of 15 gtt/mL
2. 1000 mL of 0.9% NaCl at 150 mL/hour with tubing with a drop factor of 20 gtt/mL
3. 2.5 L of lactated Ringer's to infuse over 24 hours with tubing with a drop factor of 10 gtt/min
4. 4 L of intravenous solution to infuse over 48 hours with tubing with a drop factor of 60 gtt/min
5. 100 mL of antibiotic solution to infuse at 200 mL/hour with tubing with a drop factor of 15 gtt/mL

6. 2 L of 5% dextrose in 0.45% NaCl over 20 hours with tubing with a drop factor of 20 gtt/mL
7. 800 mL of normal saline to infuse at 200 mL/hour with tubing with a drop factor of 10 gtt/mL
8. 50 mL of medication solution to infuse at 100 mL/hour with tubing with a drop factor of 60 gtt/mL
9. 1500 mL lactated Ringer's to infuse over 12 hours with tubing with a drop factor of 20 gtt/mL
10. 450 mL of solution to infuse at 75 mL/hour with tubing with a drop factor of 15 gtt/mL

Answers to Practice Problems

Practice Problem Answers 9-1

1. 250 mL of 0.9% NaCl

    Set up the problem: Remember 0.9% NaCl is equal to 0.9 g NaCl per 100 mL.

    $$\frac{0.9\ g}{100\ mL} = \frac{x\ g}{250\ mL}$$

    Cross multiply:

    $$\frac{0.9\ g}{100\ mL} \diagdown\!\!\!\!\diagup \frac{x\ g}{250\ mL}$$

    $$100x = 225$$

    Isolate x in the equation by dividing both sides by 100.

    $$\frac{100x}{100} = \frac{225}{100}$$

    $$x = \frac{225}{100}$$

    $$x = 2.25\ g$$

    The answer: In a solution of 250 mL of 0.9% NaCl, there is 2.25 g of NaCl.

2. 1000 mL 10% dextrose in 0.45% NaCl

    Set up the problem: Remember 10% dextrose is equal to 10 g dextrose per 100 mL.

    $$\frac{10\ g}{100\ mL} = \frac{x\ g}{1000\ mL}$$

    Cross multiply:

    $$\frac{10\ g}{100\ mL} \diagdown\!\!\!\!\diagup \frac{x\ g}{1000\ mL}$$

    $$100x = 10,000$$

    Isolate X in the equation by dividing both sides by 100.

    $$\frac{100x}{100} = \frac{10,000}{100}$$

    $$x = \frac{10,000}{100}$$

    $$x = 100\ g$$

    Set up the problem: Remember 0.45% NaCl is equal to 0.45 g NaCl per 100 mL.

    $$\frac{0.45\ g}{100\ mL} = \frac{x\ g}{1000\ mL}$$

    Cross multiply:

    $$\frac{0.45\ g}{100\ mL} \diagdown\!\!\!\!\diagup \frac{x\ g}{1000\ mL}$$

    $$100x = 450$$

Isolate x in the equation by dividing both sides by 100.

$$\frac{100x}{100} = \frac{450}{100}$$

$$x = \frac{450}{100}$$

$$x = 4.5 \text{ g}$$

The answer: In a solution of 1000 mL of 10% dextrose in 0.45% NaCl, there is 100 g of dextrose and 4.5 g of NaCl.

3. 500 mL of 5% dextrose in water

Set up the problem: Remember 5% dextrose is equal to 5 g dextrose per 100 mL.

$$\frac{5 \text{ g}}{100 \text{ mL}} = \frac{x \text{ g}}{500 \text{ mL}}$$

Cross multiply:

$$\frac{5 \text{ g}}{100 \text{ mL}} \diagup\!\!\!\!\diagdown \frac{x \text{ g}}{500 \text{ mL}}$$

$$100x = 2500$$

Isolate x in the equation by dividing both sides by 100.

$$\frac{100x}{100} = \frac{2500}{100}$$

$$x = \frac{2500}{100}$$

$$x = 25 \text{ g}$$

The answer: In a solution of 500 mL of 5% dextrose in water, there is 25 g of dextrose.

4. 500 mL of 0.45% NaCl

Set up the problem: Remember 0.45% NaCl is equal to 0.45 g NaCl per 100 mL.

$$\frac{0.45 \text{ g}}{100 \text{ mL}} = \frac{x \text{ g}}{500 \text{ mL}}$$

Cross multiply:

$$\frac{0.45 \text{ g}}{100 \text{ mL}} \diagup\!\!\!\!\diagdown \frac{x \text{ g}}{500 \text{ mL}}$$

$$100x = 225$$

Isolate x in the equation by dividing both sides by 100.

$$\frac{100x}{100} = \frac{225}{100}$$

$$x = \frac{225}{100}$$

$$x = 2.25 \text{ g}$$

The answer: In a solution of 500 mL of 0.45% NaCl, there is 2.25 g of NaCl.

5. 2 L of 5% dextrose in 0.45% NaCl

Set up the problem: Remember 5% dextrose is equal to 5 g dextrose per 100 mL.

$$\frac{5 \text{ g}}{100 \text{ mL}} = \frac{x \text{ g}}{2000 \text{ mL}}$$

Cross multiply:

$$\frac{5 \text{ g}}{100 \text{ mL}} \times \frac{x \text{ g}}{2000 \text{ mL}}$$

$$100x = 10,000$$

Isolate x in the equation by dividing both sides by 100.

$$\frac{100x}{100} = \frac{10,000}{100}$$

$$x = \frac{10,000}{100}$$

$$x = 100 \text{ g}$$

Set up the problem: Remember 0.45% NaCl is equal to 0.45 g NaCl per 100 mL.

$$\frac{0.45 \text{ g}}{100 \text{ mL}} = \frac{x \text{ g}}{2000 \text{ mL}}$$

Cross multiply:

$$\frac{0.45 \text{ g}}{100 \text{ mL}} \times \frac{x \text{ g}}{2000 \text{ mL}}$$

$$100x = 900$$

Isolate x in the equation by dividing both sides by 100.

$$\frac{100x}{100} = \frac{900}{100}$$

$$x = \frac{900}{100}$$

$$x = 9 \text{ g}$$

The answer: In a solution of 2000 mL of 5% dextrose in 0.45% NaCl, there is 100 g of dextrose and 9 g of NaCl.

6. 4L of 5% dextrose in 0.9% NaCl

Set up the problem: Remember 5% dextrose is equal to 5 g dextrose per 100 mL.

$$\frac{5 \text{ g}}{100 \text{ mL}} = \frac{x \text{ g}}{4000 \text{ mL}}$$

Cross multiply:

$$\frac{5 \text{ g}}{100 \text{ mL}} \times \frac{x \text{ g}}{4000 \text{ mL}}$$

$$100x = 20,000$$

Isolate x in the equation by dividing both sides by 100.

$$\frac{100x}{100} = \frac{20,000}{100}$$

$$x = \frac{20,000}{100}$$

$$x = 200 \text{ g}$$

Set up the problem: Remember 0.9% NaCl is equal to 0.9 g NaCl per 100 mL.

$$\frac{0.9\text{ g}}{100\text{ mL}} = \frac{x\text{ g}}{4000\text{ mL}}$$

Cross multiply:

$$\frac{0.9\text{ g}}{100\text{ mL}} \diagdown\!\!\!\!\diagup \frac{x\text{ g}}{4000\text{ mL}}$$

$$100x = 3600$$

Isolate x in the equation by dividing both sides by 100.

$$\frac{100x}{100} = \frac{3600}{100}$$

$$x = \frac{3600}{100}$$

$$x = 36\text{ g}$$

The answer: In a solution of 4000 mL of 5% dextrose in 0.9% NaCl, there is 200 g of dextrose and 36 g of NaCl.

Practice Problem Answers 9-2

1. $\dfrac{500\text{ mL}}{4\text{ hours}} = 125\text{ mL/hour}$

2. $\dfrac{1000\text{ mL}}{6\text{ hours}} = 166.666\text{ mL/hour}$, round to 167 mL/hour

3. $\dfrac{250\text{ mL}}{3\text{ hours}} = 83.333\text{ mL/hour}$, round to 83 mL/hour

4. Convert 3 L to milliliters. Remember 1 L = 1000 mL.

   $3 \times 1000\text{ mL} = 3000\text{ mL}$

   $\dfrac{3000\text{ mL}}{24\text{ hours}} = 125\text{ mL/hour}$

5. Convert 2 L to milliliters. 1 L = 1000 mL

   $2 \times 1000\text{ mL} = 2000\text{ mL}$

   $\dfrac{2000\text{ mL}}{24\text{ hours}} = 83.333\text{ mL/hour}$, round to 83 mL/hour

6. $\dfrac{150\text{ mL}}{45\text{ min}} = \dfrac{x\text{ mL/hour}}{60\text{ min}}$

   Cross multiply:

   $$\frac{150\text{ mL}}{45\text{ min}} \diagdown\!\!\!\!\diagup \frac{x\text{ mL/hour}}{60\text{ min}}$$

   $$9000 = 45x$$

   Isolate x in the equation by dividing both sides of the equation by 45.

   $$\frac{9000}{45} = \frac{45x}{45}$$

   $$\frac{9000}{45} = x$$

   $$200 = x$$

The answer is 200 mL/hour.

Practice Problem Answers 9-3

1. $\dfrac{150 \text{ mL}}{60 \text{ min}} \times 15 \text{ gtt/mL} = \text{gtt/min}$

    $\dfrac{150 \text{ mL}}{60 \text{ min}} \times \dfrac{15 \text{ gtt}}{1 \text{ mL}} = \text{gtt/min}$

    $\dfrac{150 \text{ mL}}{\underset{4}{\cancel{60}} \text{ min}} \times \dfrac{\overset{1}{\cancel{15}} \text{ gtt}}{1 \cancel{\text{ mL}}} = \text{gtt/min}$

    $\dfrac{150 \text{ gtt}}{4 \text{ min}} = 37.5 \text{ gtt/min, round to } 38 \text{ gtt/min}$

2. $\dfrac{100 \text{ mL}}{60 \text{ min}} \times 10 \text{ gtt/mL} = \text{gtt/min}$

    $\dfrac{100 \text{ mL}}{60 \text{ min}} \times \dfrac{10 \text{ gtt}}{1 \text{ mL}} = \text{gtt/min}$

    $\dfrac{100 \cancel{\text{ mL}}}{\underset{6}{\cancel{60}} \text{ min}} \times \dfrac{\overset{1}{\cancel{10}} \text{ gtt}}{1 \cancel{\text{ mL}}} = \text{gtt/min}$

    $\dfrac{100 \text{ gtt}}{6 \text{ min}} = 16.67 \text{ gtt/min, round to } 17 \text{ gtt/min}$

3. $\dfrac{75 \text{ mL}}{60 \text{ min}} \times 20 \text{ gtt/mL} = \text{gtt/min}$

    $\dfrac{75 \text{ mL}}{60 \text{ min}} \times \dfrac{20 \text{ gtt}}{1 \text{ mL}} = \text{gtt/min}$

    $\dfrac{75 \cancel{\text{ mL}}}{\underset{3}{\cancel{60}} \text{ min}} \times \dfrac{\overset{1}{\cancel{20}} \text{ gtt}}{1 \cancel{\text{ mL}}} = \text{gtt/min}$

    $\dfrac{75 \text{ gtt}}{3 \text{ min}} = 25 \text{ gtt/min}$

4. $\dfrac{125 \text{ mL}}{60 \text{ min}} \times 60 \text{ gtt/mL} = \text{gtt/min}$

    $\dfrac{125 \text{ mL}}{60 \text{ min}} \times \dfrac{60 \text{ gtt}}{1 \text{ mL}} = \text{gtt/min}$

    $\dfrac{125 \cancel{\text{ mL}}}{\underset{1}{\cancel{60}} \text{ min}} \times \dfrac{\overset{1}{\cancel{60}} \text{ gtt}}{1 \cancel{\text{ mL}}} = \text{gtt/min}$

    $\dfrac{125 \text{ gtt}}{1 \text{ min}} = 125 \text{ gtt/min}$

5. First find mL/hour

    $\dfrac{1000 \text{ mL}}{12 \text{ hours}} = 83.333 \text{ mL/hour, round to } 83 \text{ mL/hr}$

    $\dfrac{83 \text{ mL}}{60 \text{ min}} \times 10 \text{ gtt/mL} = \text{gtt/min}$

    $\dfrac{83 \text{ mL}}{60 \text{ min}} \times \dfrac{10 \text{ gtt}}{1 \text{ mL}} = \text{gtt/min}$

    $\dfrac{83 \cancel{\text{ mL}}}{\underset{6}{\cancel{60}} \text{ min}} \times \dfrac{\overset{1}{\cancel{10}} \text{ gtt}}{1 \cancel{\text{ mL}}} = \text{gtt/min}$

    $\dfrac{83 \text{ gtt}}{6 \text{ min}} = 13.8 \text{ gtt/min, round to } 14 \text{ gtt/min}$

6. $\dfrac{50 \text{ mL}}{60 \text{ min}} \times 15 \text{ gtt/mL} = \text{gtt/min}$

    $\dfrac{50 \text{ mL}}{60 \text{ min}} \times \dfrac{15 \text{ gtt}}{1 \text{ mL}} = \text{gtt/min}$

    $\dfrac{50 \cancel{\text{ mL}}}{\underset{4}{\cancel{60}} \text{ min}} \times \dfrac{\overset{1}{\cancel{15}} \text{ gtt}}{1 \cancel{\text{ mL}}} = \text{gtt/min}$

    $\dfrac{50 \text{ gtt}}{4 \text{ min}} = 12.5 \text{ gtt/min, round to } 13 \text{ gtt/min}$

Practice Problem Answers 9-4

1. $\dfrac{\text{Total mL}}{\text{Total hours}} = \dfrac{3000}{24} = 125 \text{ mL/hour}$

    $\dfrac{\text{mL/hour}}{\text{Constant}} = \dfrac{125 \text{ mL/hour}}{6} = 20.833 \text{ gtt/min, round to } 21 \text{ gtt/min}$

2. $\dfrac{\text{mL/hour}}{\text{Constant}} = \dfrac{75 \text{ mL/hour}}{4} = 18.75 \text{ gtt/min, round to } 19 \text{ gtt/min}$

3. $\dfrac{\text{Total mL}}{\text{Total hours}} = \dfrac{1000}{8} = 125 \text{ mL/hour}$

    $\dfrac{\text{mL/hour}}{\text{Constant}} = \dfrac{125 \text{ mL/hour}}{1} = 125 \text{ gtt/min}$

4. $\dfrac{mL/hour}{Constant} = \dfrac{50 \ mL/hour}{3} = 16.666$ gtt/min, round to 17 gtt/min

5. $\dfrac{mL/hour}{Constant} = \dfrac{200 \ mL/hour}{4} = 50$ gtt/min

6. $\dfrac{mL/hour}{Constant} = \dfrac{80 \ mL/hour}{6} = 13.333$ gtt/min, round to 13 gtt/min

Answers to Chapter Review Problems

Chapter Review Problem Answers 9-1

Use the formula: $\dfrac{mL \ of \ solution \ ordered}{Total \ hours \ ordered} = mL/hour$

1. 500 mL of 0.9% normal saline to infuse over 3 hours

   $\dfrac{500 \ mL}{3 \ hours} = 166.67$ mL/hour, round to 167 mL/hour

2. 2 L of lactated Ringer's to infuse over 24 hours

   $\dfrac{2000 \ mL}{24 \ hours} = 83.33$ mL/hour, round to 83 mL/hour

3. 1000 mL of 5% dextrose in water to infuse over 6 hours

   $\dfrac{1000 \ mL}{6 \ hours} = 166.67$ mL/hour, round to 167 mL/hour

4. 4 L of 0.45% NaCl to infuse over 36 hours

   $\dfrac{4000 \ mL}{36 \ hours} = 111.11$ mL/hour, round to 111 mL/hour

5. 250 mL of medication to infuse over 2 hours

   $\dfrac{250 \ mL}{2 \ hours} = 125$ mL/hour

6. 1.5 L of 0.9% NaCl to infuse over 10 hours

   $\dfrac{1500 \ mL}{10 \ hours} = 150$ mL/hour

7. 750 mL 5% dextrose in 0.225% NaCl to infuse over 5 hours

   $\dfrac{750 \ mL}{5 \ hours} = 150$ mL/hour

8. 100 mL of antibiotic to infuse over 30 minutes

   $\dfrac{100 \ mL}{0.5 \ hours} = 200$ mL/hour

9. 250 mL normal saline to infuse over 3 hours

   $\dfrac{250 \ mL}{3 \ hours} = 83.33$ mL/hour, round to 83 mL/hour

10. 2.5 L lactated Ringer's to infuse over 48 hours

$$\frac{2500 \text{ mL}}{48 \text{ hours}} = 52.08 \text{ mL/hour, round to 52 mL/hour}$$

Chapter Review Problem Answers 9-2

Use the formula: $\dfrac{\# \text{ g}}{100 \text{ mL}} = \dfrac{x \text{ g}}{\text{total mL solution}}$

1. 750 mL of 0.9% NaCl

Set up the problem: Remember that 0.9% NaCl is equal to 0.9 g per 100 mL.

$$\frac{0.9 \text{ g}}{100 \text{ mL}} = \frac{x \text{ g}}{750 \text{ mL}}$$

Cross multiply: $\dfrac{0.9 \text{ g}}{100 \text{ mL}} \diagdown\!\!\!\!\diagup \dfrac{x \text{ g}}{750 \text{ mL}}$

$$100x = 675$$

Isolate x in the equation by dividing both sides by 100.

$$\frac{100x}{100} = \frac{675}{100}$$

$$x = \frac{675}{100}$$

$$x = 6.75 \text{ g}$$

The answer is: In 750 mL of 0.9% NaCl there are 6.75 g of NaCl

2. 1000 mL 5% dextrose in 0.225% NaCl

Set up the problem: Remember that 5% dextrose is equal to 5 g dextrose per 100 mL.

$$\frac{5 \text{ g}}{100 \text{ mL}} = \frac{x \text{ g}}{1000 \text{ mL}}$$

Cross multiply: $\dfrac{5 \text{ g}}{100 \text{ mL}} \diagdown\!\!\!\!\diagup \dfrac{x \text{ g}}{1000 \text{ mL}}$

$$100x = 5000$$

Isolate x in the equation by dividing both sides by 100.

$$\frac{100 \, x}{100} = \frac{5000}{100}$$

$$x = \frac{5000}{100}$$

$$x = 50 \text{ g}$$

Set up the problem: Remember that 0.225% NaCl is equal to 0.225 g NaCl per 100 mL.

$$\frac{0.225 \text{ g}}{100 \text{ mL}} = \frac{x \text{ g}}{1000 \text{ mL}}$$

Cross multiply: $\dfrac{0.225 \text{ g}}{100 \text{ mL}} \diagdown\!\!\!\!\diagup \dfrac{x \text{ g}}{1000 \text{ mL}}$

$$100x = 225$$

Isolate x in the equation by dividing both sides by 100.

$$\frac{100x}{100} = \frac{225}{100}$$

$$x = \frac{225}{100}$$

$$x = 2.25 \text{ g}$$

The answer is: In 1000 mL of 5% dextrose in 0.225% NaCl, there are 50 g of dextrose and 2.25 g NaCl

3. 1000 mL of 5% dextrose in water

Set up the problem: Remember that 5% dextrose is equal to 5 g dextrose per 100 mL.

$$\frac{5 \text{ g}}{100 \text{ mL}} = \frac{x \text{ g}}{1000 \text{ mL}}$$

Cross multiply:

$$\frac{5 \text{ g}}{100 \text{ mL}} \diagdown\!\!\!\diagup \frac{x \text{ g}}{1000 \text{ mL}}$$

$$100x = 5000$$

Isolate x in the equation by dividing both sides by 100.

$$\frac{100x}{100} = \frac{5000}{100}$$

$$x = \frac{5000}{100}$$

$$x = 50 \text{ g}$$

The answer is: In 1000 mL of 5% dextrose in water there are 50 g of dextrose

4. 1000 mL of 0.45% NaCl

Set up the problem: Remember that 0.45% NaCl is equal to 0.45 g NaCl per 100 mL.

$$\frac{0.45 \text{ g}}{100 \text{ mL}} = \frac{x \text{ g}}{1000 \text{ mL}}$$

Cross multiply:

$$\frac{0.45 \text{ g}}{100 \text{ mL}} \diagdown\!\!\!\diagup \frac{x \text{ g}}{1000 \text{ mL}}$$

$$100x = 450$$

Isolate x in the equation by dividing both sides by 100.

$$\frac{100x}{100} = \frac{450}{100}$$

$$x = \frac{450}{100}$$

$$x = 4.5 \text{ g}$$

The answer is: In 1000 mL of 0.45% NaCl there are 4.5 g of NaCl

5. 2 L of 10% dextrose in 0.9% NaCl

Set up the problem: Remember that 10% dextrose is equal to 10 g dextrose per 100 mL.

$$\frac{10 \text{ g}}{100 \text{ mL}} = \frac{x \text{ g}}{2000 \text{ mL}}$$

Cross multiply:

$$\frac{10 \text{ g}}{100 \text{ mL}} \diagdown\!\!\!\diagup \frac{x \text{ g}}{2000 \text{ mL}}$$

$$100x = 20,000$$

Isolate x in the equation by dividing both sides by 100.

$$\frac{100x}{100} = \frac{20,000}{100}$$

$$x = \frac{20,000}{100}$$

$$x = 200 \text{ g}$$

Set up the problem: Remember that 0.9% NaCl is equal to 0.9 g NaCl per 100 mL.

$$\frac{0.9 \text{ g}}{100 \text{ mL}} = \frac{x \text{ g}}{1000 \text{ mL}}$$

Cross multiply:

$$\frac{0.9 \text{ g}}{100 \text{ mL}} \diagdown\diagup \frac{x \text{ g}}{1000 \text{ mL}}$$

$$100x = 900$$

Isolate x in the equation by dividing both sides by 100.

$$\frac{100x}{100} = \frac{900}{100}$$

$$x = \frac{900}{100}$$

$$x = 9 \text{ g}$$

The answer is: In 1000 mL of 10% dextrose in 0.9% NaCl there are 200 g of dextrose and 9 g of NaCl.

6. 3L of 5% dextrose in 0.45% NaCl

Set up the problem: Remember that 5% dextrose is equal to 5 g dextrose per 100 mL.

$$\frac{5 \text{ g}}{100 \text{ mL}} = \frac{x \text{ g}}{3000 \text{ mL}}$$

Cross multiply:

$$\frac{5 \text{ g}}{100 \text{ mL}} \diagdown\diagup \frac{x \text{ g}}{3000 \text{ mL}}$$

$$100x = 15,000$$

Isolate x in the equation by dividing both sides by 100.

$$\frac{100x}{100} = \frac{15,000}{100}$$

$$x = \frac{15,000}{100}$$

$$x = 150 \text{ g}$$

Set up the problem: Remember that 0.45% NaCl is equal to 0.45 g NaCl per 100 mL.

$$\frac{0.45 \text{ g}}{100 \text{ mL}} = \frac{x \text{ g}}{3000 \text{ mL}}$$

Cross multiply:

$$\frac{0.45 \text{ g}}{100 \text{ mL}} \diagdown\diagup \frac{x \text{ g}}{3000 \text{ mL}}$$

$$100x = 1350$$

Isolate x in the equation by dividing both sides by 100.

$$\frac{100x}{100} = \frac{1350}{100}$$

$$x = \frac{1350}{100}$$

$$x = 13.5 \text{ g}$$

The answer is: In 3 L of 5% dextrose in 0.45% NaCl there are 150 g of dextrose and 13.5 g NaCl

7. 4 L of 5% dextrose in water

Set up the problem: Remember that 5% dextrose is equal to 5 g dextrose per 100 mL.

$$\frac{5\text{ g}}{100\text{ mL}} = \frac{x\text{ g}}{4000\text{ mL}}$$

Cross multiply:

$$\frac{5\text{ g}}{100\text{ mL}} \diagdown\kern-1.2em\diagup \frac{x\text{ g}}{4000\text{ mL}}$$

$$100x = 20{,}000$$

Isolate x in the equation by dividing both sides by 100.

$$\frac{100x}{100} = \frac{20{,}000}{100}$$

$$x = \frac{20{,}000}{100}$$

$$x = 200\text{ g}$$

The answer is: In 4 L of 5% dextrose in water there are 200 g of dextrose

8. 1.5 L of 0.33% NaCl

Set up the problem: Remember that 0.33% NaCl is equal to 0.33 g NaCl per 100 mL.

$$\frac{0.33\text{ g}}{100\text{ mL}} = \frac{x\text{ g}}{1500\text{ mL}}$$

Cross multiply:

$$\frac{0.33\text{ g}}{100\text{ mL}} \diagdown\kern-1.2em\diagup \frac{x\text{ g}}{1500\text{ mL}}$$

$$100x = 495$$

Isolate x in the equation by dividing both sides by 100.

$$\frac{100x}{100} = \frac{495}{100}$$

$$x = \frac{495}{100}$$

$$x = 4.95\text{ g}$$

The answer is: In 1.5 L of 0.33% NaCl there are 4.95 g of NaCl

9. 2 L 50% dextrose in 0.9% NaCl

Set up the problem: Remember that 50% dextrose is equal to 50 g dextrose per 100 mL.

$$\frac{50\text{ g}}{100\text{ mL}} = \frac{x\text{ g}}{2000\text{ mL}}$$

Cross multiply:

$$\frac{50\text{ g}}{100\text{ mL}} \diagdown\kern-1.2em\diagup \frac{x\text{ g}}{2000\text{ mL}}$$

$$100x = 100{,}000$$

Isolate x in the equation by dividing both sides by 100.

$$\frac{100x}{100} = \frac{100{,}000}{100}$$

$$x = \frac{100{,}000}{100}$$

$$x = 1000\text{ g}$$

Set up the problem: Remember that 0.9% NaCl is equal to 0.9 g NaCl per 100 mL.

$$\frac{0.9\text{ g}}{100\text{ mL}} = \frac{x\text{ g}}{2000\text{ mL}}$$

Cross multiply:

$$\frac{0.9\ g}{100\ mL} \diagdown\!\!\!\!\diagup \frac{x\ g}{2000\ mL}$$

$$100x = 1800$$

Isolate x in the equation by dividing both sides by 100.

$$\frac{100x}{100} = \frac{1800}{100}$$

$$x = \frac{1800}{100}$$

$$x = 18\ g$$

The answer is: In 2 L of 50% dextrose in 0.9% NaCl there are 1000 g of dextrose and 18 g NaCl

10. 100 mL 5% dextrose in 0.45% NaCl

Set up the problem: Remember that 5% dextrose is equal to 5 g dextrose per 100 mL.

$$\frac{5\ g}{100\ mL} = \frac{x\ g}{100\ mL}$$

Cross multiply:

$$\frac{5\ g}{100\ mL} \diagdown\!\!\!\!\diagup \frac{x\ g}{100\ mL}$$

$$100x = 500$$

Isolate x in the equation by dividing both sides by 100.

$$\frac{100x}{100} = \frac{500}{100}$$

$$x = \frac{500}{100}$$

$$x = 5\ g$$

Set up the problem: Remember that 0.45% NaCl is equal to 0.45 g NaCl per 100 mL.

$$\frac{0.45\ g}{100\ mL} = \frac{x\ g}{100\ mL}$$

Cross multiply:

$$\frac{0.45\ g}{100\ mL} \diagdown\!\!\!\!\diagup \frac{x\ g}{100\ mL}$$

$$100x = 45$$

Isolate x in the equation by dividing both sides by 100.

$$\frac{100x}{100} = \frac{45}{100}$$

$$x = \frac{45}{100}$$

$$x = 0.45\ g$$

The answer is: In 100 mL of 5% dextrose in 0.45 NaCl there are 5 g of dextrose and 0.45 g NaCl

Chapter Review Problem Answers 9-3

Use the formula:

$$\frac{mL\ of\ IV\ solution}{Time\ in\ minutes} \times drop\ factor\ (gtt/mL) = gtt/min$$

1. 100 mL of antibiotic to infuse at 50 mL/hour with tubing that has a drop factor of 10 gtt/mL

$$\frac{50\ mL}{60\ min} \times 10\ gtt/mL = gtt/min$$

$$\frac{50 \text{ mL}}{60 \text{ min}} \times \frac{10 \text{ gtt}}{1 \text{ mL}} = \text{gtt/min}$$

$$\frac{50 \cancel{\text{ mL}}}{\underset{6}{\cancel{60} \text{ min}}} \times \frac{\overset{1}{\cancel{10} \text{ gtt}}}{1 \cancel{\text{ mL}}} = \text{gtt/min}$$

$$\frac{50 \text{ gtt}}{6 \text{ min}} = 8.33 \text{ gtt/min, round to 8 gtt/min}$$

2. 2 L of lactated Ringer's over 24 hours with tubing that has a drop factor of 15 gtt/mL

First calculate the mL/hour: $\dfrac{2000 \text{ mL}}{24 \text{ hours}} = 83.33$ mL/hour, round to 83 mL/hour

$$\frac{83 \text{ mL}}{60 \text{ min}} \times 15 \text{ gtt/mL} = \text{gtt/min}$$

$$\frac{83 \text{ mL}}{60 \text{ min}} \times \frac{15 \text{ gtt}}{1 \text{ mL}} = \text{gtt/min}$$

$$\frac{83 \cancel{\text{ mL}}}{\underset{4}{\cancel{60} \text{ min}}} \times \frac{\overset{1}{\cancel{15} \text{ gtt}}}{1 \cancel{\text{ mL}}} = \text{gtt/min}$$

$$\frac{83 \text{ gtt}}{4 \text{ min}} = 20.75 \text{ gtt/min, round to 21 gtt/min}$$

3. 1000 mL of 0.9% NaCl over 6 hours with tubing that has a drop factor of 60 gtt/mL

First calculate the mL/hour: $\dfrac{1000 \text{ mL}}{6 \text{ hours}} = 166.67$ mL/hour, round to 167 mL/hr

$$\frac{167 \text{ mL}}{60 \text{ min}} \times 60 \text{ gtt/mL} = \text{gtt/min}$$

$$\frac{167 \text{ mL}}{60 \text{ min}} \times \frac{60 \text{ gtt}}{1 \text{ mL}} = \text{gtt/min}$$

$$\frac{167 \cancel{\text{ mL}}}{\underset{1}{\cancel{60} \text{ min}}} \times \frac{\overset{1}{\cancel{60} \text{ gtt}}}{1 \cancel{\text{ mL}}} = \text{gtt/min}$$

$$\frac{167 \text{ gtt}}{1 \text{ min}} = 167 \text{ gtt/min}$$

4. 500 mL 0.45% NaCl over 10 hours with tubing that has a drop factor of 20 gtt/mL

First calculate the mL/hour: $\dfrac{500 \text{ mL}}{10 \text{ hours}} = 50$ mL/hour

$$\frac{50 \text{ mL}}{60 \text{ min}} \times 20 \text{ gtt/mL} = \text{gtt/min}$$

$$\frac{50 \text{ mL}}{60 \text{ min}} \times \frac{20 \text{ gtt}}{1 \text{ mL}} = \text{gtt/min}$$

$$\frac{50 \cancel{\text{ mL}}}{\underset{3}{\cancel{60} \text{ min}}} \times \frac{\overset{1}{\cancel{20} \text{ gtt}}}{1 \cancel{\text{ mL}}} = \text{gtt/min}$$

$$\frac{50 \text{ gtt}}{3 \text{ min}} = 16.67 \text{ gtt/min, round to 17 gtt/min}$$

5. 250 mL of 5% dextrose in water over 4 hours with tubing with a drop factor of 60 gtt/min

First calculate the mL/hour:

$$\frac{250 \text{ mL}}{4 \text{ hours}} = 62.5 \text{ mL/hour, round to 63 mL/hour}$$

$$\frac{63 \text{ mL}}{60 \text{ min}} \times 60 \text{ gtt/mL} = \text{gtt/min}$$

$$\frac{63 \text{ mL}}{60 \text{ min}} \times \frac{60 \text{ gtt}}{1 \text{ mL}} = \text{gtt/min}$$

$$\frac{63 \cancel{\text{mL}}}{\cancel{60} \text{ min}} \times \frac{\overset{1}{\cancel{60}} \text{ gtt}}{1 \cancel{\text{mL}}} = \text{gtt/min}$$

$$\frac{63 \text{ gtt}}{1 \text{ min}} = 63 \text{ gtt/min}$$

6. 3 L of 5% dextrose in 0.225% NaCl to run at 125 mL/hour with tubing with a drop factor of 10 gtt/mL

$$\frac{125 \text{ mL}}{60 \text{ min}} \times 10 \text{ gtt/mL} = \text{gtt/min}$$

$$\frac{125 \text{ mL}}{60 \text{ min}} \times \frac{10 \text{ gtt}}{1 \text{ mL}} = \text{gtt/min}$$

$$\frac{125 \cancel{\text{mL}}}{\underset{6}{\cancel{60}} \text{ min}} \times \frac{\overset{1}{\cancel{10}} \text{ gtt}}{1 \cancel{\text{mL}}} = \text{gtt/min}$$

$$\frac{125 \text{ gtt}}{6 \text{ min}} = 20.83 \text{ gtt/min, round to 21 gtt/min}$$

7. 1000 mL of lactated Ringer's at 83 mL/hour with tubing with a drop factor of 15 gtt/mL

$$\frac{83 \text{ mL}}{60 \text{ min}} \times 15 \text{ gtt/mL} = \text{gtt/min}$$

$$\frac{83 \text{ mL}}{60 \text{ min}} \times \frac{15 \text{ gtt}}{1 \text{ mL}} = \text{gtt/min}$$

$$\frac{83 \cancel{\text{mL}}}{\underset{4}{\cancel{60}} \text{ min}} \times \frac{\overset{1}{\cancel{15}} \text{ gtt}}{1 \cancel{\text{mL}}} = \text{gtt/min}$$

$$\frac{83 \text{ gtt}}{4 \text{ min}} = 20.75 \text{ gtt/min, round to 21 gtt/min}$$

8. 500 mL of antibiotic solution to run at 100 mL/hour with tubing with a drop factor of 20 gtt/mL

$$\frac{100 \text{ mL}}{60 \text{ min}} \times 20 \text{ gtt/mL} = \text{gtt/min}$$

$$\frac{100 \text{ mL}}{60 \text{ min}} \times \frac{20 \text{ gtt}}{1 \text{ mL}} = \text{gtt/min}$$

$$\frac{100 \cancel{\text{mL}}}{\underset{3}{\cancel{60}} \text{ min}} \times \frac{\overset{1}{\cancel{20}} \text{ gtt}}{1 \cancel{\text{mL}}} = \text{gtt/min}$$

$$\frac{100 \text{ gtt}}{3 \text{ min}} = 33.33 \text{ gtt/min, round to 33 gtt/min}$$

9. 750 mL of intravenous solution to run at 250 mL/hour with tubing with a drop factor of 15 gtt/mL

$$\frac{250 \text{ mL}}{60 \text{ min}} \times 15 \text{ gtt/mL} = \text{gtt/min}$$

$$\frac{250 \text{ mL}}{60 \text{ min}} \times \frac{15 \text{ gtt}}{1 \text{ mL}} = \text{gtt/min}$$

$$\frac{250 \text{ mL}}{\underset{4}{60} \text{ min}} \times \frac{\overset{1}{\cancel{15}} \text{ gtt}}{1 \text{ mL}} = \text{gtt/min}$$

$$\frac{250 \text{ gtt}}{4 \text{ min}} = 62.5 \text{ gtt/min, round to 63 gtt/min}$$

10. 1500 mL 0.45% NaCl with 20 mEq KCl to infuse at 150 mL/hour with tubing with a drop factor of 10 gtt/mL

$$\frac{150 \text{ mL}}{60 \text{ min}} \times 10 \text{ gtt/mL} = \text{gtt/min}$$

$$\frac{150 \text{ mL}}{60 \text{ min}} \times \frac{15 \text{ gtt}}{1 \text{ mL}} = \text{gtt/min}$$

$$\frac{150 \text{ mL}}{\underset{6}{60} \text{ min}} \times \frac{\overset{1}{\cancel{10}} \text{ gtt}}{1 \text{ mL}} = \text{gtt/min}$$

$$\frac{150 \text{ gtt}}{6 \text{ min}} = 25 \text{ gtt/min}$$

Chapter Review Problem Answers 9-4

Use the formula:

$$\frac{\text{mL/hour}}{\text{Constant}} = \text{gtt/min}$$

1. 250 mL of antibiotic solution to infuse over 2 hours with tubing with a drop factor of 15 gtt/mL

First calculate the mL/hour: $\frac{250 \text{ mL}}{2 \text{ hours}} = 125 \text{ mL/hour}$

$$\frac{125 \text{ mL/hour}}{4} = 31.25 \text{ gtt/min, round to 31 gtt/min}$$

2. 1000 mL 0.9% NaCl at 150 mL/hour with tubing with a drop factor of 20 gtt/mL

$$\frac{150 \text{ mL/hour}}{3} = 50 \text{ gtt/min}$$

3. 2.5 L of lactated Ringer's to infuse over 24 hours with tubing with a drop factor of 10 gtt/min

First calculate the mL/hour: $\frac{2500 \text{ mL}}{24 \text{ hours}} = 104.16 \text{ mL/hour, round to 104 mL/hr}$

$$\frac{104 \text{ mL/hour}}{6} = 17.33 \text{ gtt/min, round to 17 gtt/min}$$

4. 4 L of intravenous solution to infuse over 48 hours with tubing with a drop factor of 60 gtt/min

First calculate the mL/hour: $\frac{4000 \text{ mL}}{48 \text{ hours}} = 83.33 \text{ mL/hour, round to 83 mL/hour}$

$$\frac{83 \text{ mL/hour}}{1} = 83 \text{ gtt/min}$$

5. 100 mL of antibiotic solution to infuse at 200 mL/hour with tubing with a drop factor of 15 gtt/mL

$$\frac{200 \text{ mL/hour}}{4} = 50 \text{ gtt/min}$$

6. 2 L of 5% dextrose in 0.45% NaCl over 20 hours with tubing with a drop factor of 20 gtt/mL

First calculate the mL/hour: $\dfrac{2000 \text{ mL}}{20 \text{ hours}} = 100 \text{ mL/hour}$

$$\frac{100 \text{ mL/hour}}{3} = 33.33 \text{ gtt/min, round to } 33 \text{ gtt/min}$$

7. 800 mL of normal saline to infuse at 200 mL/hour with tubing with a drop factor of 10 gtt/mL

$$\frac{200 \text{ mL/hour}}{6} = 33.33 \text{ gtt/min, round to } 33 \text{ gtt/min}$$

8. 50 mL of medication solution to infuse at 100 mL/hour with tubing with a drop factor of 60 gtt/mL

$$\frac{100 \text{ mL/hour}}{1} = 100 \text{ gtt/min}$$

9. 1500 mL of lactated Ringer's to infuse over 12 hours with tubing with a drop factor of 20 gtt/mL

First calculate the mL/hour: $\dfrac{1500 \text{ mL}}{12 \text{ hours}} = 125 \text{ mL/hour}$

$$\frac{125 \text{ mL/hour}}{3} = 41.67 \text{ gtt/min, round to } 42 \text{ gtt/min}$$

10. 450 mL of solution to infuse at 75 mL/hour with tubing with a drop factor of 15 gtt/mL

$$\frac{75 \text{ mL/hour}}{4} = 18.75 \text{ gtt/min, round to } 19 \text{ gtt/min}$$

Advanced Intravenous Calculations

This chapter contains content on:

- **Dosage Ordered in Units/Hour**
- **Dosage Ordered as Flow Rate**
- **Medications Ordered in mg/hour or g/hour**
- **Medications Ordered in mg/min, mcg/min, mg/kg/min, or mcg/kg/min**

Learning Objectives

Upon completion of Chapter 10, you will be able to:

- Calculate dosages and infusion rates of medications ordered in units/hour.
- Calculate dosages and infusion rates of medications ordered in mg/hour.
- Calculate dosages and infusion rates of medications ordered in mcg/kg/min or mg/kg/hour.
- Calculate dosages and infusion rates of medications ordered in mg/min or mcg/min.

Key Terms

- Loading dose
- mcg/kg/min
- Titration

CASE STUDY

Mr. Watson, age 68, was admitted to the cardiac intensive care unit at 0600 with a diagnosis of acute myocardial infarction. He has an intravenous infusion of heparin and nitroglycerin. His orders include:

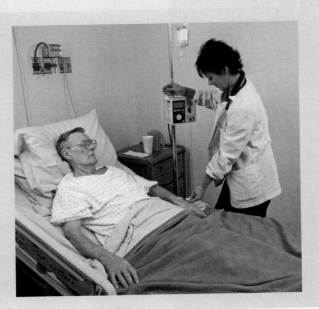

- 0.9% NaCl solution to infuse at 50 mL/hour
- Heparin infusion 25,000 units in 500 mL of 0.9% normal saline to infuse at 1,200 units/hour
- Nitroglycerin 50 mg/250 mL normal saline to infuse at 20 mcg/minute
- Morphine sulfate 2 mg IV p.r.n. for chest pain
- Acetaminophen 650 mg p.o. every 4 hours for headache
- Enteric-coated aspirin 81 mg p.o. every morning

You are providing care for Mr. Watson and need to use knowledge of advanced intravenous calculation skills.

When working in a critical care area, you will be responsible for administering medications that are ordered in dosages other than standard milligram or gram dosage. These medications may be ordered in units/hour, mcg/kg/min, mcg/min, or mg/min. These medications are potent and require close monitoring for accurate delivery rates and appearance of adverse effects for the patient.

Critical care drugs are often ordered to be administered via a process called titration. **Titration** is a process where medication dosages are ordered to be increased or decreased to achieve a specified desired effect. Titrated drugs are often started at a loading dose or initial dosage given over a specified time period to increase serum blood levels to a therapeutic level or achieve the desired effect rapidly. After the loading dose, the medications may then be given at a different dosage and time period. The physician generally orders upper and lower limits for titrating the medications. Medications that are titrated are often ordered as a specific number of micrograms based on kilograms of body weight per minute (**mcg/kg/min**). Dobutamine hydrochloride and dopamine are examples of medications commonly ordered as mcg/kg/min. Other types of medications that can have titration orders may be ordered in number of units per hour. Insulin and heparin are medications ordered in units per hour.

Close monitoring when administering these medications is essential because small changes in dosages or flow rates can seriously affect the patient. Subsequently, electronic infusion devices are used to administer these drugs. Additionally, accurate calculation of dosages and intravenous flow rates are crucial to safe patient care. This chapter provides you with the necessary skills to safely calculate medication dosage and intravenous flow rate.

DOSAGE ORDERED IN UNITS/HOUR

Medications such as heparin and insulin are prescribed in units per hour (units/hr). These medications are administered as continuous infusions to patients. For patient safety, both heparin and insulin intravenous solutions should be administered through an electronic infusion device. Patients receiving heparin need to be closely monitored for signs of bleeding. Patients receiving insulin need to be closely monitored for signs of hypoglycemia.

Flow rates can be calculated using either the formula or ratio-proportion method.

Formula Method for Heparin Ordered in Units/Hour

The formula for calculating mL/hr for medications ordered in units/hr is:

$$\frac{D}{H} \times V = \text{flow rate (mL/hour)}$$

Where: D = dosage desired in units/hr

H = total units on hand

V = volume of solution in total mL

CASE STUDY

Recall Mr. Watson's order that reads: Heparin 25,000 units in 500 mL of 0.9% NaCl to infuse at 1200 units/hour. Use the formula to calculate the mL/hour.

STEP 1: CONVERT

For Mr. Watson, conversion is not necessary because the dosage desired and the medication dosage on hand are in the same unit of measurement. They are both in units.

STEP 2: COMPUTE

Set up the problem like this:

$$\frac{1200 \text{ units/hr}}{25,000 \text{ units}} \times 500 \text{ mL} = \text{flow rate (mL/hour)}$$

Units cancel out so that mL/hr is left.

$$\frac{1200 \text{ units/hr}}{\underset{50}{25,000 \text{ units}}} \times \overset{1}{500} \text{ mL} = \text{flow rate}$$

$$\frac{1200}{50} = 24 \text{ mL/hr}$$

The answer is 24 mL/hour.

STEP 3: CRITICALLY THINK

ASK YOURSELF – *Does this answer seem logical, correct, and plausible?*

You can check yourself by evaluating whether or not this is a safe dosage of heparin. The safe dose of heparin is 20,000–40,000 units in 24 hours. To determine if this is a safe dose, multiply 1200 units/hour by 24 hours to determine the total number of units in a 24-hour period. The result is 28,800 units, which is within the safe heparin dosage.

Ratio-Proportion Method for Heparin Ordered in Units/Hour

The problem can also be done using the ratio-proportion method, which is set up as follows:

$$\frac{\text{Dosage on hand (D)}}{\text{Amount on hand (H)}} = \frac{\text{Dosage prescribed (Q)}}{x}$$

Where: D = total number of units on hand

H = volume of solution on hand in mL

Q = dosage prescribed in units/hr

X = is the mL/hour solved for in the equation

Use the ratio-proportion method for Mr. Watson's order.

STEP 1: CONVERT

No conversion is needed in this problem because the medication prescribed and the medication on hand are both in units.

STEP 2: COMPUTE

Using Mr. Watson's medication order, set up the proportion:

$$\frac{25,000 \text{ units}}{500 \text{ mL}} = \frac{1200 \text{ units/hour}}{x}$$

Cross multiply:

$$\frac{25,000 \text{ units}}{500 \text{ mL}} \diagdown\!\!\!\!\diagup \frac{1200 \text{ units/hour}}{x}$$

$$25,000x \text{ units} = 600,000 \text{ units} \times \text{mL/hour}$$

The next step is to isolate x on one side of the equation. Do this by dividing both sides of the equation by 25,000 units, or the dosage on hand. Units cancel out so that mL/hr is left.

$$\frac{25,000 \text{ units}\, x}{25,000 \text{ units}} = \frac{600,000 \text{ units} \times \text{mL/hour}}{25,000 \text{ units}}$$

You then solve for x:

$$\frac{25{,}000 \text{ units}\, x}{25{,}000 \text{ units}} = \frac{600{,}000 \text{ units} \times \text{mL/hour}}{25{,}000 \text{ units}}$$

$$x = \frac{600,000 \text{ mL/hour}}{25,000}$$

$$x = 24 \text{ mL/hr}$$

STEP 3: CRITICALLY THINK

ASK YOURSELF – *Does this answer seem logical, correct, and plausible?*

You can check yourself by evaluating whether or not this is a safe dosage of heparin for Mr. Watson. Remember the safe dose of heparin is 20,000–40,000 units in 24 hours. To determine if Mr. Watson is receiving a safe dose, multiply 1200 units/hour by 24 hours to determine the total number of units in a 24-hour period. The result is 28,800 units, which is within the safe heparin dosage.

Formula Method for Insulin Ordered in Units/Hour

Determining the units per hour for insulin involves the same process as that for heparin. Consider this example; the order reads: 100 units regular insulin in 100 mL of 0.9% NaCl to infuse at 6 units/hour.

STEP 1: CONVERT

No conversion needs to be done for this problem because the dosage ordered and the dosage on hand are both in units. The measurement unit is the same, so you can set up the problem.

STEP 2: COMPUTE

To calculate the flow rate using the formula method:

$$\frac{D}{H} \times V = \text{flow rate (mL/hour)}$$

$$\frac{6 \text{ units/hr}}{100 \text{ units}} \times 100 \text{ mL} = \text{flow rate (mL/hour)}$$

Units cancel out so that mL/hr is left.

$$\frac{6 \text{ units/hr}}{100 \text{ units}} \times 100 \text{ mL} = \text{flow rate}$$

$$\frac{6}{1} = 6 \text{ mL/hr}$$

STEP 3: CRITICALLY THINK

ASK YOURSELF – *Does this answer seem logical, correct, and plausible?*

Insulin is prescribed based on the patient's need to lower or maintain serum glucose within an acceptable range. There is not a safe dose for a 24-hour period. What you can do is to logically think about the problem. Since there are 100 units in 100 mL you recognize that there is 1 unit per each 1 mL. Knowing this, you recognize that to give 6 units/hour you would need a flow rate of 6 mL/hour.

Ratio-Proportion Method for Insulin Ordered in Units/Hour

STEP 1: CONVERT

No conversion needs to be done for this problem because the dosage ordered and the dosage on hand are both in units. The measurement unit is the same so you can set up the problem.

STEP 2: COMPUTE

Using the ratio-proportion method, set up the proportion as follows:

$$\frac{\text{Dosage on hand (U)}}{\text{Amount on hand (mL)}} = \frac{\text{Dosage prescribed (U/hr)}}{x}$$

$$\frac{100 \text{ units}}{100 \text{ mL}} = \frac{6 \text{ units/hour}}{x}$$

Cross multiply:

$$\frac{100 \text{ units}}{100 \text{ mL}} \times \frac{6 \text{ units/hour}}{x}$$

$$100 \text{ units } x = 600 \text{ units} \times \text{mL/hour}$$

The next step is to isolate x on one side of the equation. Do this by dividing both sides of the equation by 100 units. Units cancel out so that mL/hr is left.

$$\frac{100 \text{ units } x}{100 \text{ units}} = \frac{600 \text{ units} \times \text{mL/hour}}{100 \text{ units}}$$

You then solve for x:

$$\frac{100 \text{ units } x}{100 \text{ units}} = \frac{600 \text{ units} \times \text{mL/hour}}{100 \text{ units}}$$

$$x = \frac{600 \text{ mL/hour}}{100}$$

$$x = 6 \text{ mL/hr}$$

The answer is 6 mL/hr.

STEP 3: CRITICALLY THINK

ASK YOURSELF – Does this answer seem logical, correct, and plausible?

Insulin is prescribed based on the patient's need to lower or maintain serum glucose within an acceptable range. There is not a safe dose for a 24-hour period. What you can do is to logically think about the problem. Since there are 100 units in 100 mL you recognize that there is 1 unit per each 1 mL. Knowing this, you recognize that to give 6 units/hour you would need a flow rate of 6 mL/hour.

PRACTICE PROBLEMS 10-1. Practice Problems for Medications Ordered in Units/Hour

DIRECTIONS: Calculate the flow rate for each of the medications using the formula method when the dosage is ordered. The answers to the problems can be found at the end of the chapter.

1. Heparin 25,000 units in 500 mL of 0.9% NaCl to infuse at 1400 units/hour

2. Insulin 200 units in 100 mL of 0.9% NaCl to infuse at 10 units/hour

3. Heparin 25,000 units in 250 mL of 5% dextrose in water to infuse at 950 units/hour

4. Insulin 100 units in 200 mL of 0.9% NaCl to infuse at 6 units/hour

5. Heparin 50,000 units in 1000 mL of 0.9% NaCl to infuse at 1100 units/hour

PRACTICE PROBLEMS 10-2. Practice Problems for Medications Ordered in Units/Hour Using Ratio-Proportion Method

DIRECTIONS: Calculate the flow rate for each of the medications using the ratio-proportion method when the dosage is ordered. The answers to the problems can be found at the end of the chapter.

1. Insulin 100 units in 100 mL of 0.9% NaCl to infuse at 5 units/hour

2. Heparin 30,000 units in 500 mL of 0.9% NaCl to infuse at 1250 units/hour

3. Heparin 10,000 units in 100 mL of 0.9% NaCl to infuse at 750 units/hour

4. Heparin 25,000 units in 1000 mL of 0.45% NaCl to infuse at 1000 units/hour

5. Insulin 500 units in 250 mL of 0.45% NaCl to infuse at 10 units/hour

DOSAGE ORDERED AS FLOW RATE

The prescriber may order heparin or insulin to infuse at a specific mL/hour flow rate. You will then have to calculate the dosage of the medication that the patient is receiving.

Ratio-Proportion Method for Heparin Dosages as Flow Rates

Calculating the dosage will help you safely monitor the patient. To calculate dosage, use the ratio-proportion method. The formula is:

$$\frac{\text{Dosage on hand (units)}}{\text{Amount on hand (mL)}} = \frac{x\,(\text{units/hr})}{\text{mL/hour}}$$

The order reads: Heparin 25,000 units in 250 mL of 0.9% NaCl to infuse at 10 mL/hour.

STEP 1: CONVERT

No conversion is needed to solve this problem because the dosage on hand of heparin and the dosage that you are calculating are both in units. Since the two are ordered in the same measurement system, you can set up the problem.

STEP 2: COMPUTE

Use the formula:

$$\frac{\text{Dosage on hand (units)}}{\text{Amount on hand (mL)}} = \frac{x\,(\text{units/hr})}{\text{mL/hour}}$$

Putting in the numbers from the order, the formula would be:

$$\frac{25{,}000 \text{ units}}{250 \text{ mL}} = \frac{x\,(\text{units/hr})}{10 \text{ mL/hour}}$$

Cross multiply:

$$\frac{25{,}000 \text{ units}}{250 \text{ mL}} \diagup\!\!\!\!\diagdown \frac{x}{10 \text{ mL/hour}}$$

$$250 \text{ mL } x = 250{,}000 \text{ units} \times \text{mL/hour}$$

The next step is to isolate x on one side of the equation. Do this by dividing both sides of the equation by 250 mL.

$$\frac{250 \text{ mL } x}{250 \text{ mL}} = \frac{250{,}000 \text{ units} \times \text{mL/hour}}{250 \text{ mL}}$$

You then solve for x:

$$\frac{250 \text{ mL } x}{250 \text{ mL}} = \frac{250{,}000 \text{ units} \times \text{mL/hour}}{250 \text{ mL}}$$

$$x = \frac{250{,}000 \text{ units/hour}}{250}$$

$$x = 1000 \text{ units/hr}$$

The answer is 1000 units/hr.

STEP 3: CRITICALLY THINK

ASK YOURSELF – Does this answer seem logical, correct, and plausible?

You can check yourself by evaluating whether or not this is a safe dosage of heparin. The safe dose of heparin is 20,000–40,000 units in 24 hours. To determine if this is a safe dose, multiply 1000 units/hour by 24 hours to determine the total number of units in a 24-hour period. The result is 24,000 units, which is within the safe heparin dosage range.

Ratio-Proportion Method for Insulin Dosages as Flow Rates

An order reads: Regular insulin 200 units in 100 mL of 0.9% NaCl to infuse at 4 mL/hour.

STEP 1: CONVERT

No conversion needs to be done. The dosage ordered and the medication dosage on hand are both in units. Since the unit of measurement for both is the same, you can set up the problem.

STEP 2: COMPUTE

Use the formula:

$$\frac{\text{Dosage on hand (units)}}{\text{Amount on hand (mL)}} = \frac{x \, (\text{units/hr})}{\text{mL/hour}}$$

Putting in the numbers from the order, the formula would be:

$$\frac{200 \text{ units}}{100 \text{ mL}} = \frac{x \, (\text{units/hr})}{4 \text{ mL/hour}}$$

Cross multiply:

$$\frac{200 \text{ units}}{100 \text{ mL}} \diagdown\!\!\!\!\diagup \frac{x}{4 \text{ mL/hour}}$$

$$100 \text{ mL } x = 800 \text{ units} \times \text{mL/hour}$$

The next step is to isolate x on one side of the equation. Do this by dividing both sides of the equation by 100 mL. mL cancels out so that units/hr is left.

$$\frac{100 \text{ mL} x}{100 \text{ mL}} = \frac{800 \text{ units} \times \text{mL/hour}}{100 \text{ mL}}$$

You then solve for x:

$$\frac{100 \, \cancel{\text{mL}} \, x}{100 \, \cancel{\text{mL}}} = \frac{800 \text{ units} \times \cancel{\text{mL}}/\text{hour}}{100 \, \cancel{\text{mL}}}$$

$$x = \frac{800 \text{ units/hour}}{100}$$

$$x = 8 \text{ units/hr}$$

The answer is 8 units/hr.

STEP 3: CRITICALLY THINK

ASK YOURSELF – Does this answer seem logical, correct, and plausible?

Insulin is prescribed based on the patient's need to lower or maintain serum glucose within an acceptable range. There is not a safe dose for a 24-hour period. What you can do is to logically think about the problem. When you look at the problem you can see that there are 2 units for each mL. Since the order reads for 4 mL/hour you logically arrive at 8 units because $2 \times 4 = 8$.

PRACTICE PROBLEMS 10-3. Practice Problems for Medications Ordered as Flow Rate

DIRECTIONS: Calculate the units/hour for each of the medications when the flow rate of the medication is ordered. The answers to the problems can be found at the end of the chapter.

1. Heparin 25,000 units in 500 mL of 0.9% NaCl to infuse at 24 mL/hour

2. Heparin 10,000 units in 250 mL of 0.45% NaCl to infuse at 30 mL/hour

3. Insulin 500 units in 250 mL of 0.9% NaCl to infuse at 3 mL/hour

4. Heparin 40,000 units in 1000 mL of 0.45% NaCl to infuse at 20 mL/hour

5. Insulin 50 units in 100 mL of 0.9% NaCl to infuse at 10 mL/hour

MEDICATIONS ORDERED IN mg/hour OR g/hour

Patients in the critical care areas or on the general nursing units may be receiving continuous intravenous medications that are ordered in milligrams per hour (mg/hour) or grams per hour (g/hour). An example of a drug that can be given as a continuous infusion ordered in mg/hour is furosemide (Lasix). Magnesium sulfate is an example of a medication that can be ordered in g/hour. An electronic infusion device is used to administer these medications. In addition, close monitoring of the patient for possible adverse effects is important.

The flow rate of these medications can be calculated using the formula method or ratio-proportion method previously discussed.

Formula Method

When using the formula method, the formula for calculating flow rate in mg/hour is:

$$\frac{D}{H} \times V = \text{flow rate (mL/hour)}$$

Where: D = dosage desired in mg/hr or g/hour

H = total mg or g on hand

V = volume of solution in total mL

Consider the following example; the order reads: Lasix 200 mg in 100 mL of 0.9% NaCl to infuse at 6 mg/hour.

STEP 1: CONVERT

No conversion is necessary in this problem. The medication dosage ordered and the medication dosage on hand are both in milligrams.

STEP 2: COMPUTE

Set up the problem like this when using the formula method:

$$\frac{6 \text{ mg/hr}}{200 \text{ mg}} \times 100 \text{ mL} = \text{flow rate (mL/hour)}$$

Milligrams cancel out so that mL/hr is left.

$$\frac{\overset{1}{6 \text{ mg/hr}}}{\underset{2}{200 \text{ mg}}} \times 100 \text{ mL} = \text{flow rate}$$

$$\frac{6}{2} = 3 \text{ mL/hr}$$

The answer is 3 mL/hour.

STEP 3: CRITICALLY THINK

ASK YOURSELF – *Does this answer seem logical, correct, and plausible?*

The answer does seem logical and plausible. Looking at the milligrams per milliliter ratio you see that it is 2:1. Knowing this, and the fact that 6 milligrams is ordered, you see that in a 2:1 ratio, the correct answer is 3. You calculate the total milligrams of Lasix in the 24-hour period to be 144 mg. This is well within the acceptable dosage range of Lasix for 24 hours, which is 2–2.5 grams.

Ratio-Proportion Method

The ratio-proportion method can also be used to calculate the flow rate for medication ordered in mg/hour or g/hour. The equation is:

$$\frac{\text{Dosage on hand (D)}}{\text{Amount on hand (H)}} = \frac{\text{Dosage prescribed (Q)}}{x}$$

Where: D = total number of mg or g on hand

H = volume of solution on hand in mL

Q = dosage prescribed in mg/hr or g/hour

x = is the mL/hour solved for in the equation

Consider the following example. The order reads: magnesium sulfate 40 g in 1000 mL of 0.9% NaCl to infuse at 2 g/hour.

STEP 1: CONVERT

No conversion is necessary in this problem. The medication dosage ordered and the medication dosage on hand are both in grams.

STEP 2: COMPUTE

You would set up the equation:

$$\frac{40 \text{ g}}{1000 \text{ mL}} = \frac{2 \text{ g/hour}}{x}$$

Cross multiply:

$$\frac{40 \text{ g}}{1000 \text{ mL}} \diagdown\!\!\diagup \frac{2 \text{ g/hour}}{x}$$

$$40 \text{ g } x = 2000 \text{ g} \times \text{mL/hour}$$

The next step is to isolate x on one side of the equation. Do this by dividing both sides of the equation by 40 g. Cancel out g and mL/hour is left.

$$\frac{40 \text{ g} x}{40 \text{ g}} = \frac{2000 \text{ g} \times \text{mL/hour}}{40 \text{ g}}$$

You then solve for x.

$$\frac{\cancel{40\,g}\,x}{\cancel{40\,g}} = \frac{2000\,g \times mL/hour}{40\,g}$$

$$x = \frac{2000\,mL/hour}{40}$$

$$x = 50\,mL/hr$$

STEP 3: CRITICALLY THINK

ASK YOURSELF – ***Does this answer seem logical, correct, and plausible?***

The answer does seem logical and plausible. Looking at the grams per milliliter ratio, you see that it is 25:1. Knowing this, and the fact that 2 grams is ordered, you see that in a 25:1 ratio, the correct answer is 50.

PRACTICE PROBLEMS 10-4. Practice Problems for Medications Ordered in mg/hour or mcg/hour

DIRECTIONS: Use the formula method to calculate flow rate. The answers to the problems can be found at the end of the chapter.

1. Cardizem 500 mg in 250 mL of 0.9% NaCl to infuse at 8 mg/hour

2. Morphine sulfate 100 mg in 200 mL of 0.45% NaCl to infuse at 3 mg/hour

3. Magnesium sulfate 10 g in 250 mL of lactated Ringer's to infuse at 1 g/hour

DIRECTIONS: Use the ratio-proportion method to calculate flow rate. The answers to the problems can be found at the end of the chapter.

4. Lasix 250 mg in 500 mL 0.9% NaCl to infuse at 6 mg/hour

5. Ranitidine hydrochloride (Zantac) 250 mg in 500 mL 5% dextrose in water to infuse at 6.25 mg/hour

6. Aminophylline 1000 mg in 500 mL 5% dextrose in water to infuse at 20 mg/hour

MEDICATIONS ORDERED IN mg/min, mcg/min, mg/kg/min, or mcg/kg/min

Medication may be ordered at a prescribed dosage to be given in a specified time period of one minute. Typically, these include milligrams/minute (mg/min) and micrograms per minute (mcg/min). Examples of medications ordered in this manner are intravenous nitroglycerine and epinephrine, which are ordered in mcg/min, and intravenous lidocaine, which is ordered in mg/min.

Other critical care medications such as milrinone lactate, dobutamine hydrochloride, and dopamine hydrochloride are prescribed as a dosage based on kilograms of body weight over the specified time period of a minute. These are ordered as microgram per kilogram per minute (mcg/kg/min).

The prescriber may order the dosage of the medication such as lidocaine to infuse at 3 mg/min, or dopamine to infuse at 14 mcg/kg/min. Knowing the concentration of each drug, you can calculate the flow rate in mL/hour. This is the rate that is set on the electronic infusion device to safely administer the medications.

Flow Rate for Medications Ordered in mg/min

To calculate the mL/hour flow rate of medications ordered in mg/min or mcg/min, use the formula:

$$\frac{D \times 60}{C} = \text{Rate}$$

Where: D = dosage of medication prescribed in mg/min or mcg/min

C = concentration of medication in mg/mL or mcg/mL

60 = is the constant 60 minutes/hour

Rate = mL/hour

You will need to perform a calculation to obtain the concentration of the medication (C) as mg/mL or mcg/mL. Use this formula to obtain mg/mL:

$$\frac{\text{Total milligrams}}{\text{Total volume in mL}} = \text{mg/mL}$$

For example, if you had 1000 mg in 250 mL, you would set up the formula:

$$\frac{1000 \text{ mg}}{250 \text{ mL}} = 4 \text{ mg/mL}$$

Use the 3-step approach for the following order, which reads: lidocaine 2 g in 250 mL of 0.9% NaCl to infuse at 3 mg/min.

STEP 1: CONVERT

The first step in solving this problem is to convert to like units. Lidocaine is ordered in grams, but milligrams are required in the formula. Convert 2 grams to 2000 milligrams by multiplying 2 by 1000. (Remember that 1 g = 1000 mg.) Next, divide the total number of milligrams by total milliliters to get the mg/mL.

$$\frac{2000 \text{ mg}}{250 \text{ mL}} = 8 \text{ mg/mL}$$

STEP 2: COMPUTE

Set up the problem:

$$\text{Rate} = \frac{3 \text{ mg/min} \times 60 \text{ min/hour}}{8 \text{ mg/mL}}$$

The rate is in mL/hour, as mg and min are cancelled out.

$$\text{Rate (mL/hour)} = \frac{3 \text{ mg/min} \times 60 \text{ min/hour}}{8 \text{ mg/ml}}$$

$$\text{Rate (mL/hour)} = \frac{180\text{/hour}}{8\text{/mL}} = 22.5 \text{ mL/hour}$$

The correct answer is 22.5 mL/hour.

*ASK YOURSELF – **Does this answer seem logical, correct, and plausible?***

You can double check your math by using the formula:

$$\frac{\text{concentration (mg/mL)} \times \text{rate (mL/hour)}}{60 \text{ min/hour}} = \text{dosage (mg/min)}$$

$$\frac{8 \text{ mg/mL} \times 22.5 \text{ mL/hour}}{60 \text{ min/hour}} = 3 \text{ mg/min}$$

In doing the math check, you find that your answer of 22.5 mL/hour is correct.

Flow Rate for Medications Ordered in mcg/min

To calculate the mL/hour flow rate of medications ordered in mcg/min, use the formula:

$$\frac{D \times 60}{C} = \text{Rate}$$

Where: D = dosage of medication prescribed in mg/min or mcg/min
C = concentration of medication in mg/mL or mcg/mL
60 = is the constant 60 minutes/hour
Rate = mL/hour

Some drugs are ordered in concentrations of milligrams, but require administration in mcg/min. Nitroglycerine is one such drug, commonly ordered in dosages of mcg/min. It may come from the pharmacy as nitroglycerine 50 mg in 250 mL of solution. Therefore, a conversion to like units is necessary. If this is the case, you will need to use this formula to convert milligrams to micrograms:

$$\text{mcg/mL} = \frac{\text{Total milligrams}}{\text{Total volume in mL}} \times 1000 \text{ mcg/mg}$$

Remember, 1 mg = 1000 mcg, which is 1000 in the formula. Milligrams cancel and you are left with mcg/mL.

In the nitroglycerin dosage stated above, set up and solve the problem like this:

$$\text{mcg/mL} = \frac{50 \text{ mg}}{250 \text{ mL}} \times 1000 \text{ mcg/mg} = 200 \text{ mcg/mL}$$

Use the 3-step approach for the following order that reads: phenylephrine hydrochloride (Neo-Synephrine) 10 mg in 500 mL of 0.9% NaCl to infuse at 40 mcg/min.

This problem requires a conversion. The drug on hand is available in milligrams, and the prescribed dosage is in micrograms. Convert milligrams to micrograms using this formula for the conversion:

$$\text{mcg/mL} = \frac{\text{Total milligrams}}{\text{Total volume in mL}} \times 1000 \text{ mcg/mg}$$

$$\text{mcg/mL} = \frac{10 \text{ mg}}{500 \text{ mL}} \times 1000 \text{ mcg/mg} = \frac{10,000}{500} = 20 \text{ mcg/mL}$$

STEP 2: COMPUTE

Set up the problem:

$$\text{Rate} = \frac{40 \text{ mcg/min} \times 60 \text{ min/hour}}{20 \text{ mcg/mL}}$$

The rate is in mL/hour, as mcg and min are cancelled out.

$$\text{Rate (mL/hour)} = \frac{40 \text{ mcg/min} \times 60 \text{ min/hour}}{20 \text{ mcg/mL}}$$

$$\text{Rate (mL/hour)} = \frac{2400}{20} = 120 \text{ mL/hour}$$

The correct answer is 120 mL/hour.

STEP 3: CRITICALLY THINK

*ASK YOURSELF – **Does this answer seem logical, correct and plausible?***

You can double check your math by using the formula:

$$\frac{\text{concentration (mcg/mL)} \times \text{rate (mL/hour)}}{60 \text{ min/hour}} = \text{dosage (mcg/min)}$$

$$\frac{20 \text{ mcg/mL} \times 120 \text{ mL/hour}}{60 \text{ min/hour}} = 40 \text{ mcg/min}$$

In doing the math check, you find that your answer of 120 mL/hour is correct.

CASE STUDY

After priming the tubing and setting up the infusion pump, you prepare to administer Mr. Watson's nitroglycerin infusion. Remember he is receiving nitroglycerin 50 mg/250 mL normal saline to infuse at 20 mcg/minute. Calculate the infusion rate using the formula for mcg/min.

Formula: $\quad \text{Rate} = \dfrac{\text{mcg/min} \times 60}{\text{Concentration (mcg/mL)}}$

$$\text{Rate} = \frac{20 \text{ mcg/min} \times 60 \text{ min/hr}}{200 \text{ mcg/mL}}$$

$$\text{Rate} = \frac{1200}{200}$$

$$\text{Rate} = 6 \text{ mL/hour}$$

You set the infusion rate on the pump at 6 mL/hour.

Flow Rate for Medications Ordered in mcg/kg/min

The formula for calculating mcg/kg/min is similar to the one used in calculating mcg/min or mg/min. The difference is that weight is factored into the formula. The formula is:

$$\frac{D \times 60 \times W}{C} = \text{Rate}$$

Where:
- D = dosage of medication prescribed in mg/kg/min or mcg/kg/min
- C = concentration of medication in mg/mL or mcg/mL
- 60 = is the constant 60 minutes/hour
- W = weight in kilograms
- Rate = mL/hour

Medications are generally available in milligrams. You will need to perform a calculation to obtain the concentration of the medication as mcg/mL. You will need to use this formula to convert milligrams to micrograms:

$$\text{mcg/mL} = \frac{\text{Total milligrams}}{\text{Total volume in mL}} \times 1000 \text{ mcg/mg}$$

Remember, 1 mg = 1000 mcg, which is 1000 in the formula. Milligrams cancel and you are left with mcg/mL.

Use the 3-step approach for the following order, which reads: dobutamine hydrochloride 500 mg in 250 mL of 0.9% NaCl to infuse at 5 mcg/kg/min. The patient weighs 80 kg.

STEP 1: CONVERT

This problem requires a conversion. The drug on hand is available in milligrams and the prescribed dosage is in micrograms. Convert milligrams to micrograms, using this formula:

$$\text{mcg/mL} = \frac{\text{Total milligrams}}{\text{Total volume in mL}} \times 1000 \text{ mcg/mg}$$

$$\text{mcg/mL} = \frac{500 \text{ mg}}{250 \text{ mL}} \times 1000 \text{ mcg/mg} = \frac{500{,}000 \text{ mcg}}{250 \text{ mL}} = 2000 \text{ mcg/mL}$$

One other conversion that may be necessary is related to weight. Remember the formula requires that weight be in kilograms. If the patient's weight is in pounds, you will have to convert pounds to kilograms. To do this conversion, remember that 2.2 pounds equals one kilogram. Divide the total number of pounds by 2.2 to get kilograms.

STEP 2: COMPUTE

Set up the problem:

$$\frac{5 \text{ mcg/kg/min} \times 60 \text{ min/hour} \times 80 \text{ kg}}{2000 \text{ mcg/mL}} = \text{Rate (mL/hour)}$$

Micrograms, kilograms, and minutes cancel out to leave mL/hour.

$$\frac{5 \text{ mcg/kg/min} \times 60 \text{ min/hour} \times 80 \text{ kg}}{2000 \text{ mcg/mL}} = 12 \text{ mL/hour}$$

STEP 3: CRITICALLY THINK

***ASK YOURSELF** – Does this answer seem logical, correct, and plausible?*

You can double check your math by using the formula:

$$\frac{\text{concentration (mcg/mL)} \times \text{rate (mL/hour)}}{\text{weight (kg)} \times 60 \text{ min/hour}} = \text{dosage (mcg/kg/min)}$$

$$\frac{2000 \text{ mcg/mL} \times 12 \text{ mL/hour}}{80 \text{ kg} \times 60 \text{ min/hour}} = 5 \text{ mcg/kg/min}$$

In doing the math check, you find that your answer of 12 mL/hour is correct.

Dosage of Medication When Flow Rate Is Known

Medications in critical care areas may be ordered to be titrated to a specific patient parameter. For example, a patient who is in shock may have dopamine ordered to maintain blood pressure. The written order may read: dopamine to be titrated to maintain systolic blood pressure greater than 100 mm Hg. When the order is written in this manner, the nurse adjusts the flow rate on the electronic infusion device. Each time that the flow rate is adjusted, the nurse needs to recalculate the dosage of medication that the patient is receiving. To do this, use this formula for medications that are administered in mg/min or mcg/min:

$$\frac{C \times R}{60} = D$$

Where: C = concentration in mcg/mL
         R = rate in mL/hour
         60 = 60 minutes/hour
         D = dosage in mg/min or mcg/min

The formula for calculating dosage of mcg/kg/min when flow rate is known, use this formula:

$$\frac{C \times R}{60 \times W} = D$$

Where: C = concentration in mcg/mL
         R = rate in mL/hour
         W = weight in kilograms
         60 = 60 minutes/hour
         D = dosage in mcg/kg/min

Phenylephrine hydrochloride is a drug that is often titrated to maintain blood pressure. The order may read as follows: phenylephrine hydrochloride 10 mg in 250 mL of 0.9% NaCl. Adjust rate to maintain systolic blood pressure greater than 120 mm Hg. The medication is currently infusing at 12 mL/hour. Use the 3-step approach to calculate the dosage of the medication that the patient is receiving.

STEP 1: CONVERT

You know that phenylephrine hydrochloride (Neo-Synephrine) is prescribed in dosages of mcg/min. Your prescribed dosage (mcg/min) is different than the dosage on hand (mg). This requires conversion of milligram (mg) into micrograms (mcg). Remember that 1 mg = 1000 mcg. Use the formula:

$$mcg/mL = \frac{\text{Total milligrams}}{\text{Total volume in mL}} \times 1000 \text{ mcg/mg}$$

$$mcg/mL = \frac{10 \text{ mg}}{250 \text{ mL}} \times 1000 \text{ mcg/mg} = \frac{10,000}{250} = 40 \text{ mcg/mL}$$

You now the have the correct piece for the formula: 40 mcg/mL.

STEP 2: COMPUTE

Set up the problem:

$$\frac{C \text{ (mcg/mL)} \times R \text{ (mL/hour)}}{60 \text{ min/hour}} = D$$

mL and hour cancel out to leave mcg/min

$$\frac{40 \text{ mcg/mL} \times 12 \text{ mL/hour}}{60 \text{ min/hour}} = \frac{480 \text{ mcg}}{60 \text{ min}} = 8 \text{ mcg/min}$$

The patient is receiving 8 mcg/min of phenylephrine hydrochloride (Neo-Synephrine).

STEP 3: CRITICALLY THINK

ASK YOURSELF – Does this answer seem logical, correct, and plausible?

You can double check your math by using the formula previously learned to calculate rate:

$$\frac{dosage\ (mcg/min) \times 60\ min/hour}{concentration\ (mcg/mL)} = rate\ (mL/hour)$$

$$\frac{8\ mcg/min \times 60\ min/hour}{40\ mcg/mL} = 12\ mL/hour$$

In doing the math check, you find that your answer of 12 mL/hour is the correct rate that was originally ordered for the medication. Your calculation of 8 mcg/min as the dosage is correct.

CASE STUDY

As the day progresses, Mr. Watson's condition deteriorates and the physician is concerned about his cardiac output decreasing. Because of the decrease in his vital signs and urine output, the physician orders Mr. Watson to be started on a dobutamine drip.

The order is: dobutamine hydrochloride 800 mg/250 mL normal saline, infuse at 5 mcg/kg/min.

Mr. Watson's morning weight was 110 kg. Knowing that you must use an intravenous infusion pump to administer the dobutamine, you calculate the rate on pump using the previous learned formula.

Formula:

$$Rate = \frac{mcg/kg/min \times weight\ (kg) \times 60\ min/hour}{concentration\ (mcg/mL)}$$

$$Rate = \frac{5\ mcg/kg/min \times 110\ kg \times 60\ min/hour}{3200\ mcg/mL}$$

$$Rate = \frac{33,000/hour}{3200/mL}$$

$$Rate = 10.3\ mL/hour$$

Based on your calculation, you set the infusion rate on the pump at 10.3 mL/hour.

PRACTICE PROBLEMS 10-5. Practice Problems for Medications Ordered in mcg/min, mg/min, or mcg/kg/min

DIRECTIONS: Calculate the flow rate for each of the medications. The answers to the problems can be found at the end of the chapter.

Use this formula for mg/min or mcg/min:

$$\frac{D\ (mg/min\ or\ mcg/min) \times 60}{C\ (mg/mL\ or\ mcg/mL)} = Rate$$

Use this formula for mcg/kg/min:

$$\frac{D\ (mg/kg/min) \times W\ (kg) \times 60\ min/hour}{C\ (mcg/mL)} = Rate$$

1. Nitroglycerin 100 mg in 250 mL of 5% dextrose in water to infuse at 60 mcg/min

2. Nitroprusside 50 mg in 250 mL of 0.9% NaCl to infuse at 4 mcg/kg/min; patient weighs 70 kg

3. Zemuron 1 gram in 250 mL of 0.9% NaCl to infuse at 12 mcg/kg/min; patient weighs 64 kg

4. Norepinephrine 4 mg in 250 mL of 5% dextrose in water to infuse at 8 mcg/min

5. Dopamine 800 mg in 250 mL of 5% dextrose in water to infuse at 3 mcg/kg/min; patient weighs 82 kg

6. Xylocaine 2 grams in 250 mL of 0.9% NaCl to infuse at 2 mg/min

7. Epinephrine 2 mg in 250 mL of 5% dextrose in water to infuse at 6 mcg/min

8. Dobutamine 500 mg in 250 mL of 5% dextrose in water to infuse at 7.5 mcg/kg/min; patient weighs 93 kg

9. Milrinone 20 mg in 100 mL of 5% dextrose in water to infuse at 0.5 mcg/kg/min; patient weighs 100 kg

10. Neo-Synephrine 50 mg in 250 mL of 5% dextrose in water to infuse at 140 mcg/min

PRACTICE PROBLEMS 10-6. Practice Problems for Medication Dosages When Flow Rate Is Known

DIRECTIONS: Calculate the dosage of medications ordered given the flow rate. The answers to the problems can be found at the end of the chapter.

Use this formula when medication dosages are in mg/min or mcg/min:

$$\frac{C \ (mg/mL \ or \ mcg/min) \times R \ (mL/hour)}{60 \ min/hour} = D \ (mg/min \ or \ mcg/min)$$

Use this formula when medication dosages are in mcg/kg/min:

$$\frac{C \ (mcg/mL) \times R \ (mL/hour)}{W \ (kg) \times 60 \ min/hour} = D \ (mcg/kg/min)$$

1. Zemuron 1000 mg in 250 mL of 0.9% NaCl infusing at 13 mL/hour. The patient weighs 72 kg. How many mcg/kg/min is the patient receiving?

2. Dobutamine 250 mg in 250 mL of 5% dextrose in water infusing at 20.5 mL/hour. The patient weighs 68 kg. How many mcg/kg/min is the patient receiving?

3. Norepinephrine 4 mg in 250 mL of 5% dextrose in water infusing at 37 mL/hour. How many mcg/min is the patient receiving?

4. Nitroglycerine 100 mg in 250 mL of 5% dextrose in water infusing at 10.5 mL/hour. How many mcg/min is the patient receiving?

5. Nitroprusside 100 mg in 250 mL of 0.9% NaCl infusing at 65 mL/hour. The patient weighs 72 kg. How many mcg/kg/min is the patient receiving?

6. Epinephrine 2 mg in 250 mL of 5% dextrose in water infusing at 30 mL/hour. How many mcg/min is the patient receiving?

7. Xylocaine 2 grams in 250 mL of 0.9% NaCl infusing at 22.5 mL/hour. How many mg/min is the patient receiving?

8. Milrinone 20 mg in 100 mL of 5% dextrose in water infusing at 20 mL/hour. The patient weighs 91 kg. How many mcg/kg/min is the patient receiving?

9. Neo-Synephrine 50 mg in 250 mL of 5% dextrose in water infusing at 36 mL/hour. How many mcg/min is the patient receiving?

10. Dopamine 400 mg in 250 mL of 5% dextrose in water infusing at 35 mL/hour. The patient weighs 67 kg. How many mcg/kg/min is the patient receiving?

Critical Thinking/Decision Making Exercise

You are the nurse caring for a patient in the Intensive Care Unit who was admitted in hypertensive crisis. The patient's admitting blood pressure was 220/124. The patient weighs 66 kg. The physician prescribed nitroprusside sodium to lower the patient's blood pressure and maintain it at a safe level. The order reads: nitroprusside sodium (Nipride) 100 mg in 250 mL of 0.9% NaCl titrate to maintain systolic bloodpressure below 170 mm Hg.

The medication is infusing on the electronic infusion device at 99 mL/hour. The patient's blood pressure for the last hour is 182/100. The nurse increases the rate on the infusion pump to 108 mL/hour over the next hour to lower the patient's blood pressure to the prescribed level.

Did the Nurse Make the Correct Decision?

The nurse made an incorrect decision to increase the flow rate on the nitroprusside sodium. The nurse needed to calculate the dosage being administered at 99 mL/hour. Knowing the nitroprusside is ordered in mcg/kg/min, the nurse used the formula:

$$\frac{C\ (mcg/mL) \times R\ (mL/hour)}{W\ (kg) \times 60\ min/hour} = D\ (mcg/kg/min)$$

Set up the problem:

$$\frac{400\ mcg/mL \times 99\ mL/hour}{66\ kg \times 60\ min/hour} = \frac{39{,}600}{3960} = 10\ mcg/kg/min$$

When looking up nitroprusside sodium, the nurse finds that the dosage of nitroprusside should not exceed 10 mcg/kg/min. The patient was currently receiving the maximum dosage prescribed. When the nurse increased the flow rate to 108 mL/hour over the next hour, the dosage of nitroprusside was increased to 11 mcg/kg/min, which exceeds the safe dose of the medication.

What Should the Nurse Have Done?

After checking the nitroprusside order, the nurse sees that the patient's systolic blood pressure exceeds the prescribed level. The first step was to calculate how many mcg/kg/min of nitroprusside that the patient was receiving. After finding that the patient was receiving 10 mcg/kg/min of the medication, which is the maximum dosage, the nurse should call the physician and report that the patient's blood pressure is 182/100 and that the patient is receiving 10 mcg/kg/min of nitroprusside sodium. At this time, the physician prescribes additional antihypertensive medication for the patient. The physician also informs the nurse to put an order on the patient's chart that the nitroprusside sodium dosage should not exceed 8 mcg/kg/min.

CASE STUDY

Mr. Watson responds favorably to the dobutamine. His vital signs improve. His urine output increases to 30 to 40 mL/hour. Mr. Watson tells you that he has a headache and requests Tylenol. After you verified that Mr. Watson had not received any Tylenol in the last 6 hours, you give Mr. Watson acetaminophen 650 mg (Tylenol) as ordered. When you check on Mr. Watson in an hour, he tells you that his headache is gone and he feels much better.

CHAPTER REVIEW PROBLEMS

The answers to the problems can be found at the end of the chapter.

Review Problems 10-1. Calculate the flow rate for the following intravenous medications.

1. Cardizem 250 mg in 250 mL of 0.9% NaCl to infuse at 10 mg/hour

2. Nitroprusside 100 mg in 250 mL of 0.9% NaCl to infuse at 4 mcg/kg/min. The patient weighs 66 kg.

3. Heparin 25,000 units in 500 mL 0.9% NaCl to infuse at 1150 units/hour

4. Amiodarone hydrochloride 900 mg in 500 mL of 5% dextrose in water to infuse at 1 mg/min

5. Epinephrine 2 mg in 250 mL of 5% dextrose in water to infuse at 8 mcg/min

6. Insulin 200 units in 100 mL of 0.9% NaCl to infuse at 4 units/hour

7. Dopamine 800 mg in 250 mL of 5% dextrose in water to infuse at 10 mcg/kg/min. The patient weighs 83 kg.

8. Magnesium sulfate 4 grams in 250 mL of 5% dextrose in water to infuse at 5 mg/min

9. Zemuron 1 gram in 250 mL of 0.9% NaCl to infuse at 16 mcg/kg/min. The patient weighs 76 kg.

10. Lasix 200 mg in 100 mL of 0.9% NaCl to infuse at 2 mg/hour

11. Heparin 25,000 units in 250 mL of 0.9% NaCl to infuse at 900 units/hour

12. Norepinephrine 4 mg in 250 mL of 5% dextrose in water to infuse at 8 mcg/min

13. Dobutamine 250 mg in 250 mL of 5% dextrose in water to infuse at 10 mcg/kg/min. The patient weighs 62 kg.

14. Oxytocin 10 units in 1000 mL of 0.9% NaCl to infuse at 0.002 units/min

15. Procainamide hydrochloride 500 mg in 250 mL of 5% dextrose in water to infuse at 4 mg/min

Review Problems 10-2. Calculate the dosage of the medication when the flow rate is known.

1. Esmolol hydrochloride 2.5 grams in 500 mL of 0.9% NaCl infusing at 84 mL/hour. The patient weighs 70 kg. How many mcg/kg/min is the patient receiving?

2. Heparin 25,000 units in 500 mL of 0.9% NaCl infusing at 26 mL/hour. How many units/hour is the patient receiving?

3. Nitroglycerin 50 mg in 250 mL of 5% dextrose in water infusing at 24 mL/hour. How many mcg/min is the patient receiving?

4. Diltiazem hydrochloride 250 mg in 500 mL of 5% dextrose in water infusing at 30 mL/hour. How many mg/hour is the patient receiving?

5. Neo-Synephrine 50 mg in 250 mL of 5% dextrose in water infusing at 45 mL/hour. How many mcg/min is the patient receiving?

6. Dopamine 400 mg in 250 mL of 5% dextrose in water infusing at 9 mL/hour. The patient weighs 92 kg. How many mcg/kg/min is the patient receiving?

7. Magnesium sulfate 5 grams in 250 mL of 5% dextrose in water infusing at 36 mL/hour. How many mg/min is the patient receiving?

8. Morphine sulfate 100 mg in 100 mL of 0.9% NaCl infusing at 3 mL/hour. How many mg/hour is the patient receiving?

9. Amiodarone hydrochloride 540 mg in 500 mL of 5% dextrose in water infusing at 28 mL/hour. How many mg/min is the patient receiving?

10. Nitroprusside 100 mg in 250 mL of 0.9% NaCl infusing at 26 mL/hour. The patient weighs 87 kg. How many mcg/kg/min is the patient receiving?

11. Xylocaine 2 g in 250 mL of 0.9% NaCl infusing at 15 mL/hour. How many mg/min is the patient receiving?

12. Isoproterenol hydrochloride 1 mg in 500 mL of 5% dextrose in water infusing at 75 mL/hour. How many mcg/min is the patient receiving?

13. Milrinone 50 mg in 250 mL 5% dextrose in water infusing at 9 mL/hour. The patient weighs 58 kg. How many mcg/kg/min is the patient receiving?

14. Epinephrine 4 mg in 250 mL 5% dextrose in water infusing at 30 mL/hour. How many mcg/min is the patient receiving?

15. Esmolol hydrochloride 5 g in 500 mL of 0.9% NaCl infusing at 73 mL/hour. The patient weighs 81 kg. How many mcg/kg/min is the patient receiving?

Answers to Practice Problems

Practice Problem Answers 10-1

Use the formula:
$$\frac{D}{H} \times V = \text{flow rate (mL/hour)}$$

Where: D = dosage desired in Units/hr
H = total units on hand
V = volume of solution in total mL

1. Heparin 25,000 units in 500 mL of 0.9% NaCl to infuse at 1400 units/hour

$$\frac{D}{H} \times V = \frac{1400}{25,000} \times 500 = 28 \text{ mL/hour}$$

2. Insulin 200 units in 100 mL of 0.9% NaCl to infuse at 10 units/hour

$$\frac{D}{H} \times V = \frac{10}{200} \times 100 = 5 \text{ mL/hour}$$

3. Heparin 25,000 units in 250 mL of 5% dextrose in water to infuse at 950 units/hour

$$\frac{D}{H} \times V = \frac{950}{25,000} \times 250 = 9.5 \text{ mL/hour}$$

4. Insulin 100 units in 200 mL of 0.9% NaCl to infuse at 6 units/hour

$$\frac{D}{H} \times V = \frac{6}{100} \times 200 = 12 \text{ mL/hour}$$

5. Heparin 50,000 units in 1000 mL of 0.9% NaCl to infuse at 1100 units/hour

$$\frac{D}{H} \times V = \frac{1100}{50,000} \times 1000 = 22 \text{ mL/hour}$$

Practice Problem Answers 10-2

Use the formula:
$$\frac{\text{Dosage on hand (D)}}{\text{Amount on hand (H)}} = \frac{\text{Dosage prescribed (Q)}}{x}$$

Where: D = total number of Units (U) on hand
H = volume of solution on hand in mL
Q = dosage prescribed in U/hr
x = is the mL/hour solved for in the equation

1. Insulin 100 units in 100 mL of 0.9% NaCl to infuse at 5 units/hour

$$\frac{100}{100} = \frac{5}{x}$$

Cross multiply:

$$\frac{100}{100} \diagup\!\!\!\!\diagdown \frac{5}{x}$$

$$100x = 500$$

The next step is to isolate x on one side of the equation. Do this by dividing both sides of the equation by 100.

$$\frac{100x}{100} = \frac{500}{100}$$

You then solve for x.

$$\frac{1\cancel{0}\cancel{0}x}{1\cancel{0}\cancel{0}} = \frac{500}{100}$$

$$x = \frac{500}{100}$$

$$x = 5 \text{ mL/hr}$$

2.   Heparin 30,000 units in 500 mL of 0.9% NaCl to infuse at 1250 units/hour

$$\frac{30,000}{500} = \frac{1250}{x}$$

Cross multiply:

$$\frac{30,000}{500} \diagdown\!\!\!\!\diagup \frac{1250}{x}$$

$$30,000x = 625,000$$

The next step is to isolate x on one side of the equation. Do this by dividing both sides of the equation by 30,000.

$$\frac{30,000x}{30,000} = \frac{625,000}{30,000}$$

You then solve for x.

$$\frac{3\cancel{0,000}x}{3\cancel{0,000}} = \frac{625,000}{30,000}$$

$$x = \frac{625,000}{30,000}$$

$$x = 20.8 \text{ mL/hr}$$

3.   Heparin 10,000 units in 100 mL of 0.9% NaCl to infuse at 750 units/hour

$$\frac{10,000}{100} = \frac{750}{x}$$

Cross multiply:

$$\frac{10,000}{100} \diagdown\!\!\!\!\diagup \frac{750}{x}$$

$$10,000x = 75,000$$

The next step is to isolate x on one side of the equation. Do this by dividing both sides of the equation by 10,000.

$$\frac{10,000x}{10,000} = \frac{75,000}{10,000}$$

You then solve for x.

$$\frac{1\cancel{0,000}x}{1\cancel{0,000}} = \frac{75,000}{10,000}$$

$$x = \frac{75,000}{10,000}$$

$$x = 7.5 \text{ mL/hr}$$

4.   Heparin 25,000 units in 1000 mL of 0.45% NaCl to infuse at 1000 units/hour

$$\frac{25,000}{1000} = \frac{1000}{x}$$

Cross multiply:

$$\frac{25,000}{1000} \diagdown\!\!\!\!\!\diagup \frac{1000}{x}$$

$$25,000x = 1,000,000$$

The next step is to isolate x on one side of the equation. Do this by dividing both sides of the equation by 25,000.

$$\frac{25,000x}{25,000} = \frac{1,000,000}{25,000}$$

You then solve for x.

$$\frac{\cancel{25,000}x}{\cancel{25,000}} = \frac{1,000,000}{25,000}$$

$$x = \frac{1,000,000}{25,000}$$

$$x = 40 \text{ mL/hr}$$

5. Insulin 500 units in 250 mL of 0.45% NaCl to infuse at 10 units/hour

$$\frac{500}{250} = \frac{10}{x}$$

Cross multiply:

$$\frac{500}{250} \diagdown\!\!\!\!\!\diagup \frac{10}{x}$$

$$500x = 2500$$

The next step is to isolate x on one side of the equation. Do this by dividing both sides of the equation by 500.

$$\frac{500x}{500} = \frac{2500}{500}$$

You then solve for x.

$$\frac{\cancel{500}x}{\cancel{500}} = \frac{2500}{500}$$

$$x = \frac{2500}{500}$$

$$x = 5 \text{ mL/hr}$$

Practice Problem Answers 10-3

Use the formula:

$$\frac{\text{Dosage on hand (units)}}{\text{Amount on hand (mL)}} = \frac{x \, (\text{units/hr})}{\text{mL/hour}}$$

1. Heparin 25,000 units in 500 mL of 0.9% NaCl to infuse at 24 mL/hour

$$\frac{25,000 \text{ units}}{500 \text{ mL}} = \frac{x \, (\text{units/hr})}{24 \text{ mL/hour}}$$

Cross multiply:

$$\frac{25,000}{500} \diagdown\!\!\!\!\!\diagup \frac{x}{24}$$

$$500x = 600,000$$

The next step is to isolate x on one side of the equation. Do this by dividing both sides of the equation by 500.

$$\frac{500x}{500} = \frac{600,000}{500}$$

You then solve for x.

$$\frac{5\!\!\!/00x}{5\!\!\!/00} = \frac{600,000}{500}$$

$$x = \frac{600,000}{500}$$

$$x = 1200 \text{ units/hr}$$

2. Heparin 10,000 units in 250 mL of 0.45% NaCl to infuse at 30 mL/hour

$$\frac{10,000 \text{ units}}{250 \text{ mL}} = \frac{x \text{ (units/hr)}}{30 \text{ mL/hour}}$$

Cross multiply:

$$\frac{10,000}{250} \bowtie \frac{x}{30}$$

$$250x = 300,000$$

The next step is to isolate x on one side of the equation. Do this by dividing both sides of the equation by 250.

$$\frac{250x}{250} = \frac{300,000}{250}$$

You then solve for x.

$$\frac{2\!\!\!/50x}{2\!\!\!/50} = \frac{300,000}{250}$$

$$x = \frac{300,000}{250}$$

$$x = 1200 \text{ units/hr}$$

3. Insulin 500 units in 250 mL of 0.9% NaCl to infuse at 3 mL/hour

$$\frac{500 \text{ units}}{250 \text{ mL}} = \frac{x \text{ (units/hr)}}{3 \text{ mL/hour}}$$

Cross multiply:

$$\frac{500}{250} \bowtie \frac{x}{3}$$

$$250x = 1500$$

The next step is to isolate x on one side of the equation. Do this by dividing both sides of the equation by 250.

$$\frac{250x}{250} = \frac{1500}{250}$$

You then solve for x.

$$\frac{2\!\!\!/50x}{2\!\!\!/50} = \frac{1500}{250}$$

$$x = \frac{1500}{250}$$

$$x = 6 \text{ units/hr}$$

4. Heparin 40,000 units in 1000 mL of 0.45% NaCl to infuse at 20 mL/hour

$$\frac{40,000 \text{ units}}{1000 \text{ mL}} = \frac{x \text{ (units/hr)}}{20 \text{ mL/hour}}$$

Cross multiply:

$$\frac{40,000}{1000} \diagdown\!\!\!\diagup \frac{x}{20}$$

$$1000x = 800,000$$

The next step is to isolate x on one side of the equation. Do this by dividing both sides of the equation by 1000.

$$\frac{1000x}{1000} = \frac{800,000}{1000}$$

You then solve for x.

$$\frac{\cancel{1000}x}{\cancel{1000}} = \frac{800,000}{1000}$$

$$x = \frac{800,000}{1000}$$

$$x = 800 \text{ units/hr}$$

5. Insulin 50 units in 100 mL of 0.9% NaCl to infuse at 10 mL/hour

$$\frac{50 \text{ units}}{100 \text{ mL}} = \frac{x \,(\text{units/hr})}{10 \text{ mL/hour}}$$

Cross multiply:

$$\frac{50}{100} \diagdown\!\!\!\diagup \frac{x}{10}$$

$$100x = 500$$

The next step is to isolate x on one side of the equation. Do this by dividing both sides of the equation by 100.

$$\frac{100x}{100} = \frac{500}{100}$$

You then solve for x.

$$\frac{\cancel{100}x}{\cancel{100}} = \frac{500}{100}$$

$$x = \frac{500}{100}$$

$$x = 5 \text{ units/hr}$$

Practice Problem Answers 10-4

Formula method. Use the formula:

$$\frac{D}{H} \times V = \text{flow rate (mL/hour)}$$

Where: D = dosage desired in mg/hr or g/hour
          H = total mg or g on hand
          V = volume of solution in total mL

1. Cardizem 500 mg in 250 mL of 0.9% Na Cl to infuse at 8 mg/hour

$$\frac{8 \cancel{\text{mg}}/\text{hr}}{500 \cancel{\text{mg}}} \times 250 \text{ mL} = 4 \text{ mL/hour}$$

2. Morphine sulfate 100 mg in 200 mL of 0.45% NaCl to infuse at 3 mg/hour

$$\frac{3 \text{ mg/hr}}{100 \text{ mg}} \times 200 \text{ mL} = 6 \text{ mL/hour}$$

3. Magnesium sulfate 10 g in 250 mL lactated Ringer's to infuse at 1 g/hour

$$\frac{1 \text{ g/hr}}{10 \text{ g}} \times 250 \text{ mL} = 25 \text{ mL/hour}$$

Ratio-Proportion method. Use the formula:

$$\frac{\text{Dosage on hand (D)}}{\text{Amount on hand (H)}} = \frac{\text{Dosage prescribed (Q)}}{x \text{ mL/hour}}$$

Where: D = total number of mg or g on hand
H = volume of solution on hand in mL
Q = dosage prescribed in mg/hr or g/hour
x = is the mL/hour solved for in the equation

4. Lasix 250 mg in 500 mL of 0.9% NaCl to infuse at 6 mg/hour

$$\frac{250 \text{ mg}}{500 \text{ mL}} = \frac{6 \text{ mg/hour}}{x}$$

Cross multiply:

$$\frac{250 \text{ mg}}{500 \text{ mL}} \bowtie \frac{6 \text{ mg/hour}}{x}$$

$$250 \text{ mg } x = 3000 \text{ mg} \times \text{mL/hour}$$

The next step is to isolate x on one side of the equation. Do this by dividing both sides of the equation by 250.

$$\frac{250 \text{ mg } x}{250 \text{ mg}} = \frac{3000 \text{ mg} \times \text{mL/hour}}{250 \text{ mg}}$$

You then solve for x.

$$\frac{250 \text{ mg } x}{250 \text{ mg}} = \frac{3000 \text{ mg} \times \text{mL/hour}}{250 \text{ mg}}$$

$$x = \frac{3000 \text{ mL/hour}}{250}$$

$$x = 12 \text{ mL/hr}$$

5. Ranitidine hydrochloride (Zantac) 250 mg in 500 mL of 5% dextrose in water to infuse at 6.25 mg/hour

$$\frac{250 \text{ mg}}{500 \text{ mL}} = \frac{6.25 \text{ mg/hour}}{x}$$

Cross multiply:

$$\frac{250 \text{ mg}}{500 \text{ mL}} \bowtie \frac{6.25 \text{ mg/hour}}{x}$$

$$250 \text{ mg } x = 3125 \text{ mg} \times \text{mL/hour}$$

The next step is to isolate x on one side of the equation. Do this by dividing both sides of the equation by 250.

$$\frac{250 \text{ mg } x}{250 \text{ mg}} = \frac{3125 \text{ mg} \times \text{mL/hour}}{250 \text{ mg}}$$

You then solve for x.

$$\frac{250 \text{ mg } x}{250 \text{ mg}} = \frac{3125 \text{ mg} \times \text{mL/hour}}{250 \text{ mg}}$$

$$x = \frac{3125 \text{ mL/hour}}{250}$$

$$x = 12.5 \text{ mL/hr}$$

6. Aminophylline 1,000 mg in 500 mL of 5% dextrose in water to infuse at 20 mg/hour

$$\frac{1000 \text{ mg}}{500 \text{ mL}} = \frac{20 \text{ mg/hour}}{x}$$

Cross multiply:

$$\frac{1000 \text{ mg}}{500 \text{ mL}} \bowtie \frac{20 \text{ mg/hour}}{x}$$

$$1000 \text{ mg } x = 10,000 \text{ mg} \times \text{mL/hour}$$

The next step is to isolate x on one side of the equation. Do this by dividing both sides of the equation by 1000.

$$\frac{1000 \text{ mg } x}{1000 \text{ mg}} = \frac{10,000 \text{ mg} \times \text{mL/hour}}{1000 \text{ mg}}$$

You then solve for x.

$$\frac{\cancel{1000 \text{ mg}} \ x}{\cancel{1000 \text{ mg}}} = \frac{10,000 \ \cancel{\text{mg}} \times \text{mL/hour}}{1000 \ \cancel{\text{mg}}}$$

$$x = \frac{10,000 \text{ mL/hour}}{1000}$$

$$x = 10 \text{ mL/hr}$$

Practice Problem Answers 10-5

1. Nitroglycerin 100 mg in 250 mL of 5% dextrose in water to infuse at 60 mcg/min

$$\frac{60 \times 60}{400} = \frac{3600}{400} = 9 \text{ mL/hour}$$

2. Nitroprusside 50 mg in 250 mL of 0.9% NaCl to infuse at 4 mcg/kg/min. Patient weighs 70 kg.

$$\frac{4 \times 70 \times 60}{200} = \frac{16,800}{200} = 84 \text{ mL/hour}$$

3. Zemuron 1 gram in 250 mL of 0.9% NaCl to infuse at 12 mcg/kg/min. Patient weighs 64 kg.

$$\frac{12 \times 64 \times 60}{4000} = \frac{46,080}{4000} = 11.5 \text{ mL/hour}$$

4. Norepinephrine 4 mg in 250 mL of 5% dextrose in water to infuse at 8 mcg/min

$$\frac{8 \times 60}{16} = \frac{480}{16} = 30 \text{ mL/hour}$$

5. Dopamine 800 mg in 250 mL of 5% dextrose in water to infuse at 3 mcg/kg/min. Patient weighs 82 kg.

$$\frac{3 \times 82 \times 60}{3200} = \frac{14,760}{3200} = 4.6 \text{ mL/hour}$$

6. Xylocaine 2 grams in 250 mL of 0.9% NaCl to infuse at 2 mg/min

$$\frac{2 \times 60}{8} = \frac{120}{8} = 15 \text{ mL/hour}$$

7. Epinephrine 2 mg in 250 mL of 5% dextrose in water to infuse at 6 mcg/min

$$\frac{6 \times 60}{8} = \frac{360}{8} = 45 \text{ mL/hour}$$

8. Dobutamine 500 mg in 250 mL of 5% dextrose in water to infuse at 7.5 mcg/kg/min. Patient weighs 93 kg.

$$\frac{7.5 \times 93 \times 60}{2000} = \frac{41,850}{2000} = 20.9 \text{ mL/hour}$$

9. Milrinone 20 mg in 100 mL of 5% dextrose in water to infuse at 0.5 mcg/kg/min. Patient weighs 100 kg.

$$\frac{0.5 \times 100 \times 60}{200} = \frac{3000}{200} = 15 \text{ mL/hour}$$

10. Neo-Synephrine 50 mg in 250 mL of 5% dextrose in water to infuse at 140 mcg/min

$$\frac{140 \times 60}{200} = \frac{8400}{200} = 42 \text{ mL/hour}$$

Practice Problem Answers 10-6

1. Zemuron 1000 mg in 250 mL of 0.9% NaCl infusing at 13 mL/hour. The patient weighs 72 kg. How many mcg/kg/min is the patient receiving?

$$\frac{4000 \text{ mcg/mL} \times 13 \text{ mL/hour}}{72 \text{ kg} \times 60 \text{ min/hour}} = \frac{52,000}{4320} = 12 \text{ mcg/kg/min}$$

2. Dobutamine 250 mg in 250 mL of 5% dextrose in water infusing at 20.5 mL/hour. The patient weighs 68 kg. How many mcg/kg/min is the patient receiving?

$$\frac{1000 \text{ mcg/mL} \times 20.5 \text{ mL/hour}}{68 \text{ kg} \times 60 \text{ min/hour}} = \frac{20,500}{4080} = 5 \text{ mcg/kg/min}$$

3. Norepinephrine 4 mg in 250 mL of 5% dextrose in water infusing at 37 mL/hour. How many mcg/min is the patient receiving?

$$\frac{16 \text{ mcg/mL} \times 37 \text{ mL/hour}}{60 \text{ min/hour}} = \frac{592}{60} = 9.9 \text{ mcg/min}$$

4. Nitroglycerine 100 mg in 250 mL of 5% dextrose in water infusing at 10.5 mL/hour. How many mcg/min is the patient receiving?

$$\frac{400 \text{ mcg/mL} \times 10.5 \text{ mL/hour}}{60 \text{ min/hour}} = \frac{4200}{60} = 70 \text{ mcg/min}$$

5. Nitroprusside 100 mg in 250 mL of 0.9% NaCl infusing at 65 mL/hour. The patient weighs 72 kg. How many mcg/kg/min is the patient receiving?

$$\frac{400 \text{ mcg/mL} \times 65 \text{ mL/hour}}{72 \text{ kg} \times 60 \text{ min/hour}} = \frac{26,000}{4320} = 6 \text{ mcg/kg/min}$$

6. Epinephrine 2 mg in 250 mL of 5% dextrose in water infusing at 30 mL/hour. How many mcg/min is the patient receiving?

$$\frac{8 \text{ mcg/mL} \times 30 \text{ mL/hour}}{60 \text{ min/hour}} = \frac{240}{60} = 4 \text{ mcg/min}$$

7. Xylocaine 2 grams in 250 mL of 0.9% NaCl infusing at 22.5 mL/hour. How many mg/min is the patient receiving?

$$\frac{8 \text{ mg/mL} \times 22.5 \text{ mL/hour}}{60 \text{ min/hour}} = \frac{180}{60} = 3 \text{ mg/min}$$

8. Milrinone 20 mg in 100 mL of 5% dextrose in water infusing at 20 mL/hour. The patient weighs 91 kg. How many mcg/kg/min is the patient receiving?

$$\frac{200 \text{ mcg/mL} \times 20 \text{ mL/hour}}{91 \text{ kg} \times 60 \text{ min/hour}} = \frac{4000}{5460} = 0.73 \text{ mcg/kg/min}$$

9. Neo-Synephrine 50 mg in 250 mL of 5% dextrose in water infusing at 36 mL/hour. How many mcg/min is the patient receiving?

$$\frac{200 \text{ mcg/mL} \times 36 \text{ mL/hour}}{60 \text{ min/hour}} = \frac{7200}{60} = 120 \text{ mcg/min}$$

10. Dopamine 400 mg in 250 mL of 5% dextrose in water infusing at 35 mL/hour. The patient weighs 67 kg. How many mcg/kg/min is the patient receiving?

$$\frac{1600 \text{ mcg/mL} \times 35 \text{ mL/hour}}{67 \text{ kg} \times 60 \text{ min/hour}} = \frac{56,000}{4020} = 13.9 \text{ mcg/kg/min}$$

Answers to Chapter Review Problems

Chapter Review Problem Answers 10-1

Remember the flow-rate formulas:

For medications ordered in mg/hour, units/hour, or mcg/hour:

$$\frac{D \text{ (mg/hour)}}{\text{Amount on hand (total mg, mcg, or units)}} \times \text{Volume (total mL)} = R \text{ (mL/hour)}$$

For medications ordered in mg/min or mcg/min:

$$\frac{D \text{ (mg/min or mcg/min)} \times 60 \text{ min/hour}}{C \text{ (mg/mL or mcg/mL)}} = R \text{ (mL/hr)}$$

For medications ordered in mcg/kg/min:

$$\frac{D \text{ (mcg/kg/min)} \times W \text{ (kg)} \times 60 \text{ min/hour}}{C \text{ (mcg/mL)}} = R \text{ (mL/hour)}$$

1. Cardizem 250 mg in 250 mL of 0.9% NaCl to infuse at 10 mg/hour

$$\frac{10}{250} \times 250 = 10 \text{ mL/hour}$$

2. Nitroprusside 100 mg in 250 mL of 0.9% NaCl to infuse at 4 mcg/kg/min. The patient weighs 66 kg.

$$\frac{4 \times 66 \times 60}{400} = \frac{15,840}{400} = 39.6 \text{ mL/hour}$$

3. Heparin 25,000 units in 500 mL of 0.9% NaCl to infuse at 1150 units/hour

$$\frac{1150}{25,000} \times 500 = 23 \text{ mL/hour}$$

4. Amiodarone hydrochloride 900 mg in 500 mL of 5% dextrose in water to infuse at 1 mg/min

$$\frac{1 \times 60}{1.8} = \frac{60}{1.8} = 33.3 \text{ mL/hour}$$

5. Epinephrine 2 mg in 250 mL of 5% dextrose in water to infuse at 8 mcg/min

$$\frac{8 \times 60}{8} = \frac{480}{8} = 60 \text{ mL/hour}$$

6. Insulin 200 units in 100 mL of 0.9% NaCl to infuse at 4 units/hour

$$\frac{4}{200} \times 100 = 2 \text{ mL/hour}$$

7. Dopamine 800 mg in 250 mL of 5% dextrose in water to infuse at 10 mcg/kg/min. The patient weighs 83 kg.

$$\frac{10 \times 83 \times 60}{3200} = \frac{49,800}{3200} = 15.6 \text{ mL/hour}$$

8. Magnesium sulfate 4 grams in 250 mL of 5% dextrose in water to infuse at 5 mg/min

$$\frac{5 \times 60}{16} = \frac{300}{16} = 18.8 \text{ mL/hour}$$

9. Zemuron 1 gram in 250 mL of 0.9% NaCl to infuse at 16 mcg/kg/min. The patient weighs 76 kg.

$$\frac{16 \times 76 \times 60}{4000} = \frac{72,960}{4000} = 18.2 \text{ mL/hour}$$

10. Lasix 200 mg in 100 mL of 0.9% NaCl to infuse at 2 mg/hour

$$\frac{2}{200} \times 100 = 1 \text{ mL/hour}$$

11. Heparin 25,000 units in 250 mL of 0.9% NaCl to infuse at 900 units/hour

$$\frac{900}{25,000} \times 250 = 9 \text{ mL/hour}$$

12. Norepinephrine 4 mg in 250 mL of 5% dextrose in water to infuse at 8 mcg/min

$$\frac{8 \times 60}{16} = \frac{480}{16} = 30 \text{ mL/hour}$$

13. Dobutamine 250 mg in 250 mL of 5% dextrose in water to infuse at 10 mcg/kg/min. The patient weighs 62 kg.

$$\frac{10 \times 62 \times 60}{1000} = \frac{37,200}{1000} = 37.2 \text{ mL/hour}$$

14. Oxytocin 10 units in 1000 mL of 0.9% NaCl to infuse at 0.002 units/min

$$\frac{0.002 \times 60}{0.01} = \frac{0.12}{0.01} = 12 \text{ mL/hour}$$

15. Procainamide hydrochloride 500 mg in 250 mL of 5% dextrose in water to infuse at 4 mg/min

$$\frac{4 \times 60}{2} = \frac{240}{2} = 120 \text{ mL/hour}$$

Chapter Review Problem Answers 10-2

Remember the formulas for dosage calculation when flow rate is known.

For medications ordered in units/hour, mg/hour, or mcg/hour:

$$\frac{\text{Dosage on hand (units, mg, mcg)}}{\text{Amount on hand (mL)}} = \frac{x \text{ (units or mg or mcg/ hr)}}{\text{mL/hour}}$$

For medications ordered in mg/min or mcg/min:

$$\frac{C \text{ (mg/mL or mcg/mL)} \times R \text{ (mL/hour)}}{60 \text{ min/hour}} = D \text{ (mg/min or mcg/min)}$$

For medications ordered in mcg/kg/min:

$$\frac{C \text{ (mcg/mL)} \times R \text{ (mL/hour)}}{W \text{ (kg)} \times 60 \text{ min/hour}} = D \text{ (mcg/kg/min)}$$

1. Esmolol hydrochloride 2.5 grams in 500 mL of 0.9% NaCl infusing at 84 mL/ hour. The patient weighs 70 kg. How many mcg/kg/min is the patient receiving?

$$\frac{5000 \text{ mcg/mL} \times 84 \text{ mL/hour}}{70 \text{ kg} \times 60 \text{ min/hour}} = \frac{420,000}{4200} = 100 \text{ mcg/kg/min}$$

2. Heparin 25,000 units in 500 mL of 0.9% NaCl is infusing at 26 mL/hour. How many units/hour is the patient receiving?

   Set up the problem:

$$\frac{25,000 \text{ units}}{500 \text{ mL}} = \frac{x \text{ units}}{26 \text{ mL/hour}}$$

   Cross multiply:

$$\frac{25,000}{500} \quad \diagtimes \quad \frac{x}{26}$$

$$500x = 650,000$$

   The next step is to isolate x on one side of the equation. Do this by dividing both sides of the equation by 500.

$$\frac{500x}{500} = \frac{650,000}{500}$$

   You then solve for x.

$$\frac{\cancel{500}x}{\cancel{500}} = \frac{650,000}{500}$$

$$x = \frac{650,000}{500}$$

$$x = 1300 \text{ units/hr}$$

3. Nitroglycerin 50 mg in 250 mL of 5% dextrose in water is infusing at 24 mL/hour. How many mcg/min is the patient receiving?

$$\frac{200 \text{ mcg/mL} \times 24 \text{ mL/hour}}{60 \text{ min/hour}} = \frac{4800}{60} = 80 \text{ mcg/min}$$

4. Diltiazem hydrochloride 250 mg in 500 mL in 5% dextrose in water infusing at 30 mL/hour. How many mg/hour is the patient receiving?

   Set up the problem:

$$\frac{250 \text{ mg}}{500 \text{ mL}} = \frac{x \text{ mg/hour}}{30 \text{ mL/hour}}$$

   Cross multiply:

$$\frac{250}{500} \quad \diagtimes \quad \frac{x}{30}$$

$$500x = 7500$$

   The next step is to isolate x on one side of the equation. Do this by dividing both sides of the equation by 500.

$$\frac{500x}{500} = \frac{7500}{500}$$

   You then solve for x.

$$\frac{\cancel{500}x}{\cancel{500}} = \frac{7500}{500}$$

$$x = \frac{7500}{500}$$

$$x = 15 \text{ mg/hr}$$

5. Neo-Synephrine 50 mg in 250 mL of 5% dextrose in water infusing at 45 mL/hour. How many mcg/min is the patient receiving?

$$\frac{200 \text{ mcg/mL} \times 45 \text{ mL/hour}}{60 \text{ min/hour}} = \frac{9000}{60} = 150 \text{ mcg/min}$$

6. Dopamine 400 mg in 250 mL of 5% dextrose in water infusing at 9 mL/hour. The patient weighs 92 kg. How many mcg/kg/min is the patient receiving?

$$\frac{1600 \text{ mcg/mL} \times 9 \text{ mL/hour}}{92 \text{ kg} \times 60 \text{ min/hour}} = \frac{14{,}400}{5520} = 2.6 \text{ mcg/kg/min}$$

7. Magnesium sulfate 5 grams in 250 mL of 5% dextrose in water infusing at 36 mL/hour. How many mg/min is the patient receiving?

$$\frac{20 \text{ mg/mL} \times 36 \text{ mL/hour}}{60 \text{ min/hour}} = \frac{720}{60} = 12 \text{ mg/min}$$

8. Morphine sulfate 100 mg in 100 mL of 0.9% NaCl infusing at 3 mL/hour. How many mg/hour is the patient receiving?

$$\frac{100 \text{ mg}}{100 \text{ mL}} = \frac{x \text{ mg/hr}}{3 \text{ mL/hour}}$$

Cross multiply:

$$\frac{100}{100} \diagdown\!\!\!\diagup \frac{x}{3}$$

$$100x = 300$$

The next step is to isolate x on one side of the equation. Do this by dividing both sides of the equation by 100.

$$\frac{100x}{100} = \frac{300}{100}$$

You then solve for x.

$$\frac{\cancel{100}x}{\cancel{100}} = \frac{300}{100}$$

$$x = \frac{300}{100}$$

$$x = 3 \text{ mg/hr}$$

9. Amiodarone hydrochloride 540 mg in 500 mL of 5% dextrose in water infusing at 28 mL/hour. How many mg/min is the patient receiving?

$$\frac{1.08 \text{ mg/mL} \times 28 \text{ mL/hour}}{60 \text{ min/hour}} = \frac{30.2}{60} = 0.5 \text{ mg/min}$$

10. Nitroprusside 100 mg in 250 mL of 0.9% NaCl infusing at 26 mL/hour. The patient weighs 87 kg. How many mcg/kg/min is the patient receiving?

$$\frac{400 \text{ mcg/mL} \times 26 \text{ mL/hour}}{87 \text{ kg} \times 60 \text{ min/hour}} = \frac{10{,}400}{5220} = 1.99 \text{ mcg/kg/min. Round to 2 mcg/kg/min}$$

11. Xylocaine 2 g in 250 mL of 0.9% NaCl infusing at 15 mL/hour. How many mg/min is the patient receiving?

$$\frac{8 \text{ mg/mL} \times 15 \text{ mL/hour}}{60 \text{ min/hour}} = \frac{120}{60} = 2 \text{ mg/min}$$

12. Isoproterenol hydrochloride 1 mg in 500 mL of 5% dextrose in water infusing at 75 mL/hour. How many mcg/min is the patient receiving?

$$\frac{2 \text{ mcg/mL} \times 75 \text{ mL/hour}}{60 \text{ min/hour}} = \frac{150}{60} = 2.5 \text{ mcg/min}$$

13. Milrinone 50 mg in 250 mL of 5% dextrose in water infusing at 9 mL/hour. The patient weighs 58 kg. How many mcg/kg/min is the patient receiving?

$$\frac{200 \text{ mcg/mL} \times 9 \text{ mL/hour}}{58 \text{ kg} \times 60 \text{ min/hour}} = \frac{1800}{3480} = 0.52 \text{ mcg/kg/min}$$

14. Epinephrine 4 mg in 250 mL of 5% dextrose in water infusing at 30 mL/hour. How many mcg/min is the patient receiving?

$$\frac{16 \text{ mcg/mL} \times 30 \text{ mL/hour}}{60 \text{ min/hour}} = \frac{480}{60} = 8 \text{ mcg/min}$$

15. Esmolol hydrochloride 5 g in 500 mL of 0.9% NaCl infusing at 73 mL/hour. The patient weighs 81 kg. How many mcg/kg/min is the patient receiving?

$$\frac{10,000 \text{ mcg/mL} \times 73 \text{ mL/hour}}{81 \text{ kg} \times 60 \text{ min/hour}} = \frac{730,000}{4860} = 150.2 \text{ mcg/kg/min}$$

Pediatric Calculations

This chapter contains content on:

- **Calculations Using mg/kg for Weight Stated in Kilograms**
- **Calculations Using mg/kg for Weight Stated in Pounds and Ounces**
- **Calculations Using Body Surface Area**
- **Calculations With Drugs That Are in Combination**
- **Calculations for Pediatric Intravenous Administration**

Learning Objectives

Upon completion of Chapter 11, you will be able to:

- Accurately calculate pediatric dosages for 24-hour periods.
- Determine the safe dose ranges in mg/kg.
- Use BSA to determine pediatric drug dosages.
- Determine safe dosages of drugs when supplied in combination.
- Calculate reconstituted pediatric dosages.
- Critically review the calculation to determine the accuracy of the answers for safe administration.

Key Terms

- Safe Dose Range (SDR)
- Body Surface Area (BSA)

CASE STUDY

You are caring for David Anderson, age $1\frac{1}{2}$ months, who has been admitted for bronchopneumonia. He presents with fever, 102°F (39°C), and a persistent cough. He is having difficulty coughing up secretions. On auscultation, diminished breath sounds in the bases and diffuse crackles are noted. David's weight on admission was 10 lbs 2 oz. His mother is staying with David.

His orders include:

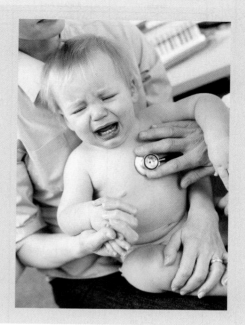

- Postural drainage and chest percussion every 4 hours
- Ceftazidime 40 mg/kg IVPB every 8 hours
- Gentamicin 2 mg/kg IVPB every 8 hours
- Amoxicillin 50 mg PO every 8 hours for 10 days
- Tylenol elixir 50 mg PO every 6 hours for temperature over 101°F (38.4°C)
- Ibuprofen liquid 10 mg/kg PO every 8 hours

Accuracy is always important when calculating and administering medications. For infants and children, accuracy takes on even greater importance. A miscalculation may be dangerous due to the small body size, weight, and body surface area of the infant or child. In addition, infants and children differ in their rate of drug absorption, distribution, metabolism, and excretion when compared to adults. Thus it is vital to follow pediatric protocols and guidelines, and use references to verify medication orders to ensure that drug dosages are correct. Make it a practice to use a calculator when determining dosages. The **safe dose range (SDR)** is the upper and lower limits of the dose range as stated by the drug manufacturer and is reported in an approved drug reference. The safe dose range is usually expressed in milligrams per kilogram (mg/kg) of body weight. When preparing to administer a drug to a child, you must first calculate the daily (24-hour) drug dose ordered by the prescriber based on kilograms of body weight, and then verify the calculated dose with the range stated in an approved drug reference. Each prescribed dose of medication for a child must be calculated, and you must check the prescribed dose against the SDR to make sure that it is an acceptable safe dosage for the child.

(!) **SAFETY ALERT:** *To ensure safe practice, always double check by comparing the prescribed dose with the recommended safe dose range (SDR) using the drug resource manual to determine the safe dose.*

Two methods are used to calculate pediatric dosages. The method most frequently used is based on body weight using mg/kg. The second method uses **body surface area (BSA)**. Calculations using BSA require the use of a chart called a nomogram, which converts the weight to square meters of BSA (see Figure 11-1). This method of dosage calculation is usually reserved for certain drugs, such as cancer chemotherapy (antineoplastic agents), whose dosages are individualized based on factors such as the severity of the illness, or the child's renal and liver function, and that are often given in sequence with other drugs. Always verify large or megadoses with the prescriber and document the verification.

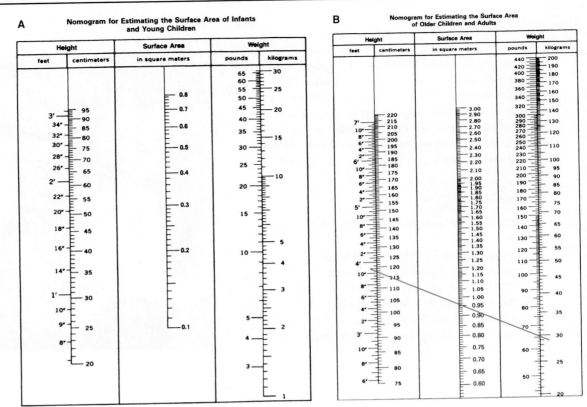

Figure 11-1. Nomograms for determining BSA. **A.** Nomogram for infants and young children. **B.** Nomogram for older children and adults. The red line indicates the BSA for a child who weighs 75 pounds and is 4 feet, 2 inches tall.

CALCULATIONS USING mg/kg FOR WEIGHT STATED IN KILOGRAMS

Using mg/kg is the most common way for calculating pediatric dosages. Pediatric drug references indicate the safe dosage of the drug using mg/kg. The references typically provide the SDR for a 24-hour period of administration of a single dose or as divided doses. The drug references may also show the dosage calculated as mcg/kg for the therapeutic dose when unusually small amounts are to be used for a particular medication.

When calculating drug dosage using mg/kg, the key to this calculation is determining the child's weight in kilograms. Once this is determined, you can then determine the safe dosage and evaluate your calculation for accuracy.

Formula Method

Consider this example: Your patient weighs 22 pounds and the prescriber has ordered ranitidine (Zantac) 50 mg by mouth two times per day.

STEP 1: CONVERT

First, convert the child's weight into kilograms by dividing the child's weight in pounds by 2.2. The formula is:

$$2.2 \text{ lbs} = 1 \text{ kg}$$

It is safest to use a calculator. The child's weight is 22 lbs, so divide:

$$22 \text{ lb} \div 2.2 \text{ lbs/kg} = 10 \text{ kg}$$

If the weight of the infant or child is in ounces, then convert the ounces to the nearest tenth of a pound, add this to the total pounds, and then convert the total pounds to kilograms to the nearest tenth. (See Chapter 1 for more information on rounding.)

STEP 2: COMPUTE

Now determine the medication dose for the SDR using a calculator and the current pediatric recommendations. Multiply the minimum dose by the weight of the child in kilograms to determine the medication dose. Then, take the maximum dose times the weight of the child in kilograms to get the safe range. Finally, compare the 24-hour prescribed dose with the recommended SDR found in an approved drug reference.

For the child in the example, determine the data you need to set up the problem accurately. The drug ordered for this patient is ranitidine (Zantac) 50 mg by mouth two times a day. For this drug order, the drug reference identifies the safe dose as 5 to 10 mg/kg daily in two divided doses. Set up the problem:

$$10 \text{ kg} \times 5 \text{ mg} = 50 \text{ mg} \qquad \text{(minimum safe range)},$$

and

$$10 \text{ kg} \times 10 \text{ mg} = 100 \text{ mg} \qquad \text{(maximum safe range)}$$

Now you have determined that the order for 50 mg two times a day is within the safe range. An easy way to remember these steps is:

- Convert weight to kilograms
- Compute the SDR
- Compare the calculation with the prescribed dose
- Calculate the dose to determine if safe for administration

 SAFETY ALERT: *Be certain when determining the safe range that you make the comparison for the same time frame.*

The drug preparation from the pharmacy provides Ranitidine 15 mg/mL. Set up the problem using the formula method:

$$\frac{D}{H} \times V = A$$

Recall that in the formula method:

    D = desired or prescribed dosage of the medication

    H = dosage of medication available or on hand

    V = volume that the medication is available in, such as one tablet or milliliters

    A = amount of medication to administer

Set up the problem as follows:

$$\frac{50 \text{ mg}}{15 \text{ mg}} \times 1 \text{ mL}$$

In this problem because mg appears in both the numerator and denominator, they cancel each other out. You are left with mL as the volume of medication in the answer.

$$\frac{50 \cancel{\text{ mg}}}{15 \cancel{\text{ mg}}} \times 1 \text{ mL} = 3.3 \text{ mL}$$

The answer is 3.3 mL. For accuracy in administration, this dose is best prepared using an oral syringe.

STEP 3: CRITICALLY THINK

After determining the SDR, calculate the actual dose for administration by using the formula method. Then ask yourself if the dose is within the 24-hour safe range as identified by a reliable drug reference. The range you calculated is 50 to 100 mg in two divided doses per day.

ASK YOURSELF – *Does this answer seem logical, correct, and plausible?*

This answer is reasonable and plausible in that it meets the safe standard for the number of mL given at one time. Three mL is not unusually large or small for a safe dose. It is correct. Think that 50 mg is approximately three times as much as 15 mg. Therefore, a dose of 3 mL is correct. To verify this step, have another nurse check your math.

Ratio-Proportion Method

When the medication dosage ordered by the prescriber is different from the dosage of the medication available, the ratio-proportion method can be used to calculate the needed dose. This method solves for an unknown *x* in the equation. The equation is:

$$\frac{\text{Dosage on hand}}{\text{Amount on hand}} = \frac{\text{Dosage desired}}{\text{Amount desired}}$$

Consider this example: A child who weighs 27 pounds is to receive ibuprofen suspension 65 mg every 6 hours for pain or fever. You have ibuprofen 100 mg/5 mL available. You recognize the need to calculate the correct dosage of ibuprofen for your patient.

 SAFETY ALERT: *Remember to always check the volume of the unit dosage in which the medication is supplied. Using the correct volume will prevent dosage errors from occurring.*

STEP 1: CONVERT

First, calculate the patient's weight in kilograms. The patient weighs 27 lbs. To convert the weight in lbs to kg, divide by 2.2 (recall that 2.2 lbs = 1 kg):

$$27 \text{ lbs} \div 2.2 \text{ lbs/kg} = 12.27 \text{ kg}$$

The child weighs 12.27 kg.

For this example, both the ordered dose and the dose available are in the same units—mg. Therefore, you do not need to perform additional conversions for this calculation.

STEP 2: COMPUTE

The ordered drug is ibuprofen suspension 65 mg every 6 hours for pain or fever. The recommended SDR for ibuprofen is 5 to 10 mg/kg every 6 to 8 hours, for a maximum of 40 mg/kg per day.

Set up the problem to determine the safe dose range:

12.27 kg × 5 mg = 61.35 mg × 4 doses = 245 mg   (minimum safe dose per day)

12.27 kg × 10 mg = 122.7 mg × 4 doses = 490.8 mg   (maximum safe dose per day)

The safe range of medication per day is 245 to 490.8 mg. You have determined that the order for ibuprofen suspension 65 mg every 6 hours is within the safe range.

Now compute the dosage for administration. Determine what data you need and set up the problem correctly. The ratio-proportion method requires you to know what medication dose is ordered and what the available dosage is. The equation is:

$$\frac{\text{Dosage on hand}}{\text{Amount on hand}} = \frac{\text{Dosage desired}}{\text{Amount desired}}$$

Cross multiply:

$$\frac{100 \text{ mg}}{5 \text{ mL}} \diagup\kern-1.5em\diagdown \frac{65 \text{ mg}}{x}$$

$$100 \text{ mg } x = 325 \text{ mg} \times \text{mL}$$

Isolate the x by dividing both sides by 100 mg. Milligrams (mg) in the numerator and denominator cancel each other out and you are left with mL as the volume of medication in the answer.

$$\frac{\cancel{100 \text{ mg}} \, x}{\cancel{100 \text{ mg}}} = \frac{325 \cancel{\text{ mg}} \times \text{mL}}{100 \cancel{\text{ mg}}}$$

Solve for x:

$$x = \frac{325 \text{ mL}}{100} = 3.25 \text{ mL}$$

Therefore, the answer to the problem is 3.25 mL.

STEP 3: CRITICALLY THINK

ASK YOURSELF – *Does this answer seem logical, correct, and plausible?*

This answer is reasonable and plausible in that it meets the safe standard for the amount of liquid medication given at one time. It is not unusually large or small for a safe dose. Think that 5 mL contains 100 mg of ibuprofen, and 3.25 mL contains 65 mg. Therefore, 3.25 mL is the correct amount when the dosage ordered is 65 mg. To verify this step, have another nurse check your math.

CALCULATIONS USING mg/kg FOR WEIGHT STATED IN POUNDS AND OUNCES

There are times when the weight is stated as pounds and ounces. In these situations, the pounds and ounces must be accurately converted to kilograms.

Formula Method

Consider this example: A child who weights 9 lbs 2 oz is prescribed amoxicillin 50 mg orally every 8 hours for 10 days. You recognize the need to change the child's weight to kilograms.

STEP 1: CONVERT

First change the ounces to pounds, being careful to use 16 ounces in the equation:

$$2 \text{ oz} \div 16 \text{ oz} = 0.125 \text{ pound (lbs)} \quad \text{(Round to 0.13)}$$

Add the computed pounds amount to the total pounds as follows:

$$9 \text{ lbs} + 0.13 \text{ lbs} = 9.13 \text{ lbs}$$

Therefore, the child weighs 9.125 lbs. Next, convert the total weight to kg:

$$9.13 \text{ lbs} \div 2.2 \text{ lbs/kg} = 4.15 \text{ kg}$$

The child's weight in kilograms is 4.15.

⚠ **SAFETY ALERT:** *Use care when converting ounces to part of a pound and remember to add the answer to the pounds. Do not forget to add, to get the total pounds before converting to kilograms.*

STEP 2: COMPUTE

Recall that the prescriber ordered amoxicillin 50 mg orally every 8 hours for 10 days. With the above calculation, the child's weight is 4.15 kg. The drug reference states that the dose for children is 40 mg/kg/24 hours. You must determine the safe dose per day and per dose.

Set up the problem:

$$4.15 \text{ kg} \times 40 \text{ mg} = 166 \text{ mg} \qquad \text{per day}$$

$$166 \text{ mg} \div 3 \text{ doses/day} = 55.33 \text{ mg} \qquad \text{per dose}$$

Therefore, 50 mg per dose is within the SDR.

After finding the SDR, calculate the actual dose for administration. The pharmacy supplies amoxicillin as 250 mg/5mL. Recall the formula method:

$$\frac{D}{H} \times V = A$$

Where: D = desired or prescribed dosage of the medication

H = dosage of medication available or on hand

V = volume that the medication is available in, such as one tablet or milliliters

A = amount of medication to administer

Set up the problem:

$$\frac{50 \text{ mg}}{250 \text{ mg}} \times 5 \text{ mL}$$

In this problem, because mg appears in both the numerator and denominator, they cancel each other out. You are left with mL as the volume of medication in the answer.

Next, reduce the fraction as follows:

$$\frac{50 \text{ mg}}{250 \text{ mg}} = \frac{1}{5}$$

$$\frac{1}{5} \times 5 \text{ mL} = 1 \text{ mL}$$

Therefore, you would administer 1 mL.

STEP 3: CRITICALLY THINK

ASK YOURSELF – Does this answer seem logical, correct, and plausible?

Is the dose within the 24-hour safe range as identified by a reliable drug reference? Review the safe dose as indicated in the drug reference and recalculate your math. Think about the calculated dose and volume. Is the answer logical, accurate, and safe? Think about the available medication, and notice that for every dose there is 50 mg/1 mL. Therefore, you are administering only one-fifth of the total volume. More importantly, the ordered dose is within the SDR as you determined in our calculations. To verify this step, have another nurse check your math.

 CASE STUDY

You notice that David has a temperature of 102.2°F (39°C). He has an order for acetaminophen elixir 50 mg every 6 hours for a temperature over 101°F (38.4°C). David's weight was 10 lbs, 2 oz. You need to administer the acetaminophen.

Ratio-Proportion Method

STEP 1: CONVERT

David's weight is recorded in pounds, but SDRs are most commonly are reported in mg/kg. So you must convert David's weight to kilograms.

First, set up the problem to convert ounces to pounds:

$$2 \text{ oz} \div 16 \text{ oz/lb} = 0.125 \text{ lb} \qquad \text{(Round to } 0.13)$$

Then, add this amount to determine the total pounds:

$$10 + 0.13 = 10.13 \text{ lbs}$$

Next, convert the pounds to kilograms:

$$10.13 \text{ lbs} \div 2.2 \text{ lbs/kg} = 4.60 \text{ kg}$$

STEP 2: COMPUTE

The ordered drug is acetaminophen 50 mg every 6 hours for pain or fever. The recommended SDR for acetaminophen is 10 to 15 mg/kg/dose. Set up the problem to determine the safe dose range:

$$4.6 \text{ kg} \times 10 \text{ mg/kg} = 46 \text{ mg} \qquad \text{(minimum safe dose)}$$
$$4.6 \text{ kg} \times 15 \text{ mg/kg} = 69 \text{ mg} \qquad \text{(maximum safe dose)}$$

The order is for 50 mg, which is within the SDR; therefore, the order is safe.

Next, determine the dose. The drug supplied is acetaminophen elixir 160 mg/teaspoon. Remember from Chapter 2 that 1 teaspoon is equal to 5 mL.

Recall the ratio-proportion method:

$$\frac{\text{Dosage on hand}}{\text{Amount on hand}} = \frac{\text{Dosage desired}}{\text{Amount desired}}$$

To solve the problem using the ratio-proportion method, set up the problem as follows:

$$\frac{160 \text{ mg}}{5 \text{ mL}} = \frac{50 \text{ mg}}{x}$$

Cross multiply:

$$\frac{160 \text{ mg}}{5 \text{ mL}} \diagup\!\!\!\!\diagdown \frac{50 \text{ mg}}{x}$$

$$160 \text{ mg } x = 250 \text{ mg} \times \text{mL}$$

Isolate the x by dividing both sides by 160 mg. Milligrams (mg) in the numerator and denominator cancel each other out and you are left with mL as the volume of medication in the answer.

$$\frac{\cancel{160 \text{ mg}} \, x}{\cancel{160 \text{ mg}}} = \frac{250 \cancel{\text{mg}} \times \text{mL}}{160 \cancel{\text{mg}}}$$

Solve for x:

$$x = \frac{250 \text{ mL}}{160} = 1.56 \text{ mL}$$

Therefore, the answer to the problem is 1.56 mL.

STEP 3: CRITICALLY THINK

ASK YOURSELF – Does this answer seem logical, correct, and plausible?

As you are thinking about the calculated dose, you can immediately think about the fact that there are 160 mg in 5 mL. Therefore, in 2.5 mL (which is one-half of 5 mL) there would be 80 mg, and in 1.25 mL there would be 40 mg. So looking at your answer of 1.56 mL for 50 mg sounds right. Remember, if you enter wrong numbers in the calculator you will get an answer, but you will get the wrong dose. To verify this step, have another nurse check your math.

PRACTICE PROBLEMS 11-1. Practice Problems Using mg/kg

DIRECTIONS: Solve the following problems using mg/kg and the formula method to calculate the medication dosage. The answers to the problems can be found at the end of the chapter.

1. **Medication Ordered:** Ceclor suspension 200 mg orally every 8 hours
   Medication Available: Ceclor suspension 125 mg/5 mL
   (Child weighs 40 pounds)
   The SDR is 6.7 to 13.4 mg/kg every 8 hours. Calculate the SDR.

   Calculation:

2. **Medication Ordered:** Furosemide liquid 15 mg PO daily
   Medication Available: Furosemide liquid 40 mg/5 mL
   (Child weighs 30 pounds)
   The SDR is 2 mg/kg PO daily.

   Calculation:

3. **Medication Ordered:** Ampicillin suspension 200 mg PO every 6 hours
   Medication Available: Ampicillin suspension 125 mg/5 mL
   (Child weighs 47 pounds)
   The SDR is 25 to 50 mg/kg/day equally divided every 6 hours.

   Calculation:

4. **Medication Ordered:** Lasix 10 mg PO three times a day
   Medication Available: Lasix 15 mg/mL
   (Child weighs 18 pounds 4 ounces)
   The SDR is 1 to 2 mg/kg every 6 to 8 hours not to exceed 6 mg/kg/day.

   Calculation:

5. **Medication Ordered:** Ibuprofen 60 mg PO every 6 hours
   Medication Available: Ibuprofen suspension 100 mg/5 mL
   (Child weighs 26 pounds)
   The SDR is 5 to 10 mg/kg every 6 to 8 hours for a maximum of 40 mg/kg/day.

   Calculation:

6. **Medication Ordered:** Biaxin liquid 200 mg PO two times a day
   Medication Available: Biaxin 125 mg/5 mL
   (Child weighs 68 pounds)
   The SDR is 7.5 mg/kg every 12 hours.

   Calculation:

PRACTICE PROBLEMS 11-2. Practice Problems Using Ratio-Proportion Method

DIRECTIONS: Solve the following medication dosage problems using the ratio-proportion method. The answers to the problems can be found at the end of the chapter.

1. **Medication Ordered:** Clindamycin 150 mg PO every 6 hours
   Medication Available: Clindamycin suspension 75 mg/5 mL
   (Child weighs 76 pounds)
   The SDR is 8 to 25 mg/kg/day.

   Calculation:

2. **Medication Ordered:** Zantac 50 mg PO every 12 hours   **Calculation:**
   Medication Available: Zantac 15 mg/mL
   (Child weighs 28 pounds 6 ounces)
   The SDR is 5 to 10 mg/kg/day in two divided doses.

3. **Medication Ordered:** Penicillin V suspension 0.2 g PO every 8 hours   **Calculation:**
   Medication Available: Penicillin V suspension 125 mg/5 mL
   (Child weighs 42 pounds)
   The SDR is 15 to 62.5 mg/kg daily divided every 4 to 8 hours.

4. **Medication Ordered:** Phenobarbital 10 mg PO every 12 hours   **Calculation:**
   Medication Available: Phenobarbital 15 mg/5 mL
   (Child weighs 38 pounds)
   The SDR is 1 to 6 mg/kg in two divided doses not to exceed 100 mg/day.

5. **Medication Ordered:** Morphine 2 mg subcutaneous every 6 hours   **Calculation:**
   Medication Available: Morphine 1 mg/mL for subcutaneous injection
   (Child weighs 46 pounds)
   The SDR is 0.1 mg to 0.2 mg/kg/day in 4 divided doses.

CALCULATIONS USING BODY SURFACE AREA

A second method for calculating pediatric drug dosages is the body surface area (BSA) method, which uses a nomogram chart. The BSA is considered the most accurate way to determine the amount of drug to administer. This method involves the use of a chart (see Figure 11-1 earlier in the chapter) that allows you to convert the weight and height to square meters (m^2) of BSA. The chart shows the height on the left in centimeters and feet, and it shows the weight on the right column in both pounds and kilograms. To determine the BSA in m^2, draw a straight line from the height on the left to the weight on the right. The point at which the line intersects the column marked m^2 is the BSA. This number is used to calculate the drug dosage.

SAFETY ALERT: *Remember to use the nomogram appropriate to the height and weight of the child or adult. For example, use the "Nomogram for Estimating the Surface Area of Infants and Young Children" when the child weighs less than 65 pounds and is less than 3 feet tall. Use the "Nomogram for Estimating the Surface Area of Older Children and Adults" for individuals who weigh more than 65 pounds and are more than 3 feet tall.*

The BSA is usually used to determine safe dosages for certain drugs such as oncology drugs, new drugs, and those that are extremely potent and require a precise amount. For example, drug references may list the SDR as mg/m^2. The BSA method may also be used for persons who are either over- or underweight.

CASE STUDY

You determine that David, who weighs 10 lbs 2 oz, is 23 inches in height. You need to determine his BSA to compute a drug dosage. You recognize the need to convert his weight in pounds and ounces to kilograms.

First, convert ounces to pounds:

$$\frac{2 \text{ oz}}{16 \text{ oz/lb}} = 0.125 \text{ lb}, \quad \text{rounded to } 0.13 \text{ lb}.$$

Then, add this amount to determine the total pounds:

$$10 \text{ lbs} + 0.13 \text{ lb} = 10.13 \text{ lbs}$$

Next, convert the pounds to kilograms:

$$\frac{10.13 \text{ lb}}{2.2 \text{ lbs/kg}} = 4.60 \text{ kg}$$

Lastly, determine the surface area by using the chart for infants and children. Draw a straight line between the height on the left and the weight in kilograms on the right. You determine the m² to be 0.26 m².

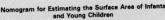

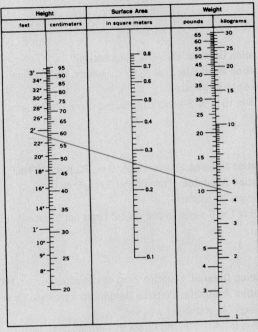

Nomogram for Estimating the Surface Area of Infants and Young Children

Once you determine the BSA, you can use this information to determine if the dosage is within the SDR, just as you would for any other dosage calculation. Once you determine the dosage is within the safe range, you would apply the 3-Step Approach, using the formula or ratio-proportion method to determine the correct dosage.

Consider this example: A child who weighs 18 lbs and is 70 cm in height is prescribed daunorubicin 15 mg IV today. The pharmacy supplies daunorubicin 5 mg/mL. First, convert the child's weight in pounds to kilograms:

$$18 \text{ lbs} \div 2.2 \text{ lbs/kg} = 8.18 \text{ kg}$$

Next, determine the surface area by using the nomogram for infants and children. Draw a straight line between the height in centimeters on the left and the weight in kilograms on the right. You determine the m² to be 0.38 m² (see Figure 11-2).

The drug reference indicates the SDR to be 30 to 60 mg/m² on one day. To determine the safe dose per day, set up the problem:

$$\text{The minimum SDR} = 30 \text{ mg} \times 0.38 \text{ m}^2 = 11.4 \text{ mg/day}$$

$$\text{The maximum SDR} = 60 \text{ mg} \times 0.38 \text{ m}^2 = 22.8 \text{ mg/day}$$

The SDR is 12 to 23 mg. Therefore, the ordered dose of 15 mg IV today is within the SDR. Then, apply the formula or ratio-proportion method to calculate the correct dose to administer based on the drug supplied by the pharmacy.

Due to differences in growth and body size, there are nomograms available for use depending on the weight and height of the child. One, used in the previous examples, is specifically for infants and young children (see Figure 11-1A earlier in the chapter). The other is for older children

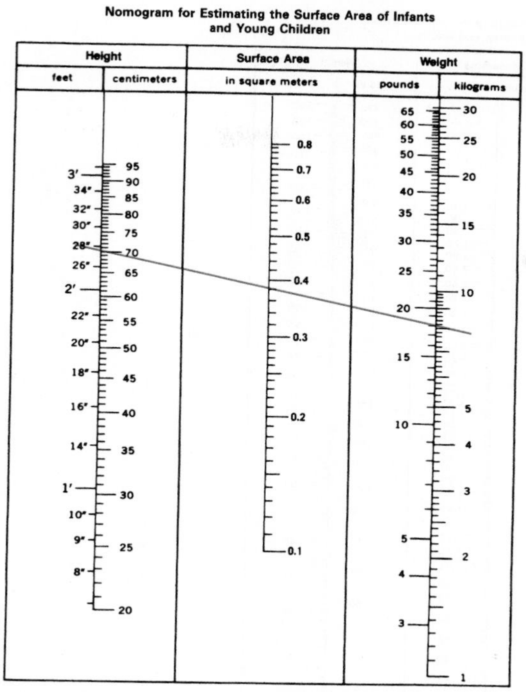

Figure 11-2. Nomogram depicting a BSA of 0.38 m².

and adults, and uses a different scale and is appropriate for children who weigh over 65 pounds or are more than 3 feet tall (see Figure 11-1B earlier in the chapter). When using the nomogram for older children and adults, you must calculate the estimated child's dose. This involves determining the BSA (m²) of the child, dividing this by 1.73 (the average adult BSA), and then multiplying the answer by the average adult dose.

Consider this example: You have a 7-year-old child who weighs 55 pounds and is 48 inches in height. The prescriber orders cytarabine 80 mg IV one time per day. First, convert the child's weight in pounds to kilograms:

$$55 \text{ lbs} \div 2.2 \text{ lbs/kg} = 25 \text{ kg}$$

Next, determine the surface area by using the chart for older children and adults. Draw a straight line between the height on the left and the weight in kilograms on the right. You determine the BSA to be 0.91 m² (see Figure 11-3).

According to the drug reference, the SDR for a normal adult dose is 100 to 200 mg/m² as a single dose. So you must determine the estimated child's dose by using the following formula:

$$\frac{\text{Child's BSA (m}^2)}{\text{Average adult's BSA (1.73 m}^2)} \times \text{Average adult dose of drug} = \text{Estimated child's dose}$$

$$\text{The minimum SDR} = \frac{0.91 \text{ m}^2}{1.73 \text{ m}^2} \times 100 \text{ mg} = 53 \text{ mg}$$

$$\text{The maximum SDR} = \frac{0.91 \text{ m}^2}{1.73 \text{ m}^2} \times 200 \text{ mg} = 105 \text{ mg}$$

The SDR is 53 to 105 mg, so the child's ordered dose is safe.

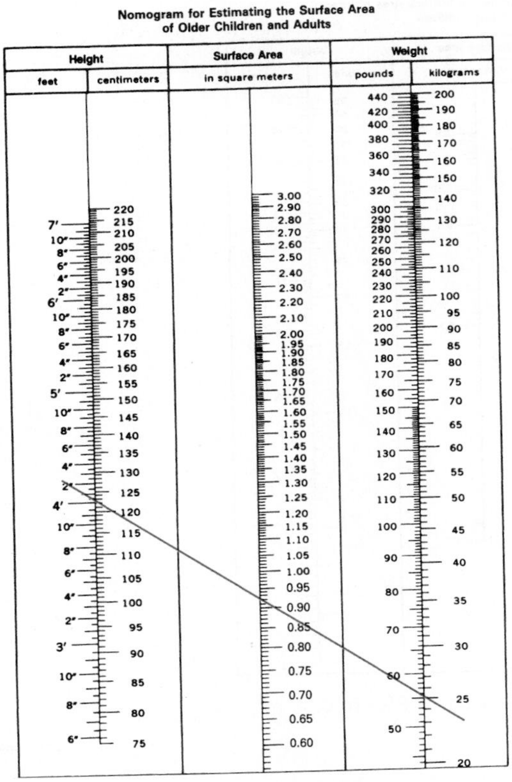
Nomogram for Estimating the Surface Area of Older Children and Adults
Height
feet
centimeters
Surface Area
in square meters
Weight
pounds
kilograms

Figure 11-3. Nomogram depicting a BSA of 0.91 m^2.

You have available 100 mg/5 mL. Set up the problem using the formula method:

$$\frac{D}{H} \times V = A$$

In the formula or rule method:

D = desired or prescribed dosage of the medication

H = dosage of medication available or on hand

V = volume that the medication is available in, such as one tablet or milliliters

A = amount of medication to administer

The problem is set up:

$$\frac{80 \text{ mg}}{100 \text{ mg}} \times 5 \text{ mL}$$

In this problem, because mg appears in both the numerator and denominator, mg is cancelled out and mL is left as the volume of medication in the answer.

Reduce the fraction:

$$\frac{80 \cancel{\text{mg}}}{100 \cancel{\text{mg}}} \times 5 \text{ mL} = \frac{8}{10} \times 5 \text{ mL} = 4 \text{ mL}$$

ASK YOURSELF – Does this answer seem logical, correct, and plausible?

This answer is reasonable and plausible in that it meets the safe standard for the amount of medication given at one time. It is not unusually large or small for a safe dose. It is correct.

Think that the average adult dose is 150 mg, and this estimated child's dose is slightly over half (80 mg) of the adult dose of 150 mg. Therefore, the ordered amount of 80 mg is calculated to be safe.

Then ask yourself if the dose is within the 24-hour safe range as identified by a reliable drug reference. Review the safe dose as indicated in the drug reference and recalculate your math. Think about the calculated dose and volume. Is the answer logical, accurate, and safe? Think about the available medication and notice that there is 20 mg/1mL. You are administering 80 mg, which would equal 4 mL of total volume. More importantly, the ordered dose is within the SDR as you previously determined. To verify these steps, have another nurse check your math.

PRACTICE PROBLEMS 11-3. Practice Problems Using BSA

DIRECTIONS: Using the appropriate nomogram, determine the BSA for each of the following and provide the calculated safe dose. The answers to the problems can be found at the end of the chapter.

1. **Medication Ordered:** Fludarabine 5 mg IV one-time bolus
   Medication Available: Fludarabine 50 mg/2mL
   (Child weighs 25 lbs and is 34 inches tall)
   The SDR is 10 mg/m²/one-time dose.

   Calculation:

Nomogram for Estimating the Surface Area of Infants and Young Children

Nomogram for Estimating the Surface Area of Older Children and Adults

2. **Medication Ordered:** Mitomycin 4 mg IV one time today
   Medication Available: Mitomycin 5 mg/10 mL
   (Child weighs 24 kg and is 30 inches tall)
   The SDR is 10 to 20 mg/m²/one-time dose.

Calculation:

Nomogram for Estimating the Surface Area of Infants and Young Children

Nomogram for Estimating the Surface Area of Older Children and Adults

3. **Medication Ordered:** Methotrexate 15 mg IV weekly
   Medication Available: Methotrexate 25 mg/mL
   (Child weighs 92 lbs and is 60 inches tall)
   The SDR is 20 to 40 mg.

Calculation:

Nomogram for Estimating the Surface Area of Infants and Young Children

Nomogram for Estimating the Surface Area of Older Children and Adults

CALCULATIONS WITH DRUGS THAT ARE IN COMBINATION

There are times when a medication is prescribed for a patient and it is supplied as a combination drug. That means that you must determine the safe dose for both drugs prior to calculating the dose to administer to the patient. Primarily there is one commonly used medication that is supplied as a combination medication, and that is acetaminophen (Tylenol) with codeine.

Formula Method

Consider this example: The prescriber orders acetaminophen (Tylenol) with codeine 1 teaspoon by mouth every 6 hours as necessary for pain. The child's weight is 36 pounds.

STEP 1: CONVERT

First, set up the problem to convert the child's weight to kilograms:

$$36 \text{ lbs} \div 2.2 \text{ lb/kg} = 16.4 \text{ kg}$$

STEP 2: COMPUTE

Next, compute the safe dose for each drug. Since there are two drugs, you must look up the safe dose for acetaminophen (Tylenol) and the safe dose for codeine. For this drug order, the drug reference identifies the safe dose for acetaminophen as 10 to 15 mg/kg/dose every 4 hours, and the safe dose for codeine as 0.5 to 1 mg/kg/dose every 4 hours.

Determine the safe dose per dose of acetaminophen (Tylenol):

$$16.4 \text{ kg} \times 10 \text{ mg/kg} = 164 \text{ mg} \quad \text{(for the minimum safe dose)}$$
$$16.4 \text{ kg} \times 15 \text{ mg/kg} = 246 \text{ mg} \quad \text{(for the maximum safe dose)}$$

Now determine the safe dose for codeine:

$$16.4 \text{ kg} \times 0.5 \text{ mg/kg} = 8.2 \text{ mg} \quad \text{(for the minimum safe dose)}$$
$$16.4 \text{ kg} \times 1 \text{ mg/kg} = 16.4 \text{ mg} \quad \text{(for the maximum safe dose)}$$

The drug is supplied in a unit dose system as 360 mg acetaminophen and 36 mg codeine in 15 mL. The question is: How much acetaminophen and how much codeine is in 1 mL? And how much is in one teaspoon? Remember that 1 teaspoon = 5 mL. Use the formula method to answer these questions.

For acetaminophen, set up the problem:

$$\frac{360 \text{ mg}}{15 \text{ mL}} = 24 \text{ mg/mL}$$

Therefore, there are 24 mg of acetaminophen (Tylenol) in 1 mL. The order is for 1 teaspoon. So multiply:

$$24 \text{ mg/mL} \times 5 \text{ mL/1 teaspoon} = 120 \text{ mg of acetaminophen (Tylenol)/1 teaspoon}$$

For codeine, set up the problem:

$$\frac{36 \text{ mg}}{15 \text{ mL}} = 2.4 \text{ mg/mL}$$

The order is for 1 teaspoon (5 mL). So multiply:

$$2.4 \text{ mg/mL} \times 5 \text{ mL/1 tsp} = 12 \text{ mg of codeine/tsp}$$

Previously, you calculated the safe doses for a child weighing 16.4 kg to be:

$$\text{Acetaminophen (Tylenol)} = 164 \text{ mg to } 246 \text{ mg}$$

$$\text{Codeine} = 8.2 \text{ mg to } 16.4 \text{ mg}$$

Based on your calculations and the dose available, you determine the dose to be acetaminophen (Tylenol) 120 mg with codeine 12 mg per teaspoon (5 mL). Therefore, 1 teaspoon (5 mL) of the combined drug is within the calculated safe dose ranges for each drug.

STEP 3: CRITICALLY THINK

Review the safe dose for both drugs as indicated in the drug reference and recalculate your math. Think about the calculated dose and volume: does the answer make sense and is the answer logical, accurate, and safe? Think about the available medication and remember that for every dose you are administering two medications.

(!) **SAFETY ALERT:** *Whenever possible, use an oral medication syringe to accurately measure the dose, especially when the dose is small. Doing so reduces the chance that the medication will be given intravenously, because an oral syringe will not fit IV tubing.*

Ratio-Proportion Method

Consider this example: The prescriber orders acetaminophen (Tylenol) with codeine 4 mL by mouth every 4 hours as necessary for pain. The child weighs 38 pounds. Use the ratio-proportion method to determine the dose.

STEP 1: CONVERT

First, set up the problem to convert the child's weight to kilograms:

$$38 \text{ lbs} \div 2.2 \text{ lbs/kg} = 17.3 \text{ kg}$$

STEP 2: COMPUTE

Next, compute the safe dose for each drug. Look up the safe dose for acetaminophen (Tylenol) and codeine in a drug reference. For this drug order, the drug reference identifies the safe dose for acetaminophen (Tylenol) as 10 to 15 mg/kg/dose every 4 hours, and the safe dose for codeine as 0.5 to 1 mg/kg/dose every 4 hours for pain.

First, determine the safe dose per dose of acetaminophen (Tylenol):

$$17.3 \text{ kg} \times 10 \text{ mg/kg} = 173 \text{ mg} \qquad \text{(for the minimum safe dose)}$$
$$17.3 \text{ kg} \times 15 \text{ mg/kg} = 260 \text{ mg} \qquad \text{(for the maximum safe dose)}$$

Now determine the safe dose for codeine:

$$17.3 \text{ kg} \times 0.5 \text{ mg/kg} = 8.7 \text{ mg} \qquad \text{(for the minimum safe dose)}$$
$$17.3 \text{ kg} \times 1 \text{ mg/kg} = 17.3 \text{ mg} \qquad \text{(for the maximum safe dose)}$$

The drug is available as acetaminophen (Tylenol) 360 mg with codeine 36 mg/15 mL. Using the ratio-proportion method, calculate the acetaminophen (Tylenol) dose per mL as follows:

$$\frac{360 \text{ mg}}{15 \text{ mL}} = \frac{x}{1}$$

Cross multiply: 15 mL x = 360 mg

Solve for x: x = 24 mg/mL

The desired dose is 4 mL. Therefore,

24 mg $\times$ 4 mL = 96 mg

Using the ratio-proportion method, calculate the codeine dose per mL as follows:

$$\frac{36 \text{ mg}}{15 \text{ mL}} = \frac{x}{1}$$

Cross multiply: 15 mL x = 36 mg

Solve for x: x = 2.4 mg/mL

The desired dose is 4 mL. Therefore,

2.4 mg $\times$ 4 mL = 9.6 mg

The safe range for acetaminophen (Tylenol) is 173 to 260 mg. The safe range for codeine is 8.7 to 17.3 mg. Both drugs are within the SDR.

STEP 3: CRITICALLY THINK

Review the safe dose range for both drugs as indicated in the drug reference and recalculate your math. Think about the calculated dose and volume. Does the answer make sense and is the answer logical, accurate, and safe? Think about the available medication and remember that for every dose you are administering two medications.

CALCULATIONS FOR PEDIATRIC INTRAVENOUS ADMINISTRATION

Chapter 9 describes the equipment, principles, and guidelines for administering intravenous medication. Refer to that chapter for additional information related to intravenous administration.

When preparing to administer a medication by the intravenous route, follow your agency's guidelines and drug reference for the correct dilution and the rate of administration. Adhere to the same procedure when determining the SDR for the prescribed dose. For example, you want to:

- Convert weight to kilograms
- Compute the SDR
- Compare the calculation with the prescribed dose
- Calculate the dose to determine if it is safe for administration
- Critically think and make a decision based on the calculation

Calculation of Pediatric Intravenous Flow Rates

For pediatric patients, intravenous flow rates are calculated in micro-drops. Generally, micro-drip tubing is used delivering 60 micro-drops, which equal 1 mL of solution. Use the following formulas when calculating the flow rate:

$$\text{Drops (gtt)/minute} = \frac{\text{Total mL of IV solution}}{\text{Total infusion time (minutes)}} \times \text{drop factor (gtt/mL)}$$

For example, if 500 mL of fluid were to be administered by micro-drip over 8 hours, the drops/minute would be calculated as follows: First, convert the 8 hours to minutes by multiplying 8 $\times$ 60. The answer is 480 minutes.

Then, use the formula above to calculate the flow rate:

$$\text{Drops/minute} = \frac{500 \text{ mL}}{480 \text{ min}} \times 60 \text{ gtt/mL}$$

$$= \frac{30,000}{480} = 62.5 \text{ gtt/minute} \quad \text{(Round to 63 gtt/min)}$$

Count the drops in the micro-drip tubing chamber to achieve 63 gtt/minute.

Another formula to use with microdriptubing, which is easier to use, is:

$$\frac{500 \text{ mL}}{8 \text{ hours}} \text{ (ordered)} = 62.5 \text{ gtt/minute} \quad \text{(Round to 63 gtt/minute)}$$

(!) **SAFETY ALERT:** *Always double check that you have accurately set the pump for both the volume to infuse per hour and per minute. Pumps are designed to calculate the required flow in milliliters per hour. Therefore, the pump can be set at the precise rate per minute. Use intravenous pumps routinely with children to ensure safety.*

Consider this example; the prescriber has ordered clindamycin (Cleocin) 150 mg IV every 8 hours. The child weighs 11.6 kg. Use the 3-step method to calculate the dose.

STEP 1: CONVERT

The child's weight is already in kilograms, so you do not need to convert pounds to kilograms.

STEP 2: COMPUTE

The drug reference indicates the SDR of clindamycin to be 25 to 50 mg/kg/8 hours not to exceed 6 grams/24 hours. First, determine the safe dosage per day and per dose. Set up the problem:

Minimum SDR:	25 mg/kg × 11.6 kg = 290 mg/day
Maximum SDR:	50 mg/kg × 11.6 kg = 580 mg/day

The safe range is 290 to 580 mg/day.

The ordered dose is   150 mg × 3 doses = 450 mg/day

Therefore, the order for clindamycin (Cleocin) 150 mg is within the SDR.

Next, calculate the actual dose for administration by using the formula method. The preparation supplied by the pharmacy provides the medication as 150 mg/mL. Set up the problem using the formula method:

$$\frac{150 \text{ mg}}{150 \text{ mg}} \times 1 \text{ mL}$$

In this problem, because mg appears in both the numerator and denominator, mg is cancelled out and mL is left as the volume of medication in the answer.

$$\frac{150 \ \cancel{\text{mg}}}{150 \ \cancel{\text{mg}}} = 1 \text{ mL}$$

$$\frac{1}{1} \times 1 \text{ mL} = 1 \text{ mL}$$

Therefore, you are to administer 1 mL of the drug.

The reference also states that the drug must be diluted. According to the reference, each 18 mg must be diluted with 1 mL of sodium chloride (NaCl) for safe dilution. Since the child is to receive 150 mg, set up the problem as follows:

$$150 \text{ mg} \div 18 \text{ mg/mL} = 8.33 \text{ mL}$$

Dilute with 8.33 mL + 1 mL (previously calculated) = 9.33 mL to be administered over 1/2 hour by infusion pump. Doing this would require setting the pump at 18.7 mL/hour to administer 9.33 mL in 30 minutes.

CRITICALLY THINK

ASK YOURSELF – Is the dose within the 24-hour safe range as identified by a reliable drug reference?

Review the safe dose as indicated in the drug reference and recalculate your math. Think about the calculated dose and volume. Is the answer logical, accurate, and safe? Think about the available medication and notice that there is 150 mg/1 mL. Therefore, you are administering 150 mg, which would equal 1 mL. It is important that the ordered dose is within the SDR as you determined, and that you have set the pump at the accurate setting. As always, have another nurse check your math.

 ## CASE STUDY

You are preparing to administer David's ceftazidime, ordered as 40 mg/kg intravenously every 8 hours.

STEP 1: CONVERT

Recall from a previous calculation that you determined David's weight to be 4.6 kg. If you hadn't converted his weight in pounds earlier, you would convert it now.

STEP 2: COMPUTE

The drug reference indicates that the SDR for ceftazidime for infants and children IM or IV is 90 to 150 mg/kg/24 hours to be given in divided doses every 8 hours.

The recommended concentration is 40 mg/mL in 5% dextrose and water (D5W), normal saline (NS), or Ringer's lactate (RL) by intermittent infusion over 10 to 30 minutes.

Determine the minimum and maximum safe dose:

$$4.6 \text{ kg} \times 90 \text{ mg/kg/day} = 414 \text{ mg/day} \quad \text{(for the minimum dose)}$$

$$4.6 \text{ kg} \times 150 \text{ mg/kg/day} = 690 \text{ mg/day} \quad \text{(for the maximum dose)}$$

If David receives ceftazidime 200 mg, 3 times per day, that would be:

$$200 \text{ mg} \times 3 \text{ doses} = 600 \text{ mg/day}; \quad \text{therefore, the dose is safe.}$$

The vial of ceftazidime contains 500 mg. The directions are to mix 5 mL NS into the vial so there is 90 mg/1 mL.

$$\frac{D}{H} \times V = A$$

$$\frac{200 \text{ mg}}{90 \text{ mg}} \times 1 \text{ mL}$$

In this problem, because mg appears in both the numerator and denominator, mg is cancelled out and mL is left as the volume of medication in the answer.

$$\frac{200 \; \cancel{mg}}{90 \; \cancel{mg}} \times 1 \; mL = 2.2 \; mL$$

Therefore, there are 200 mg/2.2 mL. However, the dose is concentrated, so for intermittent IV infusion you need to add 50 mL of 0.9% NaCl to the 2.2 mL and administer over $\frac{1}{2}$ hour for safe administration. When you add 50 mL + 2.2 mL, that will bring the total volume to 52.2 mL. To infuse over $\frac{1}{2}$ hour, you would set the infusion pump at 104.4 mL/hr.

STEP 3: CRITICALLY THINK

ASK YOURSELF – Does this answer seem logical, correct, and plausible?

This answer is reasonable and plausible in that it meets the safe standard for the amount of medication given at one time. It is not unusually large or small for a safe dose. Think that after you did the calculation the drug is to be further diluted and be sure that you added the original calculated answer of 2.2 mL to the 50 mL so you can administer the correct amount of medication over the correct amount of time. To verify the calculation, have another nurse check your math.

Critical Thinking/Decision Making Exercise

A child weighs 40 lbs 7 oz and has pneumonia. His breathing is rapid and he is congested, but he has no history of any fever. The prescriber orders ceftriaxone sodium (Rocephin) 900 mg IV every 12 hours. The dose on hand is ceftriaxone sodium (Rocephin) 1 gm. The label on the bottle states to dilute 1 gram of powdered ceftriaxone sodium (Rocephin) with 9.6 mL of NS to equal 100 mg/mL.

What Should the Nurse Do First?

First, the nurse needs to convert the child's weight to kg and remember to determine the ounces as a part of the pounds by dividing the 7 ounces by 16 ounces.

Next, calculate the drug dosages to determine the SDR and the safety of the dose to administer. Then, the nurse would need to calculate the total mL to use to reconstitute the drug and to administer it once he or she has determined the safety of the dose ordered.

What Actions Are Necessary to Ensure Accuracy and Safety?

To ensure accuracy and safety, use the 3-step method.

STEP 1: CONVERT

Convert the pounds to kilograms.

Child weighs 40 lbs 7 oz.

$$7 \; oz \div 16 \; oz/lb = 0.4375 \; lb \quad \text{(Round to 0.44 lb)}$$

$$40 \; lbs + 0.44 \; lb = 40.44 \; lbs$$

$$40.44 \; lbs \div 2.2 \; kg/lb = 18.4 \; kg$$

STEP 2: COMPUTE

The order reads: ceftriaxone sodium (Rocephin) 900 mg IV every 12 hours. The drug reference states that neonates to children younger than 12 years should receive 50 to 75 mg/kg for a maximum of

2 g daily given in two divided doses every 12 hours. First, determine the safe dosage per day and per dose. Set up the problem:

$$\text{Minimum SDR} = 18.4 \text{ kg} \times 50 \text{ mg/kg/day} = 920 \text{ mg/day}$$

$$\text{Divide } 920 \text{ mg/day by 2 doses/day} = 460 \text{ mg/dose}$$

$$\text{Maximum SDR} = 18.4 \text{ kg} \times 75 \text{ mg/kg/day} = 1380 \text{ mg/day}$$

$$\text{Divide } 1{,}380 \text{ mg/day by 2 doses/day} = 690 \text{ mg/dose}$$

Therefore, the ordered dose of 900 mg every 12 hours would be a total per day of 1,800 mg/day. You recognize that the dose ordered is larger than the maximum SDR for this patient. It is important that you clarify the ordered dose with the prescriber.

The prescriber changes the dose ordered to 500 mg/dose to be given IV every 12 hours. You now determine that the dose is within the SDR.

You have available Rocephin 1 g, which must be reconstituted according to the label directions. You follow the label directions and add 9.6 mL of normal saline to the medication, resulting in 100 mg/mL. Remember that the powder takes up space, so the actual total volume is 10 mL.

Then use the formula method:

$$\frac{D}{H} \times V = A$$

$$\frac{500 \text{ mg}}{100 \text{ mg}} \times 1 \text{ mL} = 5 \text{ mL} \qquad \text{(which is concentrated)}$$

$$\frac{500 \text{ mg}}{1000 \text{ mg}} \times 10 \text{ mL}$$

In this problem, because mg appears in both the numerator and denominator, mg is cancelled out and mL is left as the volume of medication in the answer.

Reduce the fraction:

$$\frac{500 \text{ mg}}{1000 \text{ mg}} = \frac{5}{10}$$

$$\frac{5 \text{ mg}}{10 \text{ mg}} \times 10 \text{ mL}$$

$$\frac{5}{10} \times 10 \text{ mL} = 5 \text{ mL}$$

Therefore, you would administer 5 mL.

The drug reference states that you are to have a concentration of 10 to 40 mg/mL in D5W, NS with a maximum concentration of 40 mg/mL. Administer by intermittent infusion over 10 to 30 minutes.

Next, divide $\qquad$ $500 \text{ mg} \div 40 \text{ mg/mL} = 12.5 \text{ mL}$

Therefore, dilute the ceftriaxone sodium (Rocephin) concentrate with 12.5 mL:

$$5 \text{ mL} + 12.5 \text{ mL} = 17.5 \text{ mL}$$

The answer is to administer 17.5 mL and, according to the drug reference, to give this over $\frac{1}{2}$ hour.

STEP 3: CRITICALLY THINK

ASK YOURSELF *– Did you calculate the pounds and ounces correctly, and does this answer seem logical, correct, and plausible?*

This answer is reasonable and plausible since the prescriber adjusted the dose to be within the SDR and this changed dose meets the safe standard for the amount of medication given at one time. It is important to dilute this medication further so it would not be too concentrated to administer by intermittent infusion. Think that through careful calculation you were able to prevent an overdose from being administered to this child. Therefore, the ordered amount of 500 mg is calculated to be safe. To verify this step, have another nurse check your math.

CHAPTER REVIEW PROBLEMS

1. The order reads: ibuprofen 330 mg every 6 hours orally as needed for pain or fever. The child's weight is 33 kg. The drug reference states the safe dose as 5 to 10 mg/kg/dose.
   a. Calculate the minimum and maximum safe dose to determine if the ordered dose is safe.
   b. If the pharmacy supplies the ibuprofen 100 mg/teaspoon, how many mL will you administer?

2. The child's weight is 10 lbs 6 oz and the doctor orders Valium 2 mg by mouth every 6 hours as needed for agitation. The SDR for ages 6 months to 12 years is 0.12 to 0.8 mg/kg/24 hrs in divided doses every 6-8 hours.
   a. Calculate the SDR and calculate the child's weight in kg.
   b. What is the appropriate action after determining the SDR and comparing it with the ordered dose for this child?

3. A child's weight is 11 lbs 5 oz. The child is to receive ceftazidime 250 mg every 8 hours. Calculate the SDR for this child and the amount of dilution for administration of the drug. The dilution is 10 mL NS so that 1 mL = 100 mg. The SDR for infants and children is 90 to 150 mg/kg/24 hours in divided doses every 8 hours.

4. A child weighs 31.7 kg and is to receive valproate 250 mg every 6 hours. The drug is supplied as 250 mg/mL. The SDR is 15 to 60 mg/kg/24 hours. Determine the safe dose and the amount to be given.

5. A child weighs 30 lbs 5 oz. Convert the child's weight to kg, and then calculate the SDR for the order of morphine sulfate 1 to 2 mg IV as needed every 2 to 4 hours for pain. The SDR for IV administration is 0.1 to 0.2 mg/kg/dose every 2 to 4 hours. The recommended concentration for IV administration is 5 mg/mL of D5W over 4 to 5 minutes. The dose available is 10 mg/mL.

Answers to Practice Problems

Practice Problem Answers 11-1

1. **Medication Ordered:** Ceclor suspension 200 mg orally every 8 hours

   Medication Available: Ceclor suspension 125 mg/5 mL

   The safe range for Ceclor is 6.7 to 13.4 mg/kg every 8 hours. Calculate the safe dose range.

   Child weighs 40 lbs

   $$40 \text{ lbs} \div 2.2 \text{ lbs/kg} = 18.2 \text{ kg}$$

   $$18.2 \text{ kg} \times 6.7 \text{ mg/kg/8 hours} = 121.94 \text{ mg/8 hours is the minimum safe dose.}$$

   $$18.2 \text{ kg} \times 13.4 \text{ mg/kg/8 hours} = 243.88 \text{ mg/8 hours is the maximum safe dose.}$$

   The safe dose range is 121.94 to 243.88 mg every 8 hours. Therefore, 200 mg every 8 hours is a safe dose.

   To calculate the medication dose using the available Ceclor suspension, 125 mg/5 mL:

   $$\frac{D}{H} \times V = \frac{200 \text{ mg}}{125 \text{ mg}} \times 5 \text{ mL} = \frac{1000 \text{ mL}}{125} = 8 \text{ mL}$$

   You would give 8 mL.

2. **Medication Ordered:** Furosemide liquid 15 mg PO daily

   Medication Available: Furosemide liquid 40 mg/5 mL

   Child weighs 30 lbs

   The safe dose for furosemide is 2 mg/kg PO daily.

   Convert weight to kg: $30 \text{ lbs} \div 2.2 \text{ lbs/kg} = 13.6 \text{ kg}$

   Calculate the SDR:

   $$13.6 \text{ kg} \times 2 \text{ mg/kg} = 27.2 \text{ mg daily is the safe dose range of furosemide.}$$

   Therefore, 15 mg PO daily is safe.

   To calculate the medication dosage using the available furosemide liquid 40 mg/5 mL:

   $$\frac{D}{H} \times V = \frac{15 \text{ mg}}{40 \text{ mg}} \times 5 \text{ mL} = 1.87 \text{ mL} \quad \text{(Round to 1.9 mL)}$$

3. **Medication Ordered:** Ampicillin 200 mg every 6 hours

   Medication Available: Ampicillin suspension 125 mg/5 mL

   Safe range = 25 to 50 mg/kg/day equally divided every 6 hours.

   Child weighs 47 lbs

   Convert weight to kg: $47 \text{ lb} \div 2.2 \text{ lb/kg} = 21.4 \text{ mkg}$

   Minimum SDR: $21.4 \text{ kg} \times 25 \text{ mg/kg/day} = 535 \text{ mg/day/4 doses} = 133.8 \text{ mg/dose}$

   Maximum SDR: $21.4 \text{ kg} \times 50 \text{ mg/kg/day} = 1{,}070 \text{ mg/day/4 doses} = 267.5 \text{ mg/dose}$

   Therefore, 200 mg is within the safe range.

   $$\frac{200 \text{ mg}}{125 \text{ mg}} \times 5 \text{ mL} = \frac{1000 \text{ mL}}{125} = 8 \text{ mL}$$

4. **Medication Ordered:** Lasix 10 mg PO 3 times a day

   Medication Available: Lasix 15 mg/mL

   Child weighs 18 lbs 4 ounces

   The safe range is 1 to 2 mg/kg every 6 to 8 hours not to exceed 6 mg/kg/day.

   Convert the weight to kg.

Convert ounces to pounds:

$$4 \text{ oz} \div 16 \text{ oz/lb} = 0.25 \text{ lb}$$

Then, add to determine the total pounds:

$$18 + 0.25 = 18.25 \text{ lbs}$$

Next, convert the pounds to kilograms:

$$18.25 \text{ lbs} \div 2.2 \text{ lbs/kg} = 8.3 \text{ kg}$$

Minimum safe dose: $8.3 \text{ kg} \times 1 \text{ mg} = 8.3 \text{ mg} \times 3 \text{ doses} = 24.9 \text{ mg/day}$

Maximum safe dose: $8.3 \text{ kg} \times 2 \text{ mg} = 16.6 \text{ mg} \times 3 \text{ doses} = 49.8 \text{ mg/day}$

Therefore, 10 mg/dose is within the safe range.

$$\frac{10 \text{ mg}}{15 \text{ mg}} \times 1 \text{ mL} = 0.67 \text{ mL} \quad \text{(Round to 0.7 mL every 8 hours)}$$

5. **Medication Ordered:** Ibuprofen 60 mg PO every 6 hours

   Medication Available: Ibuprofen suspension 100 mg/5 mL

   Child weighs 26 lbs

   The safe range is 5 to 10 mg/kg every 6 to 8 hours for a maximum of 40 mg/kg/day.

   Convert weight to kg:

$$26 \text{ lbs} \div 2.2 \text{ lbs/kg} = 11.8 \text{ kg}$$

   Minimum SDR: $11.8 \text{ kg} \times 5 \text{ mg/kg} = 59 \text{ mg} \times 4 \text{ doses/day} = 236 \text{ mg/day}$

   Maximum SDR: $11.8 \text{ kg} \times 10 \text{ mg/kg} = 118 \text{ mg} \times 4 \text{ doses/day} = 472 \text{ mg/day}$

   Dose ordered = 60 mg × 4 doses = 240 mg. Dose is safe.

$$\frac{60 \text{ mg}}{100 \text{ mg}} \times 5 \text{ mL} = \frac{300 \text{ mL}}{100} = 3 \text{ mL/dose}$$

6. **Medication Ordered:** Biaxin 200 mg twice a day

   Medication Available: Biaxin 125 mg/5 mL

   Child weighs 68 lbs

   The safe dose range is 7.5 mg/kg every 12 hours.

   Convert weight to kg:

$$68 \text{ lbs} \div 2.2 \text{ lbs/kg} = 30.9 \text{ kg}$$

   Compute safe dose:

$$30.9 \text{ kg} \times 7.5 \text{ mg/kg/12 hours} = 231.75 \text{ mg/12 hours} \times 2 = 463.5 \text{ mg/day}$$

   Ordered dose of 200 mg, twice per day is safe.

$$\frac{200 \text{ mg}}{125 \text{ mg}} \times 5 \text{ mL} = \frac{1000 \text{ mL}}{125} = 8 \text{ mL}$$

   Answer = 8 mL

Practice Problem Answers 11-2

1. **Medication Ordered:** Clindamycin 150 mg PO every 6 hours

   Medication Available: Clindamycin suspension 75 mg/5 mL

   Child weighs 76 lbs

   The safe dose range is 8 to 25 mg/kg/day.

Convert weight to kg:

$$76 \text{ lbs} \div 2.2 \text{ lbs/kg} = 34.5 \text{ kg}$$

Minimum SDR: $34.5 \text{ kg} \times 8 \text{ mg/kg/day} = 276 \text{ mg/day}$

Maximum SDR: $34.5 \text{ kg} \times 25 \text{ mg/kg/day} = 862.5 \text{ mg/day}$

Drug order: $150 \text{ mg/dose} \times 4 \text{ doses/day} = 600 \text{ mg/day}$

The dose is safe.

$$\frac{75 \text{ mg}}{5 \text{ mL}} = \frac{150 \text{ mg}}{x} = \frac{75 \text{ mg}}{5 \text{ mL}} \quad\rlap{$\times$}\quad \frac{150 \text{ mg}}{x} = 75 \text{ mg } x = 750 \text{ mg} \times \text{mL}$$

$$\frac{75 \text{ mg } x}{75 \text{ mg}} = \frac{750 \text{ mg} \times \text{mL}}{75 \text{ mg}} = \frac{750 \text{ mL}}{75} = 10 \text{ mL}$$

Answer = 10 mL

2. **Medication Ordered:** Zantac 50 mg PO every 12 hours

   Medication Available: Zantac 15 mg/mL

   Child weighs 28 lbs 6 oz

   The safe range is 5 to 10 mg/kg/day divided into two doses.

   Convert the weight to kg; convert ounces to pounds:

   $$6 \text{ oz} \div 16 \text{ oz/lb} = 0.375 \text{ lb}$$

   Then, add to determine the total pounds:

   $$28 + 0.375 = 28.375 \text{ lbs}$$

   Next, convert the pounds to kilograms:

   $$28.375 \text{ lbs} \div 2.2 \text{ lbs/kg} = 12.9 \text{ kg}$$

   Minimum SDR: $12.9 \text{ kg} \times 5 \text{ mg/kg/day} = 64.5 \text{ mg/day/2 doses} = 32.25 \text{ mg/dose}$

   Maximum SDR: $12.9 \text{ kg} \times 10 \text{ mg/kg/day} = 129 \text{ mg/day/2 doses} = 64.5 \text{ mg/dose}$

   Therefore, the dose of 50 mg is safe.

   $$\frac{15 \text{ mg}}{1 \text{ mL}} = \frac{50 \text{ mg}}{x \text{ mL}} = \frac{15 \text{ mg}}{1 \text{ mL}} \quad\rlap{$\times$}\quad \frac{50 \text{ mg}}{x} = 15 \text{ mg } x = 50 \text{ mg} \times 1 \text{ mL}$$

   $$\frac{15 \text{ mg } x}{15 \text{ mg}} = \frac{50 \text{ mg}}{15 \text{ mg}} = 3.3 \text{ mL}$$

3. **Medication Ordered:** Penicillin V suspension 0.2 g PO every 8 hours

   Medication Available: Penicillin V suspension 125 mg/5 mL

   Child weighs 42 lbs

   The safe range is 15 to 62.5 mg/kg daily divided every 4 to 8 hours.

   First, convert grams to mg by moving the decimal 3 places to the right: 0.2 g becomes 200 mg. Remember there are 1,000 mg in 1 gram.

   Convert weight to kg:

   $$42 \text{ lb} \div 2.2 \text{ lbs/kg} = 19.1 \text{ kg}$$

   Minimum SDR: $19.1 \text{ kg} \times 15 \text{ mg/kg/day} = 286.5 \text{ mg/day/3 doses} = 95.5 \text{ mg/dose}$

   Maximum SDR: $19.1 \text{ kg} \times 62.5 \text{ mg/kg/day} = 1193.75 \text{ mg/day/3 doses} = 397.9 \text{ mg/dose}$

   The dose is safe.

   $$\frac{125 \text{ mg}}{5 \text{ mL}} = \frac{200 \text{ mg}}{x} = \frac{125 \text{ mg}}{5 \text{ mL}} \quad\rlap{$\times$}\quad \frac{200 \text{ mg}}{x} = 125 \text{ mg } x = 1000 \text{ mg} \times \text{mL}$$

   $$\frac{125 \text{ mg } x}{125 \text{ mg}} = \frac{1000 \text{ mg} \times \text{mL}}{125 \text{ mg}} = \frac{1000 \text{ mL}}{125} = 8 \text{ mL}$$

4. **Medication Ordered:** Phenobarbital 10 mg PO every 12 hours

   Medication Available: Phenobarbital 15 mg/5 mL

   Child's Weight: 38 lbs

   Safe dosage range is 1 to 6 mg/kg in two divided doses, not to exceed 100 mg/day.

   Convert weight to kg:

   $$38 \text{ lbs} \div 2.2 \text{ lbs/kg} = 17.3 \text{ kg}$$

   Minimum SDR: 17.3 kg × 1 mg/kg = 17.3 mg/2 doses = 8.65 mg/dose

   Maximum SDR: 17.3 kg × 6 mg/kg = 103.8 mg/2 doses = 51.9, mg/dose

   The dose is safe.

   $$\frac{15 \text{ mg}}{5 \text{ mL}} = \frac{10 \text{ mg}}{x} = \frac{15 \text{ mg}}{5 \text{ mL}} \diagdown\!\!\!\!\diagup \frac{10 \text{ mg}}{x} = 15 \text{ mg } x = 50 \text{ mg} \times \text{mL}$$

   $$\frac{15 \text{ mg } x}{15 \text{ mg}} = \frac{50 \text{ mg} \times \text{mL}}{15 \text{ mg}} = \frac{50 \text{ mL}}{15} = 3.3 \text{ mL}$$

5. **Medication Ordered:** Morphine 2 mg subcutaneous every 6 hours

   Medication Available: Morphine 1 mg/mL for subcutaneous injection

   Child weighs 46 lbs.

   The safe range is 0.1 to 0.2 mg/kg/day in 4 divided doses.

   Convert weight to kg:

   $$46 \text{ lbs} \div 2.2 \text{ lbs/kg} = 20.9 \text{ kg}$$

   Minimum SDR: 20.9 kg × 0.1 mg/kg = 2.09 mg × 4 = 8.36   (Round to 8.4 mg/day)

   Maximum SDR: 20.9 kg × 0.2 mg/kg = 4.18 mg × 4 = 16.72   (Round to 16.7 mg/day)

   The ordered dose of 2 mg is safe.

   $$\frac{1 \text{ mg}}{1 \text{ mL}} = \frac{2 \text{ mg}}{x} = \frac{1 \text{ mg}}{1 \text{ mL}} \diagdown\!\!\!\!\diagup \frac{2 \text{ mg}}{x} = 1 \text{ mg } x = 2 \text{ mg} \times \text{mL}$$

   $$\frac{1 \text{ mg } x}{1 \text{ mg}} = \frac{2 \text{ mg} \times \text{mL}}{1 \text{ mg}} = 2 \text{ mL subcutaneous}$$

Practice Problem Answers 11-3

1. **Medication Ordered:** Fludarabine 5 mg IV one time

   Medication Available: Fludarabine 50 mg/2 mL

   Child weighs 25 lbs and is 34 inches tall.

   Convert the pounds to kilograms: 25 lbs ÷ 2.2 lbs/kg = 11.4 kg

   Determine the surface area by using the chart for infants and children. Draw a straight line between the height on the left and the weight in kilograms on the right. You determine the BSA to be 0.5 m².

Nomogram for Estimating the Surface Area of Infants and Young Children

The drug reference indicates the SDR to be 10 mg/m²/one-time dose. The safe dose according to the drug reference is

$$10 \text{ mg/m}^2 \times 0.5 \text{ m}^2 = 5 \text{ mg/day}$$

Therefore, the ordered dose of 5 mg/day is safe.

$$\frac{5 \text{ mg}}{50 \text{ mg}} \times 2 \text{ mL} = \frac{10 \text{ mL}}{50} = 0.2 \text{ mL}$$

Give 0.2 mL.

2. **Medication Ordered:** Mitomycin 4 mg IV today

Medication Available: Mitomycin 5 mg/10 mL

Child weighs 24.0 kg and is 30 inches tall.

Using the nomogram for infants and young children, you determine the BSA to be 0.64 m^2.

Nomogram for Estimating the Surface Area of Infants and Young Children

Height		Surface Area	Weight	
feet	centimeters	in square meters	pounds	kilograms

The drug reference indicates the SDR to be 10 to 20 mg/m^2/one-time dose.

Minimum SDR: 10 mg/m^2 × 0.64 m^2 = 6.4 mg/day.

Maximum SDR: 20 mg/m^2 × 0.64 m^2 = 12.8 mg/day.

Therefore, the ordered dose of 4 mg as a one-time dose is safe.

$$\frac{4\ mg}{5\ mg} \times 10\ mL = \frac{4}{5} \times 10\ mL = 8\ mL$$

Give 8 mL.

3. **Medication Ordered:** Methotrexate 15 mg IV weekly

   Medication Available: Methotrexate 25 mg/mL

Child weighs 92 lbs and is 60 inches tall.

The SDR is 20 to 40 mg.

Use the nomogram for older children and adults to determine BSA, which would be 1.33 m^2.

**Nomogram for Estimating the Surface Area
of Older Children and Adults**

Height		Surface Area	Weight	
feet	centimeters	in square meters	pounds	kilograms

$$\frac{\text{Child's BSA (m}^2)}{\text{Average adult's BSA (1.73 m}^2)} \times \text{Average adult dose of drug} = \text{Estimated child's dose}$$

Minimum SDR: $\dfrac{1.33 \text{ m}^2}{1.73 \text{ m}^2} \times 20 \text{ mg} = 15.4 \text{ mg}$

Maximum SDR: $\dfrac{1.33 \text{ m}^2}{1.73 \text{ m}^2} \times 40 \text{ mg} = 30.8 \text{ mg}$

The order for 15 mg is less than the minimum SDR and is therefore safe.

$$\frac{15 \text{ mg}}{25 \text{ mg}} \times 1 \text{ mL} = 0.6 \text{ mL}$$

Give 0.6 mL.

Answers to Chapter Review Problems

Chapter Review Problem Answers 11-1

1. The order reads: ibuprofen 330 mg every 6 hours orally as needed for pain or fever. The child's weight is 33 kg. The drug reference states the safe dose as 5 to 10 mg/kg/dose.

   a. Calculate the minimum and maximum safe dose to determine if the ordered dose is safe.

   Minimum SDR: 33 kg $\times$ 5 mg/kg = 165 mg/dose

   Maximum SDR: 33 kg $\times$ 10 mg/kg = 330 mg/dose

   The order is for 330 mg, so the dose is safe.

   b. Ibuprofen is supplied as 100 mg/teaspoon

   1 tsp = 5 mL, so set up the problem as follows:

   $$\frac{330 \text{ mg}}{100 \text{ mg}} \times 5 \text{ mL} = 16.5 \text{ mL}$$

   The correct answer is 16.5 mL.

2. The child's weight is 10 lbs 6 oz and the doctor orders Valium 2 mg by mouth every 6 hours as needed for agitation.

   a. Calculate the SDR and child's weight in kilograms.

   Convert the child's weight to kg: 6 oz $\div$ 16 oz/lb = 0.375 lb. + 10 lbs = 10.375 lbs

   10.375 lbs $\div$ 2.2 lbs/kg = 4.716, or 4.72 kg

   The drug ordered is diazepam (Valium) 2 mg. The drug reference indicates that SDR for diazepam (Valium) for ages 6 months to 12 years should be 0.12 to 0.8 mg/kg/24 hours in divided doses every 6 to 8 hours. Calculate the safe range for this child:

   4.72 kg $\times$ 0.12 = 0.566 minimum

   4.72 kg $\times$ 0.8 = 3.776 maximum

   Therefore, the safe range based on this order is 0.57 to 3.78 mg/day.

   Administering every 6 hours would equal 4 times within a 24-hour period, so calculate the SDR/dose:

   0.57 mg/4 = 0.14 mg minimum

   3.78 mg/4 = 0.944 mg maximum

   b. What is the appropriate action after you have determined the SDR and compared it with the ordered dose for this child?

   The ordered dose exceeds the SDR of 0.12 to 0.8 mg/kg/24 hours in divided doses every 6 to 8 hours. So the order for diazepam (Valium) 2 mg is a high dose, and the nurse needs to notify the physician.

3. A child's weight is 11 lbs 5 oz. The child is to receive ceftazidime 250 mg every 8 hours. Calculate the SDR for this child and the amount of dilution for administration of the drug.

   The SDR for ceftazidime IM or IV for infants and children is 90 to 150 mg/kg/24 hours in divided doses every 8 hours. The dilution is for the dose to be 40 mg/mL.

   Convert weight to kg: 5 oz $\div$ 16 oz/lb = 0.3125 + 11 = 11.3125 lbs $\div$ 2.2 lbs/kg = 5.14 kg

   Minimum SDR: 5.14 kg $\times$ 90 mg/kg/day = 462.6 mg/day

   Maximum SDR: 5.14 kg $\times$ 150 mg/kg/day = 771 mg/day

   The child receives 250 mg three times/day, which equals 750 mg/day.

   Critically think: The dose is safe.

   Next: dilute ceftazidime $\dfrac{250 \text{ mg}}{40 \text{ mg}} \times 1 \text{ mL} = 6.25 \text{ mL}$

Mix 10 mL NS so that 1 mL = 100 mg

$$\frac{D}{H} \times V = A$$

$$\frac{250 \text{ mg}}{100 \text{ mg}} \times 1 \text{ mL} = 2.5 \text{ mL}$$

Therefore, dilute 6.25 mL + 2.5 mL = 8.75 mL, and give over $\frac{1}{2}$ hour.

4. A child weighs 31.7 kg and is to receive valproate 250 mg every 6 hours. The SDR according to the drug reference is: children and adults 15 to 60 mg/kg/24 hours. Calculate the SDR for this child based on weight.

   Minimum SDR: 31.7 kg × 15 mg/kg/24 hours = 475.5 mg/24 hours

   Maximum SDR: 31.7 kg × 60 mg/kg/24 hours = 1902 mg/24 hours

   The child is to receive valproate 250 mg 4 times per day.

   250 mg × 4 = 1000 mg,   so the total dose falls within the safe range.

$$\frac{D}{H} \times V = A$$

$$\frac{250 \text{ mg}}{250 \text{ mg}} \times 1 \text{ mL} = 1 \text{ mL to be given}$$

5. A child weighs 30 lbs 5 oz. Convert the child's weight to kg, and then calculate the SDR for the order of morphine sulfate 1 to 2 mg IV as needed every 2 to 4 hours for pain. The recommended concentration for IV administration is 5 mg/mL of D5W over 4 to 5 minutes. The dose available is 10 mg/mL.

   Convert the weight: 5 oz ÷ 16 oz/lb = 0.3125 lbs + 30 lbs = 30.3125 lbs ÷ 2.2 lbs/kg = 13.78 kg

   The reference indicates the SDR for IV administration is 0.1 to 0.2 mg/kg/dose every 2 to 4 hours.

   Minimum SDR: 13.78 kg × 0.1 mg/kg = 1.378 mg

   Maximum SDR: 13.78 kg × 0.2 mg/kg = 2.756 mg

   The SDR is 1.4 to 2.8 mg; it is safe.

   Since the dosage on hand (10 mg/mL) is twice as strong as the recommended dosage (5 mg/mL), you need to mix it with another mL of D5W to achieve the recommended concentration.

   Set up the problem using the formula method:

$$\frac{2 \text{ mg}}{10 \text{ mg}} \times 2 \text{ mL} = 0.4 \text{ mL}$$

   In this problem, because mg appears in both the numerator and denominator, mg is cancelled out and mL is left as the volume of medication in the answer. Therefore, you would administer 0.4 mL of the diluted medication over 4 to 5 minutes.

   To calculate this problem using the ratio-proportion method, set up the problem as follows:

$$\frac{10 \text{ mg}}{1 \text{ mL}} = \frac{2 \text{ mg}}{x}$$

   Cross multiply:

$$\frac{10 \text{ mg}}{1 \text{ mL}} \diagdown \frac{2 \text{ mg}}{x}$$

$$10 \text{ mg } x = 2 \text{ mg} \times 1 \text{ mL}$$

   Isolate the x by dividing both sides by 10 mg. Milligrams (mg) in the numerator and denominator cancel each other out and mL is left as the volume of medication in the answer.

$$\frac{10 \text{ mg } x}{10 \text{ mg}} = \frac{2 \text{ mg} \times \text{mL}}{10 \text{ mg}}$$

   Solve for x.

$$x = \frac{2 \text{ mL}}{10} = 0.2 \text{ mL}$$

The answer is to give 0.2 mL, which is to be diluted in 1 mL D5W and administered over 4 to 5 minutes.

Comprehensive Practice Test

The answers to the problems can be found at the end of the test.

DIRECTIONS: Solve the problem and reduce any fractions to lowest terms.

1. $6\frac{7}{8} \div \frac{4}{5}$

2. $\frac{5}{6} + \frac{7}{8} + \frac{1}{4}$

3. $\frac{7}{9} \times \frac{3}{5}$

4. $\frac{6}{11} \div \frac{3}{4}$

5. 2.86×0.45

6. $10.64 \div 4.2$

7. Convert the Roman numeral to an Arabic number: XXVIII

8. Convert the fraction to a mixed number: $\frac{57}{6}$

9. Convert the fraction to a decimal: $\frac{11}{13}$

10. Solve for x: $\frac{24}{32} = \frac{x}{12}$

DIRECTIONS: Convert the following.

11. 2,000 mg = _____ g

12. 2.75 L = _____ mL

13. 1,450 mcg = _____ mg

14. 480 mg = gr _____

15. 450 mL = _____ L

16. 1.5 kg = _____ g

17. 360 mL = _____ ounces

18. 4 teaspoons = _____ mL

19. 75 mL = _____ tablespoons

20. gr X = _____ mg

DIRECTIONS: Mark each syringe at the prescribed level of medication.

21. 21 units of insulin

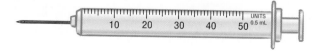

22. 36 units of insulin

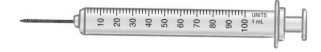

23. 0.44 mL

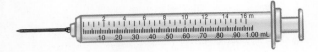

24. 0.8 mL

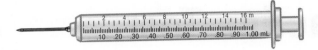

25. 2.7 mL

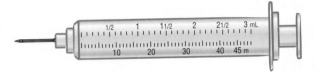

26. 1.3 mL

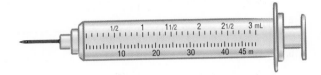

DIRECTIONS: Identify how much medication is in each syringe.

27.

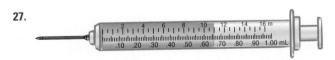

28.

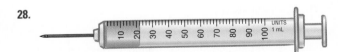

29.

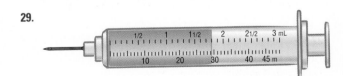

30.

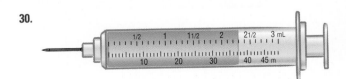

DIRECTIONS: Give the correct term for each abbreviation.

31. prn

32. q.i.d.

33. O.D.

34. noc

DIRECTIONS: Give the correct abbreviation for each term.

35. before meals

36. every 3 hours

37. intramuscular

DIRECTIONS: Identify which part of the medication order is missing from each drug order.

38. July 24, 2006
Susannah Jordan
furosemide (Lasix) 40 mg PO
Dr. Thomlinson

39. February 2, 2005
Coumadin 2 mg PO daily
Dr. Allen

40. September 4, 2006
Stanley Jameson
Robitussin every 4 hours prn for cough
Dr. Wilking

DIRECTIONS: Use the medication labels to identify the components requested.

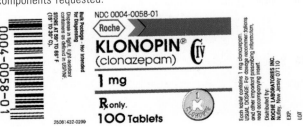

Hoffman-La Roche, Inc. Used with permission.

41. Generic name

42. National Drug Code Number

43. Storage

44. Medication form

45. Medication dose

ROMAZICON®
(flumazenil)
INJECTION Multiple Use Vial
0.5 mg/5 mL
(0.1 mg/mL) 5 mL Vial
Sterile.
For I.V. Use.
USUAL DOSAGE:
See Package Insert.
STORE AT 59° TO 86° F
(15° TO 30° C).
Roche Laboratories Inc.
Nutley, New Jersey 07110
24992712-0798

EXP.
LOT

Hoffman-La Roche, Inc. Used with permission.

46. Brand name

47. Medication strength

48. Medication quantity

49. Manufacturer's name

50. Generic name

51. Identify the six rights of medication administration.

  1. _____

  2. _____

  3. _____

  4. _____

  5. _____

  6. _____

DIRECTIONS: Calculate the medication dosage for the oral medications using the formula method.

52. Medication Ordered: Levodopa 0.5 g
   Medication Available: Levodopa 250 mg/1 tablet

53. Medication Ordered: Lasix 120 mg
   Medication Available: Lasix 40-mg tablets

54. Medication Ordered: Zebeta 2.5 mg
   Medication Available: Zebeta 5 mg/1 tablet

55. Medication Ordered: Valium 20 mg
   Medication Available: Valium 5 mg/5 mL

56. Medication Ordered: Micro-K 40 mEq
   Medication Available: Micro-K 10 mEq capsule

57. Medication Ordered: Ibuprofen 600 mg
   Medication Available: Ibuprofen 100 mg/2.5 mL

58. Medication Ordered: Zyrtec liquid 2.5 mg
   Medication Available: Zyrtec liquid 5 mg/5 mL

59. Medication Ordered: Bumex 1 mg
   Medication Available: Bumex 0.5 mg/1 tablet

60. Medication Ordered: Pravachol 10 mg
   Medication Available: Pravachol 20 mg/1 tablet

DIRECTIONS: Calculate the medication dosage for the oral medications using the ratio-proportion method.

61. **Medication Ordered:** Benadryl 100 mg
    Medication Available: Benadryl 12.5 mg/ 5 mL

62. **Medication Ordered:** Diuril 1500 mg
    Medication Available: Diuril 500 mg/1 tablet

63. **Medication Ordered:** Erythromycin suspension 750 mg
    Medication Available: Erythromycin suspension 250 mg/5 mL

64. **Medication Ordered:** Parafon Forte 500 mg
    Medication Available: Parafon Forte 250 mg per caplet

65. **Medication Ordered:** Prednisone 30 mg
    Medication Available: Prednisone 10 mg tablet

66. **Medication Ordered:** Valproic acid 750 mg
    Medication Available: Valproic acid 250 mg capsule

67. **Medication Ordered:** Amiodarone 600 mg
    Medication Available: Amiodarone 400 mg/1 tablet

68. **Medication Ordered:** Dynapen 250 mg
    Medication Available: Dynapen 62.5 mg/mL

69. **Medication Ordered:** Ibuprofen 800 mg
    Medication Available: Ibuprofen 200 mg/1 caplet

70. **Medication Ordered:** Pseudoephedrine drops 30 mg
    Medication Available: Pseudoephedrine drops 7.5 mg/0.8 mL

DIRECTIONS: Calculate the correct medication dosage for each parenteral medication. Use the formula method.

71. **Medication Ordered:** Heparin 6000 units
    Medication Available: Heparin 10,000 units/1 mL

72. **Medication Ordered:** Toradol 45 mg
    Medication Available: Toradol 30 mg/1 mL

73. **Medication Ordered:** Morphine sulfate 3 mg IV
    Medication Available: Morphine sulfate 10 mg/mL injection

74. **Medication Ordered:** Demerol 60 mg IM
    Medication Available: Demerol 100 mg/1 mL injection

75. **Medication Ordered:** Ranitidine hydrochloride 50 mg IV
    Medication Available: Ranitidine hydrochloride 25 mg/1 mL injection

DIRECTIONS: Calculate the correct medication dosage for each parenteral medication. Use the ratio-proportion method.

76. **Medication Ordered:** Digoxin 0.125 mg IV
    Medication Available: Digoxin 0.25 mg/1 mL injection

77. **Medication Ordered:** Haldol 3 mg IM
    Medication Available: Haldol 5 mg/1 mL IM

78. **Medication Ordered:** Lupron 1 mg SubQ
    Medication Available: Lupron 5 mg/1 mL injection

79. **Medication Ordered:** Atropine sulfate 0.6 mg SubQ
    Medication Available: Atropine sulfate 0.8 mg/1 mL injection

80. **Medication Ordered:** Fentanyl 0.25 mg IV
    Medication Available: Fentanyl 0.1 mg/1 mL

DIRECTIONS: Calculate the mL/hour flow rate for each IV solution.

81. 4 L lactated Ringer's to infuse over 24 hours

82. 500 mL of 0.9% NaCl to infuse over 3 hours

83. 1000 mL of 0.45% NaCl to infuse over 8 hours

84. 250 mL of 0.9% NaCl to infuse over 4 hours

85. 2 L lactated Ringer's to infuse over 15 hours

DIRECTIONS: Calculate the gtt/min for each of the ordered intravenous solutions. The drop factor is given for each problem. Use the formula method. The formula is:

$$\frac{\text{mL of IV solution}}{\text{Time in minutes}} \times \text{drop factor (gtt/mL)} = \text{gtt/min}$$

86. 750 mL 5% dextrose in 0.45% NaCl to infuse over 3 hours with tubing that has a drop factor of 15 gtt/mL

87. 100 mL antibiotic to infuse at 100 mL/hour with tubing that has a drop factor of 20 gtt/mL

88. 1000 mL lactated Ringer's to infuse over 6 hours with tubing that has a drop factor of 15 gtt/mL

DIRECTIONS: Calculate the gtt/min for each of the ordered intravenous solutions. The drop factor is given for each problem. Use the "quick method." The formula is:

$$\frac{\text{mL/hour}}{\text{Constant}} = \text{gtt/min}$$

89. 500 mL of 0.9% NaCl to infuse at 50 mL/hour with tubing that has a drop factor of 10 gtt/mL

90. 2 L of 5% dextrose in 0.45% NaCl to infuse over 24 hours with tubing that has a drop factor of 20 gtt/mL

DIRECTIONS: Solve the problems to determine rate or dosage of medication.

91. The patient has ordered nitroglycerine 100 mg in 250 mL of 5% dextrose in water to infuse at 60 mcg/min. What is the mL/hour rate to set on the pump?

92. Infusing is norepinephrine 4 mg in 250 mL of 5% dextrose in water at a rate of 45 mL/hour. How many mcg/min of norepinephrine is the patient receiving?

93. The patient is to receive dopamine 400 mg in 250 mL of 5% dextrose in water to infuse at 3 mcg/kg/min. The patient weighs 92 kg. What is the mL/hour rate to set on the pump?

94. Infusing is Nipride 100 mg/250 mL in 0.9% normal saline at a rate of 56 mL/hour. The patient weighs 75 kg. How many mcg/kg/min of Nipride is the patient receiving?

95. Xylocaine 2 g in 250 mL of 0.9% NaCl is ordered to infuse at 3 mg/min. What mL/hour rate should be set on the pump?

96. Neo-Synephrine 50 mg in 250 mL of 5% dextrose in water is infusing at a rate of 30 mL/hour. How many mcg/min of Neo-Synephrine is the patient receiving?

97. Zemuron 1 g in 250 mL of 0.9% NaCl is ordered to infuse at 6 mcg/kg/min. The patient weighs 66 kg. What mL/hour rate should be set on the pump?

98. The patient is to receive dobutamine 500 mg in 250 mL of 0.9% NaCl at 5 mcg/kg/min. The patient weighs 76 kg. What mL/hour rate should be set on the pump?

99. The patient is receiving epinephrine 2 mg in 250 mL of 5% dextrose in water at a rate of 45 mL/hour. How many mcg/min of epinephrine is the patient receiving?

100. The patient is to receive milrinone 20 mg in 100 mL of 5% dextrose in water at 0.5 mcg/kg/min. The patient weighs 55 kg. What mL/hour rate should be set on the pump?

DIRECTIONS: Calculate the correct dosages of medication for each pediatric patient.

101. Medication Ordered: Mysoline suspension 100 mg every 8 hours
Medication Available: Mysoline suspension 250 mg/5 mL
The child weighs 28 kg.
The recommended safe dose is 10 mg to 25 mg/kg.
Use the formula method to calculate the minimum and maximum safe doses.

102. Medication Ordered: Gentamicin 15 mg IM every 8 hours
Medication Available: Gentamicin 10 mg/mL IM
The child weighs 46 pounds.
The recommended safe dose is 2 to 2.5 mg/kg.
Calculate this dosage using the ratio-proportion method.

103. Medication Ordered: Ceftriaxone 1000 mg IV every 12 hours
Medication Available: Ceftriaxone 100 mg/mL IV
The child weighs 40 kg.
The recommended safe dose is 50 to 75 mg/kg.
Use the formula method to calculate the minimum and maximum safe doses.

104. Medication Ordered: Phenytoin 100 mg oral suspension every 8 hours
Medication Available: Phenytoin 125 mg/5 mL suspension
The child is 8 years old
The recommended safe dose is 300 mg daily.
Use the formula method to calculate the minimum and maximum safe doses.

105. Medication Ordered: Erythromycin ethylsuccinate 250 mg oral suspension every 6 hours
Medication Available: Erythromycin ethylsuccinate 200 mg/ 5 mL suspension
The child weighs 38 kg.
The recommended safe dose is 30 to 50 mg/kg.
Calculate the correct dosage using the ratio-proportion method.

DIRECTIONS: Calculate the correct dosage for each parenteral medication.

106. Medication Ordered: Toradol 20 mg IV twice a day
Medication Available: Toradol 15 mg/mL
Give _____ mL. Calculate the correct dosage using the ratio-proportion method.

107. Medication Ordered: Iron dextran 35 mg Z-track method IM
Medication Available: Iron dextran 50 mg/mL
Give _____ mL. Calculate the correct dosage using the formula method.

108. Medication Ordered: Dilaudid 2.5 mg IV
Medication Available: Dilaudid 4 mg/mL
You would administer _____ mL. Calculate the correct dosage using the formula method.

109. Medication Ordered: Hydrocortisone 20 mg IM as an initial dose
Medication Available: Hydrocortisone 50 mg/mL
You would administer _____ mL. Calculate the correct dosage using the formula method.

110. Medication Ordered: Clindamycin 0.2 g IV
Medication Available: Clindamycin 150 mg/mL
You would administer _____ mL. Calculate the correct dosage using the formula method.

Answers to Comprehensive Practice Test

DIRECTIONS: Solve the problem and reduce any fractions to lowest terms.

1. $6\frac{7}{8} \div \frac{4}{5} = \frac{55}{8} \div \frac{4}{5} = \frac{55}{8} \times \frac{5}{4} = \frac{275}{32} = 8\frac{19}{32}$

2. $\frac{5}{6} + \frac{7}{8} + \frac{1}{4} = \frac{20}{24} + \frac{21}{24} + \frac{6}{24} = \frac{47}{24} = 1\frac{23}{24}$

3. $\frac{7}{9} \times \frac{3}{5} = \frac{21}{45} = \frac{7}{15}$

4. $\frac{6}{11} \div \frac{3}{4} = \frac{6}{11} \times \frac{4}{3} = \frac{24}{33} = \frac{8}{11}$

5. 2.86×0.45

$$
\begin{array}{r}
2.86 \\
\times\ 0.45 \\
\hline
1430 \\
+\ 11440 \\
\hline
1.2870
\end{array}
$$

6. $10.64 \div 4.2$

$$
\begin{array}{r}
2.53 \\
4.2\overline{)10.64} \quad \text{Remainder 14} \\
\rightarrow \quad \rightarrow \\
84 \\
\hline
224 \\
210 \\
\hline
140 \\
126 \\
\hline
14
\end{array}
$$

7. Convert the Roman numeral to an Arabic number: XXVIII

   $10 + 10 + 5 + 1 + 1 + 1 = 28$

8. Convert the fraction to a mixed number:

   $\frac{57}{6} = 9\frac{3}{6} = 9\frac{1}{2}$

9. Convert the fraction to a decimal: $\frac{11}{13}$

$$
\begin{array}{r}
0.846 \\
13\overline{)11.000} \quad \text{Remainder 2} \\
104 \\
\hline
60 \\
52 \\
\hline
80 \\
78 \\
\hline
2
\end{array}
$$

10. Solve for x: $\dfrac{24}{32} = \dfrac{x}{12}$

Cross multiply: $\dfrac{24}{32} \times \dfrac{x}{12}$

$32x = 288$

Isolate x: $\dfrac{\cancel{32}x}{\cancel{32}} = \dfrac{288}{32}$

$x = \dfrac{288}{32}$

$x = 9$

DIRECTIONS: Convert the following

11. 2,000 mg = __2__ g

12. 2.75 L = __2,750__ mL

13. 1,450 mcg = __1.450__ mg

14. 480 mg = gr __8__

15. 450 mL = __0.450__ L

16. 1.5 kg = __1,500__ g

17. 360 mL = __12__ ounces

18. 4 teaspoons = __20__ mL

19. 75 mL = __5__ tablespoons

20. gr X = __600__ mg

DIRECTIONS: Mark each syringe at the prescribed level of medication.

21. 21 units of insulin

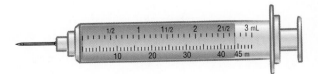

22. 36 units of insulin

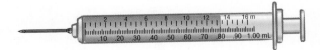

23. 0.44 mL

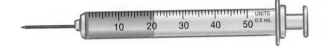

24. 0.8 mL

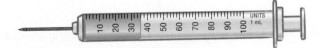

25. 2.7 mL

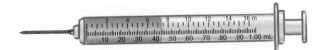

26. 1.3 mL

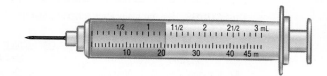

DIRECTIONS: Identify how much medication is in each syringe.

27. <u>0.66 mL</u>

28. <u>22 units</u>

29. <u>1.8 mL</u>

30. <u>2.3 mL</u>

DIRECTIONS: Give the correct term for each abbreviation.

31. prn   <u>as needed</u>

32. q.i.d.   <u>four times a day</u>

33. O.D.   <u>right eye</u>

34. noc   <u>night</u>

DIRECTIONS: Give the correct abbreviation for each term.

35. before meals   <u>ac</u>

36. every 3 hours   <u>q3h</u>

37. intramuscular   <u>IM</u>

DIRECTIONS: Identify which part of the medication order is missing from each drug order.

38. <u>Frequency of medication</u>

    July 24, 2006
      Susannah Jordan
      furosemide (Lasix) 40 mg p.o.
       Dr. Thomlinson

39. <u>Patient name</u>

    February 2, 2005
      Coumadin 2 mg p.o. daily
       Dr. Allen

40. <u>Medication dosage</u>

    September 4, 2006
      Stanley Jameson
      Robitussin every 4 hours prn for cough
       Dr. Wilking

DIRECTIONS: Use the medication labels to identify the components requested.

41. Generic name   <u>clonazepam</u>

42. National Drug Code Number   <u>NDC 0004-0058-01</u>

43. Storage   <u>Store at 59°F to 86°F (15°C to 30°C)</u>

44. Medication form   <u>tablet</u>

45. Medication dose   <u>1 mg</u>

46. Brand name   <u>Romazicon</u>

47. Medication strength   <u>0.1 mg/mL</u>

48. Medication quantity   <u>0.5 mg/5 mL</u>

49. Manufacturer's name   <u>Roche Laboratories, Inc</u>

50. Generic name   <u>flumazenil</u>

51. Identify the six rights of medication administration.

     1.   <u>Right patient</u>

     2.   <u>Right medication</u>

     3.   <u>Right dosage</u>

     4.   <u>Right route</u>

     5.   <u>Right time</u>

     6.   <u>Right documentation</u>

DIRECTIONS: Calculate the medication dosage for the oral medications using the formula method.

$$\frac{D}{H} \times V = A$$

Use the formula:

Where: D = desired or prescribed dosage of the medication

           H = dosage of medication available or on hand

           V = volume that the medication is available in, such as one tablet or milliliters

           A = amount of medication to administer

52. **Medication Ordered:** Levodopa 0.5 g
     Medication Available: Levodopa 250 mg/1 tablet
     Convert 0.5 g to 500 mg

$$\frac{500 \text{ mg}}{250 \text{ mg}} \times 1 \text{ tablet} = 2 \text{ tablets}$$

53. **Medication Ordered:** Lasix 120 mg
     Medication Available: Lasix 40-mg tablet

$$\frac{120 \text{ mg}}{40 \text{ mg}} \times 1 \text{ tablet} = 3 \text{ tablets}$$

54. **Medication Ordered:** Zebeta 2.5 mg
    Medication Available: Zebeta 5 mg/1 tablet

$$\frac{2.5 \text{ mg}}{5 \text{ mg}} \times 1 \text{ tablet} = \frac{1}{2} \text{ tablet}$$

55. **Medication Ordered:** Valium 20 mg
    Medication Available: Valium 5 mg/5 mL

$$\frac{20 \text{ mg}}{5 \text{ mg}} \times 5 \text{ mL} = 20 \text{ mL}$$

56. **Medication Ordered:** Micro-K 40 mEq
    Medication Available: Micro-K 10 mEq capsule

$$\frac{40 \text{ mEq}}{10 \text{ mEq}} \times 1 \text{ casule} = 4 \text{ capsules}$$

57. **Medication Ordered:** Ibuprofen 600 mg
    Medication Available: Ibuprofen 100 mg/2.5 mL

$$\frac{600 \text{ mg}}{100 \text{ mg}} \times 2.5 \text{ mL} = 15 \text{ mL}$$

58. **Medication Ordered:** Zyrtec liquid 2.5 mg
    Medication Available: Zyrtec liquid 5 mg/5 mL

$$\frac{2.5 \text{ mg}}{5 \text{ mg}} \times 5 \text{ mL} = 2.5 \text{ mL}$$

59. **Medication Ordered:** Bumex 1 mg
    Medication Available: Bumex 0.5 mg/1 tablet

$$\frac{1 \text{ mg}}{0.5 \text{ mg}} \times 1 \text{ tablet} = 2 \text{ tablets}$$

60. **Medication Ordered:** Pravachol 10 mg
    Medication Available: Pravachol 20 mg/1 tablet

$$\frac{10 \text{ mg}}{20 \text{ mg}} \times 1 \text{ tablet} = \frac{1}{2} \text{ tablet}$$

DIRECTIONS: Calculate the medication dosage for the oral medications using the ratio-proportion method.

Set up the problem: $\dfrac{\text{Dosage on hand}}{\text{Amount on hand}} = \dfrac{\text{Dosage desired}}{x\ \text{Amount desired}}$

61. **Medication Ordered:** Benadryl 100 mg
    Medication Available: Benadryl 12.5 mg/ 5 mL

$$\frac{12.5 \text{ mg}}{5 \text{ mL}} = \frac{100 \text{ mg}}{x}$$

Cross multiply:

$$\frac{12.5 \text{ mg}}{5 \text{ mg}} \diagdown\!\!\!\diagup \frac{100 \text{ mg}}{x}$$

$$12.5 \text{ mg } x = 500 \text{ mg} \times \text{mL}$$

Isolate x in the equation by dividing both sides of the equation by 12.5. Cancel out like units.

$$\frac{\cancel{12.5 \text{ mg}} \, x}{\cancel{12.5 \text{ mg}}} = \frac{500 \, \cancel{\text{mg}} \times \text{mL}}{12.5 \, \cancel{\text{mg}}}$$

$$x = \frac{500 \text{ mL}}{12.5}$$

$$x = 40 \text{ mL}$$

The correct answer for this problem is 40 mL.

62. **Medication Ordered:** Diuril 1500 mg
Medication Available: Diuril 500 mg/1 tablet

$$\frac{500 \text{ mg}}{1 \text{ tablet}} = \frac{1500 \text{ mg}}{x}$$

Cross multiply:

$$\frac{500 \text{ mg}}{1 \text{ tablet}} \diagdown\!\!\!\!\diagup \frac{1500 \text{ mg}}{x}$$

$$500 \text{ mg } x = 1500 \text{ mg} \times \text{tablet}$$

Isolate x in the equation by dividing both sides of the equation by 500. Cancel out like units.

$$\frac{\cancel{500 \text{ mg}} \, x}{\cancel{500 \text{ mg}}} = \frac{1500 \, \cancel{\text{mg}} \times \text{tablet}}{500 \, \cancel{\text{mg}}}$$

$$x = \frac{1500 \text{ tablet}}{500}$$

$$x = 3 \text{ tablets}$$

The correct answer for this problem is 3 tablets.

63. **Medication Ordered:** Erythromycin suspension 750 mg
Medication Available: Erythromycin suspension 250 mg/5 mL

$$\frac{250 \text{ mg}}{5 \text{ mL}} = \frac{750 \text{ mg}}{x}$$

Cross multiply:

$$\frac{250 \text{ mg}}{5 \text{ mL}} \diagdown\!\!\!\!\diagup \frac{750 \text{ mg}}{x}$$

$$250 \text{ mg } x = 3750 \text{ mg} \times \text{mL}$$

Isolate x in the equation by dividing both sides of the equation by 250. Cancel out like units.

$$\frac{\cancel{250 \text{ mg}} \, x}{\cancel{250 \text{ mg}}} = \frac{3750 \, \cancel{\text{mg}} \times \text{mL}}{250 \, \cancel{\text{mg}}}$$

$$x = \frac{3750 \text{ mL}}{250}$$

$$x = 15 \text{ mL}$$

The correct answer for this problem is 15 mL.

64. **Medication Ordered:** Parafon Forte 500 mg
Medication Available: Parafon Forte 250 mg/caplet

$$\frac{250 \text{ mg}}{1 \text{ caplet}} = \frac{500 \text{ mg}}{x}$$

Cross multiply:

$$\frac{250 \text{ mg}}{1 \text{ caplet}} \diagdown\!\!\!\!\diagup \frac{500 \text{ mg}}{x}$$

$$250 \text{ mg } x = 500 \text{ mg} \times \text{caplet}$$

Isolate x in the equation by dividing both sides of the equation by 250. Cancel out like units.

$$\frac{\cancel{250 \text{ mg}} \, x}{\cancel{250 \text{ mg}}} = \frac{500 \, \cancel{\text{mg}} \times \text{caplet}}{250 \, \cancel{\text{mg}}}$$

$$x = \frac{500 \text{ caplet}}{250}$$

$$x = 2 \text{ caplets}$$

The correct answer for this problem is 2 caplets.

---

65. Medication Ordered: Prednisone 30 mg
Medication Available: Prednisone 10 mg/1 tablet

$$\frac{10 \text{ mg}}{1 \text{ tablet}} = \frac{30 \text{ mg}}{x}$$

Cross multiply:

$$\frac{10 \text{ mg}}{1 \text{ tablet}} \diagup\!\!\!\!\diagdown \frac{30 \text{ mg}}{x}$$

$$10 \text{ mg } x = 30 \text{ mg} \times \text{tablet}$$

Isolate x in the equation by dividing both sides of the equation by 10. Cancel out like units.

$$\frac{\cancel{10 \text{ mg}} \, x}{\cancel{10 \text{ mg}}} = \frac{30 \, \cancel{\text{mg}} \times \text{tablet}}{10 \, \cancel{\text{mg}}}$$

$$x = \frac{30 \text{ tablet}}{10}$$

$$x = 3 \text{ tablets}$$

The correct answer for this problem is 3 tablets.

---

66. Medication Ordered: Valproic acid 750 mg
Medication Available: Valproic acid 250 mg capsule

$$\frac{250 \text{ mg}}{1 \text{ capsule}} = \frac{750 \text{ mg}}{x}$$

Cross multiply:

$$\frac{250 \text{ mg}}{1 \text{ capsule}} \diagup\!\!\!\!\diagdown \frac{750 \text{ mg}}{x}$$

$$250 \text{ mg } x = 750 \text{ mg} \times \text{capsule}$$

Isolate x in the equation by dividing both sides of the equation by 250. Cancel out like units.

$$\frac{\cancel{250 \text{ mg}} \, x}{\cancel{250 \text{ mg}}} = \frac{750 \, \cancel{\text{mg}} \times \text{capsule}}{250 \, \cancel{\text{mg}}}$$

$$x = \frac{750 \text{ capsule}}{250}$$

$$x = 3 \text{ capsules}$$

The correct answer for this problem is 3 capsules.

---

67. Medication Ordered: Amiodarone 600 mg
Medication Available: Amiodarone 400 mg/1 tablet

$$\frac{400 \text{ mg}}{1 \text{ tablet}} = \frac{600 \text{ mg}}{x}$$

Cross multiply:

$$\frac{400 \text{ mg}}{1 \text{ tablet}} \diagup\!\!\!\!\diagdown \frac{600 \text{ mg}}{x}$$

$$400 \text{ mg } x = 600 \text{ mg} \times \text{tablet}$$

Isolate x in the equation by dividing both sides of the equation by 400. Cancel out like units.

$$\frac{\cancel{400 \text{ mg}} \, x}{\cancel{400 \text{ mg}}} = \frac{600 \cancel{\text{ mg}} \times \text{tablet}}{400 \cancel{\text{ mg}}}$$

$$x = \frac{600 \text{ tablet}}{400}$$

$$x = 1.5 \text{ tablets}$$

The correct answer for this problem is 1.5 tablets.

68. Medication Ordered: Dynapen 250 mg
Medication Available: Dynapen 62.5 mg/mL

$$\frac{62.5 \text{ mg}}{1 \text{ mL}} = \frac{250 \text{ mg}}{x}$$

Cross multiply:

$$\frac{62.5 \text{ mg}}{1 \text{ mL}} \diagup\!\!\!\!\!\diagdown \frac{250 \text{ mg}}{x}$$

$$62.5 \text{ mg } x = 250 \text{ mg} \times \text{mL}$$

Isolate x in the equation by dividing both sides of the equation by 62.5. Cancel out like units.

$$\frac{\cancel{62.5 \text{ mg}} \, x}{\cancel{62.5 \text{ mg}}} = \frac{250 \cancel{\text{ mg}} \times \text{mL}}{62.5 \cancel{\text{ mg}}}$$

$$x = \frac{250 \text{ mL}}{62.5}$$

$$x = 4 \text{ mL}$$

The correct answer for this problem is 4 mL.

69. Medication Ordered: Ibuprofen 800 mg
Medication Available: Ibuprofen 200 mg/1 caplet

$$\frac{200 \text{ mg}}{1 \text{ caplet}} = \frac{800 \text{ mg}}{x}$$

Cross multiply:

$$\frac{200 \text{ mg}}{1 \text{ caplet}} \diagup\!\!\!\!\!\diagdown \frac{800 \text{ mg}}{x}$$

$$200 \text{ mg } x = 800 \text{ mg} \times \text{caplet}$$

Isolate x in the equation by dividing both sides of the equation by 200. Cancel out like units.

$$\frac{\cancel{200 \text{ mg}} \, x}{\cancel{200 \text{ mg}}} = \frac{800 \cancel{\text{ mg}} \times \text{caplet}}{200 \cancel{\text{ mg}}}$$

$$x = \frac{800 \text{ caplet}}{200}$$

$$x = 4 \text{ caplets}$$

The correct answer for this problem is 4 caplets.

70. Medication Ordered: Pseudoephedrine drops 30 mg
Medication Available: Pseudoephedrine drops 7.5 mg/0.8 mL

$$\frac{7.5 \text{ mg}}{0.8 \text{ mL}} = \frac{30 \text{ mg}}{x}$$

Cross multiply:

$$\frac{7.5 \text{ mg}}{0.8 \text{ mL}} \diagup\!\!\!\!\!\diagdown \frac{30 \text{ mg}}{x}$$

$$7.5 \text{ mg } x = 24 \text{ mg} \times \text{mL}$$

Isolate x in the equation by dividing both sides of the equation by 7.5. Cancel out like units.

$$\frac{\cancel{7.5 \text{ mg}}\ x}{\cancel{7.5 \text{ mg}}} = \frac{24\ \cancel{\text{mg}} \times \text{mL}}{7.5\ \cancel{\text{mg}}}$$

$$x = \frac{24\ \text{mL}}{7.5}$$

$$x = 3.2\ \text{mL}$$

The correct answer for this problem is 3.2 mL.

DIRECTIONS: Calculate the correct medication dosage for each parenteral medication. Use the formula method.

71. **Medication Ordered:** Heparin 6000 units
    Medication Available: Heparin 10,000 units/1 mL

$$\frac{6000\ \text{units}}{10{,}000\ \text{units}} \times 1\ \text{mL} = 0.6\ \text{mL}$$

72. **Medication Ordered:** Toradol 45 mg
    Medication Available: Toradol 30 mg/1 mL

$$\frac{45\ \text{mg}}{30\ \text{mg}} \times 1\ \text{mL} = 1.5\ \text{mL}$$

73. **Medication Ordered:** Morphine sulfate 3 mg IV
    Medication Available: Morphine sulfate 10 mg/mL injection

$$\frac{3\ \text{mg}}{10\ \text{mg}} \times 1\ \text{mL} = 0.3\ \text{mL}$$

74. **Medication Ordered:** Demerol 60 mg IM
    Medication Available: Demerol 100 mg/1 mL injection

$$\frac{60\ \text{mg}}{100\ \text{mg}} \times 1\ \text{mL} = 0.6\ \text{mL}$$

75. **Medication Ordered:** Ranitidine hydrochloride 50 mg IV
    Medication Available: Ranitidine hydrochloride 25 mg/1 mL injection

$$\frac{50\ \text{mg}}{25\ \text{mg}} \times 1\ \text{mL} = 2\ \text{mL}$$

DIRECTIONS: Calculate the correct medication dosage for each parenteral medication. Use the ratio-proportion method.

76. **Medication Ordered:** Digoxin 0.125 mg IV
    Medication Available: Digoxin 0.25 mg/1 mL injection

$$\frac{0.25\ \text{mg}}{1\ \text{mL}} = \frac{0.125\ \text{mg}}{x}$$

Cross multiply:

$$\frac{0.25\ \text{mg}}{1\ \text{mL}} \bowtie \frac{0.125\ \text{mg}}{x}$$

$$0.25\ \text{mg}\ x = 0.125\ \text{mg} \times \text{mL}$$

Isolate x in the equation by dividing both sides of the equation by 0.25. Cancel out like units.

$$\frac{0.25 \text{ mg } x}{0.25 \text{ mg}} = \frac{0.125 \text{ mg} \times \text{mL}}{0.25 \text{ mg}}$$

$$x = \frac{0.125 \text{ mL}}{0.25}$$

$$x = 0.5 \text{ mL}$$

The correct answer for this problem is 0.5 mL.

77. **Medication Ordered:** Haldol 3 mg IM
    Medication Available: Haldol 5 mg/1 mL IM

$$\frac{5 \text{ mg}}{1 \text{ mL}} = \frac{3 \text{ mg}}{x}$$

Cross multiply:

$$\frac{5 \text{ mg}}{1 \text{ mL}} \diagdown \frac{3 \text{ mg}}{x}$$

$$5 \text{ mg } x = 3 \text{ mg} \times \text{mL}$$

Isolate x in the equation by dividing both sides of the equation by 5. Cancel out like units.

$$\frac{5 \text{ mg } x}{5 \text{ mg}} = \frac{3 \text{ mg} \times \text{mL}}{5 \text{ mg}}$$

$$x = \frac{3 \text{ mL}}{5}$$

$$x = 0.6 \text{ mL}$$

The correct answer for this problem is 0.6 mL.

78. **Medication Ordered:** Lupron 1 mg SubQ
    Medication Available: Lupron 5 mg/1 mL injection

$$\frac{5 \text{ mg}}{1 \text{ mL}} = \frac{1 \text{ mg}}{x}$$

Cross multiply:

$$\frac{5 \text{ mg}}{1 \text{ mL}} \diagdown \frac{1 \text{ mg}}{x}$$

$$5 \text{ mg } x = 1 \text{ mg} \times \text{mL}$$

Isolate x in the equation by dividing both sides of the equation by 5. Cancel out like units.

$$\frac{5 \text{ mg } x}{5 \text{ mg}} = \frac{1 \text{ mg} \times \text{mL}}{5 \text{ mg}}$$

$$x = \frac{1 \text{ mL}}{5}$$

$$x = 0.2 \text{ mL}$$

The correct answer for this problem is 0.2 mL.

79. **Medication Ordered:** Atropine sulfate 0.6 mg SubQ
    Medication Available: Atropine sulfate 0.8 mg/1 mL injection

$$\frac{0.8 \text{ mg}}{1 \text{ mL}} = \frac{0.6 \text{ mg}}{x}$$

Cross multiply:

$$\frac{0.8 \text{ mg}}{1 \text{ mL}} \diagdown \frac{0.6 \text{ mg}}{x}$$

$$0.8 \text{ mg } x = 0.6 \text{ mg} \times \text{mL}$$

Isolate x in the equation by dividing both sides of the equation by 0.8. Cancel out like units.

$$\frac{\cancel{0.8\ mg}\ x}{\cancel{0.8\ mg}} = \frac{0.6\ \cancel{mg} \times mL}{0.8\ \cancel{mg}}$$

$$x = \frac{0.6\ mL}{0.8}$$

$$x = 0.75\ mL$$

The correct answer for this problem is 0.75 mL.

80. Medication Ordered: Fentanyl 0.25 mg IV
Medication Available: Fentanyl 0.1 mg/1 mL

$$\frac{0.1\ mg}{1\ mL} = \frac{0.25\ mg}{x}$$

Cross multiply:

$$\frac{0.1\ mg}{1\ mL} \diagdown\diagup \frac{0.25\ mg}{x}$$

$$0.1\ mg\ x = 0.25\ mg \times mL$$

Isolate x in the equation by dividing both sides of the equation by 0.1. Cancel out like units.

$$\frac{\cancel{0.1\ mg}\ x}{\cancel{0.1\ mg}} = \frac{0.25\ \cancel{mg} \times mL}{0.1\ \cancel{mg}}$$

$$x = \frac{0.25\ mL}{0.1}$$

$$x = 2.5\ mL$$

The correct answer for this problem is 2.5 mL.

DIRECTIONS: Calculate the mL/hour flow rate for each IV solution.

Use the formula: $\dfrac{mL\ of\ solution\ ordered}{Total\ hours\ ordered} = mL/hour$

81. 4 L lactated Ringer's to infuse over 24 hours

$$\frac{4000\ mL}{24\ hours} = 166.7\ mL/hour$$

82. 500 mL of 0.9% NaCl to infuse over 3 hours

$$\frac{500\ mL}{3\ hours} = 166.7\ mL/hour$$

83. 1,000 mL of 0.45% NaCl to infuse over 8 hours

$$\frac{1000\ mL}{8\ hours} = 125\ mL/hour$$

84. 250 mL of 0.9% NaCl to infuse over 4 hours

$$\frac{250\ mL}{4\ hours} = 62.5\ mL/hour$$

85. 2 L lactated Ringer's to infuse over 15 hours

$$\frac{2000\ mL}{15\ hours} = 133.3\ mL/hour$$

DIRECTIONS: Calculate the gtt/min for each of the ordered intravenous solutions. The drop factor is given for each problem. Use the formula method. The formula is:

$$\frac{\text{mL of IV solution}}{\text{Time in minutes}} \times \text{drop factor (gtt/mL)} = \text{gtt/min}$$

86. 750 mL 5% dextrose in 0.45% NaCl to infuse over 3 hours with tubing that has a drop factor of 15 gtt/mL

First, calculate mL/hour: $\dfrac{750 \text{ mL}}{3 \text{ hours}} = 250 \text{ mL/hour}$

$$\frac{250 \text{ mL}}{60 \text{ min}} \times 15 \text{ gtt/mL} = \text{gtt/min}$$

$$\frac{250 \text{ mL}}{60 \text{ min}} \times \frac{15 \text{ gtt}}{1 \text{ mL}} = \text{gtt/min}$$

$$\frac{250 \ \cancel{\text{mL}}}{\underset{4}{\cancel{60}} \text{ min}} \times \frac{\overset{1}{\cancel{15}} \text{ gtt}}{1 \ \cancel{\text{mL}}} = \text{gtt/min}$$

$$\frac{250 \text{ gtt}}{4 \text{ min}} = 62.5 \qquad \text{(Round to 63 gtt/min)}$$

87. 100 mL antibiotic to infuse at 100 mL/hour with tubing that has a drop factor of 20 gtt/mL

$$\frac{100 \text{ mL}}{60 \text{ min}} \times 20 \text{ gtt/mL} = \text{gtt/min}$$

$$\frac{100 \text{ mL}}{60 \text{ min}} \times \frac{20 \text{ gtt}}{1 \text{ mL}} = \text{gtt/min}$$

$$\frac{100 \ \cancel{\text{mL}}}{\underset{3}{\cancel{60}} \text{ min}} \times \frac{\overset{1}{\cancel{20}} \text{ gtt}}{1 \ \cancel{\text{mL}}} = \text{gtt/min}$$

$$\frac{100 \text{ gtt}}{3 \text{ min}} = 33.33 \qquad \text{(Round to 33 gtt/min)}$$

88. 1,000 mL lactated Ringer's to infuse over 6 hours with tubing that has a drop factor of 15 gtt/mL

First, calculate mL/hour: $\dfrac{1000 \text{ mL}}{6 \text{ hours}} = 167 \text{ mL/hour}$

$$\frac{167 \text{ mL}}{60 \text{ min}} \times 15 \text{ gtt/mL} = \text{gtt/min}$$

$$\frac{167 \text{ mL}}{60 \text{ min}} \times \frac{15 \text{ gtt}}{1 \text{ mL}} = \text{gtt/min}$$

$$\frac{167 \ \cancel{\text{mL}}}{\underset{4}{\cancel{60}} \text{ min}} \times \frac{\overset{1}{\cancel{15}} \text{ gtt}}{1 \ \cancel{\text{mL}}} = \text{gtt/min}$$

$$\frac{167 \text{ gtt}}{4 \text{ min}} = 41.75 \qquad \text{(Round to 42 gtt/min)}$$

DIRECTIONS: Calculate the gtt/min for each of the ordered intravenous solutions. The drop factor is given for each problem. Use the "quick method." The formula is:

$$\frac{\text{mL/hour}}{\text{Constant}} = \text{gtt/min}$$

89. 500 mL of 0.9% NaCl to infuse at 50 mL/hour with tubing that has a drop factor of 10 gtt/mL

$$\frac{50}{6} = 8.33 \qquad \text{(Round to 8 gtt/min)}$$

90. 2 L of 5% dextrose in 0.45% NaCl to infuse over 24 hours with tubing that has a drop factor of 20 gtt/mL

First, calculate mL/hour: $\qquad \dfrac{2000 \text{ mL}}{24 \text{ hours}} = 83.33, \qquad$ round to 83 mL/hour

$$\frac{83}{3} = 27.66 \qquad \text{(Round to 28 gtt/min)}$$

DIRECTIONS: Solve the problems to determine rate or dosage of medication.

91. The prescriber has ordered nitroglycerine 100 mg in 250 mL of 5% dextrose in water to infuse at 60 mcg/min. What is the mL/hour rate to set on the pump?

Convert mg/mL to mcg/mL: $\quad \dfrac{100 \text{ mg}}{250 \text{ mL}} \times \dfrac{1000 \text{ mcg}}{1 \text{ mg}} = \dfrac{100{,}000 \text{ mcg}}{250 \text{ mL}} = 400 \text{ mcg/mL}$

$$\frac{60 \text{ mcg/min} \times 60 \text{ min/hour}}{400 \text{ mcg/mL}} = 9 \text{ mL/hour}$$

92. Infusing is norepinephrine 4 mg in 250 mL of 5% dextrose in water at a rate of 45 mL/hour. How many mcg/min of norepinephrine is the patient receiving?

Convert mg/mL to mcg/mL: $\quad \dfrac{4 \text{ mg}}{250 \text{ mL}} \times \dfrac{1000 \text{ mcg}}{1 \text{ mg}} = \dfrac{4000 \text{ mcg}}{250 \text{ mL}} = 16 \text{ mcg/mL}$

$$\frac{16 \text{ mcg/mL} \times 45 \text{ mL/hour}}{60 \text{ min/hour}} = 12 \text{ mcg/min}$$

93. The patient is to receive dopamine 400 mg in 250 mL of 5% dextrose in water to infuse at 3 mcg/kg/min. The patient weighs 92 kg. What is the mL/hour rate to set on the pump?

$$\frac{3 \text{ mcg/kg/min} \times 60 \text{ min/hour} \times 92 \text{ kg}}{1600 \text{ mcg/mL}} = 10.35 \qquad \text{(Round to 10.4 mL/hour)}$$

94. Infusing is Nipride 100 mg/250 mL of 0.9% normal saline at a rate of 56 mL/hour. The patient weighs 75 kg. How many mcg/kg/min of Nipride is the patient receiving?

$$\frac{400 \text{ mcg/mL} \times 56 \text{ mL/hour}}{60 \text{ min/hour} \times 75 \text{ kg}} = 4.98 \qquad \text{(Round to 5 mcg/kg/min)}$$

95. Xylocaine 2 g in 250 mL of 0.9% NaCl is ordered to infuse at 3 mg/min. What mL/hour rate should be set on the pump?

$$\frac{3 \text{ mg/min} \times 60 \text{ min/hour}}{8 \text{ mg/mL}} = 22.5 \text{ mL/hour}$$

96. Neo-Synephrine 50 mg in 250 mL of 5% dextrose in water is infusing at a rate of 30 mL/hour. How many mcg/min of Neo-Synephrine is the patient receiving?

$$\frac{200 \text{ mcg/mL} \times 30 \text{ mL/hour}}{60 \text{ min/hour}} = 100 \text{ mcg/min}$$

97. Zemuron 1 g in 250 mL of 0.9% NaCl is ordered to infuse at 6 mcg/kg/min. The patient weighs 66 kg. What mL/hour rate should be set on the pump?

$$\frac{6 \text{ mcg/kg/min} \times 60 \text{ min/hour} \times 66 \text{ kg}}{4000 \text{ mcg/mL}} = 5.94 \qquad \text{(Round to 5.9 mL/hour)}$$

98. The patient is to receive dobutamine 500 mg in 250 mL of 0.9% NaCl at 5 mcg/kg/min. The patient weighs 76 kg. What mL/hour rate should be set on the pump?

$$\frac{5 \text{ mcg/kg/min} \times 60 \text{ min/hour} \times 76 \text{ kg}}{2000 \text{ mcg/mL}} = 11.4 \text{ mL/hour}$$

99. The patient is receiving epinephrine 2 mg in 250 mL of 5% dextrose in water at a rate of 45 mL/hour. How many mcg/min of epinephrine is the patient receiving?

$$\frac{8 \text{ mcg/mL} \times 45 \text{ mL/hour}}{60 \text{ min/hour}} = 6 \text{ mcg/min}$$

100. The patient is to receive milrinone 20 mg in 100 mL of 5% dextrose in water at 0.5 mcg/kg/min. The patient weighs 55 kg. What mL/hour rate should be set on the pump?

$$\frac{0.5 \text{ mcg/kg/min} \times 60 \text{ min/hour} \times 55 \text{ kg}}{200 \text{ mcg/mL}} = 8.25 \qquad \text{(Round to 8.3 mL/hour)}$$

DIRECTIONS: Calculate the correct dosages of medication for each pediatric patient.

101. **Medication Ordered:** Mysoline 100 mg every 8 hours
   Medication Available: Mysoline suspension 250 mg/5 mL

   The child weighs 28 kg.

   The recommended safe dose is 10 to 25 mg/kg

   First, calculate the minimum and maximum safe dose:

   Minimum SDR: 28 kg × 10 mg/kg = 280 mg/day in 3 divided doses = 93 mg/dose

   Maximum SDR: 28 kg × 25 mg/kg = 700 mg/day in 3 divided doses = 233 mg/dose

   The order is for 100 mg/dose, or 300 mg/day, which is within the safe dose range.

   To calculate the medication dose using the available Mysoline suspension 250 mg/5 mL, set up the problem using the formula method:

   $$\frac{D}{H} \times V = A$$

   $$\frac{100 \text{ mg}}{250 \text{ mg}} \times 5 \text{ mL}$$

   In this problem, because mg appears in both the numerator and denominator, mg is cancelled out and mL is left as the volume of medication in the answer.

   $$\frac{100 \text{ mg}}{250 \text{ mg}} \times 5 \text{ mL} = 2 \text{ mL}$$

   Therefore, you would administer 2 mL.

102. **Medication Ordered:** Gentamicin 15 mg IM every 8 hours
   Medication Available: Gentamicin 10 mg/mL IM

   The child weighs 46 pounds.

   The recommended safe dose is 2 to 2.5 mg/kg

   First, calculate the minimum and maximum safe dose:

   Convert weight to kg: 46 lbs ÷ 2.2 lbs/kg = 20.9 kg

   Minimum SDR: 20.9 kg × 2 mg/kg = 41.8 mg/day in 3 doses = 13.9 mg/dose

   Maximum SDR: 20.9 kg × 2.5 mg/kg = 52.3 mg/day in 3 doses = 17.4 mg/dose

   The order is for 15 mg/dose, or 45 mg/day, so the dose is safe.

To calculate the medication dose using the ratio-proportion method, set up the problem like this:

$$\frac{10\ \text{mg}}{1\ \text{mL}} = \frac{15\ \text{mg}}{x}$$

Cross multiply:

$$\frac{10\ \text{mg}}{1\ \text{mL}} \diagdown\diagup \frac{15\ \text{mg}}{x}$$

$$10\ \text{mg}\ x = 15\ \text{mg} \times 1\ \text{mL}$$

Isolate the x by dividing both sides by 10. Milligrams (mg) in the numerator and denominator cancel each other out, and mL is left as the volume of medication in the answer.

$$\frac{\cancel{10\ \text{mg}}\ x}{\cancel{10\ \text{mg}}} = \frac{15\ \cancel{\text{mg}} \times \text{mL}}{10\ \cancel{\text{mg}}}$$

Solve for x:

$$x = \frac{15\ \text{mL}}{10} = 1.5\ \text{mL}$$

Therefore, the answer to the problem is 1.5 mL.

103. **Medication Ordered:** Ceftriaxone 1000 mg IV every 12 hours
Medication Available: Ceftriaxone 100 mg/mL IV

The child weighs 40 kg.

The recommended safe dose is 50 to 75 mg/kg

First, calculate the minimum and maximum safe dose:

Minimum SDR: 40 kg × 50 mg/kg = 2000 mg/day in 2 doses = 1000 mg/dose

Maximum SDR: 40 kg × 75 mg/kg = 3000 mg/day in 2 doses = 1500 mg/dose

The reference states that one should not exceed 2 g for children weighing less than 45 kg. The order is for 1000 mg/dose, or 2,000 mg/day, which is within the safe dose range.

Ceftriaxone after reconstitution equals 100 mg/mL. To calculate the medication dose using the available ceftriaxone 100 mg/mL IV, set up the problem using the formula method:

$$\frac{D}{H} \times V = A$$

$$\frac{1000\ \text{mg}}{100\ \text{mg}} \times 1\ \text{mL}$$

In this problem, because mg appears in both the numerator and denominator, mg is cancelled out and mL is left as the volume of medication in the answer.

$$\frac{1000\ \cancel{\text{mg}}}{100\ \cancel{\text{mg}}} \times 1\ \text{mL} = 10\ \text{mL}$$

Therefore, you would administer 10 mL.

104. **Medication Ordered:** Phenytoin 100 mg orally every 8 hours
Medication Available: Phenytoin 125 mg/5 mL oral suspension

The recommended safe dose is 300 mg daily

The child is 8 years old, and the approved drug reference states that a child over 6 years may receive the minimum adult dose of 300 mg/day. The recommended safe dose is 300 mg daily; therefore, the order for 100 mg/dose, or 300 mg/day, is within the safe dose range.

To calculate the medication dose using the available phenytoin 125 mg/5 mL suspension, set up the problem using the formula method:

$$\frac{D}{H} \times V = A$$

$$\frac{100\ \text{mg}}{125\ \text{mg}} \times 5\ \text{mL}$$

In this problem, because mg appears in both the numerator and denominator, mg is cancelled out and mL is left as the volume of medication in the answer.

$$\frac{100 \cancel{mg}}{125 \cancel{mg}} \times 5\ mL = 4\ mL$$

Therefore, you would administer 4 mL.

105. Medication Ordered: Erythromycin ethylsuccinate 250 mg every 6 hours
Medication Available: Erythromycin ethylsuccinate 200 mg/5 mL suspension

The child weighs 38 kg.

The recommended safe dose is 30 to 50 mg/kg

First, calculate the minimum and maximum safe dose:

Minimum SDR: 38 kg × 30 mg/kg = 1140 mg/day in 6 divided doses = 190 mg/dose

Maximum SDR: 38 kg × 50 mg/kg = 1900 mg/day in 6 divided doses = 317 mg/dose

The order is for 250 mg/dose, or 1500 mg/day, which is within the safe range.

To calculate this problem using the ratio-proportion method, set up the problem like this:

$$\frac{200\ mg}{5\ mL} = \frac{250\ mg}{x}$$

Cross multiply:

$$\frac{200\ mg}{5\ mL} \diagdown\!\!\!\!\diagup \frac{250\ mg}{x}$$

$$200\ mg\ x = 250\ mg \times 5\ mL$$

Isolate the x by dividing both sides by 200. Milligrams (mg) in the numerator and denominator cancel each other out and mL is left as the volume of medication in the answer.

$$\frac{200\ \cancel{mg}\ x}{200\ \cancel{mg}} = \frac{250\ \cancel{mg} \times 5\ mL}{200\ \cancel{mg}}$$

Solve for x:

$$x = \frac{250 \times 5\ mL}{200} = \frac{1250\ mL}{200} = 6.25\ mL$$

Therefore, the answer to the problem is 6.25 mL.

DIRECTIONS: Calculate the correct dosage for each parenteral medication.

106. Medication Ordered: Toradol 20 mg IV twice a day
Medication Available: Toradol 15 mg/mL

Give _____ mL. Calculate the correct dosage using the ratio-proportion method.

$$\frac{15\ mg}{1\ mL} = \frac{20\ mg}{x}$$

Cross multiply: 15 mg x = 20 mg × mL

Isolate x in the equation by dividing by 15; like units cancel each other out:

$$\frac{15\ \cancel{mg}\ x}{15\ \cancel{mg}} = \frac{20\ \cancel{mg} \times mL}{15\ \cancel{mg}}$$

$$x = 1.33\ mL$$

After rounding, the answer is to administer 1.3 mL.

107. **Medication Ordered:** Iron dextran 35 mg Z-track method IM
Medication Available: Iron dextran 50 mg/mL

Give _____ mL. Calculate the correct dosage using the formula method.

$$\frac{35 \text{ mg}}{50 \text{ mg}} \times 1 \text{ mL}$$

$$\frac{35 \text{ \cancel{mg}}}{50 \text{ \cancel{mg}}} \times 1 \text{ mL} = 0.7 \text{ mL}$$

Administer 0.7 mL.

108. **Medication Ordered:** Dilaudid 2.5 mg IV
Medication Available: Dilaudid 4 mg/mL.

You would administer _____ mL. Calculate the correct dosage using the formula method.

$$\frac{2.5 \text{ mg}}{4 \text{ mg}} \times 1 \text{ mL}$$

$$\frac{2.5 \text{ \cancel{mg}}}{4 \text{ \cancel{mg}}} \times 1 \text{ mL} = 0.625 \qquad \text{(Round to 0.63 mL)}$$

Administer 0.6 mL.

109. **Medication Ordered:** Hydrocortisone 20 mg IM as an initial dose
Medication Available: Hydrocortisone 50 mg/mL

You would administer _____ mL. Calculate the correct dosage using the formula method.

$$\frac{20 \text{ mg}}{50 \text{ mg}} \times 1 \text{ mL}$$

$$\frac{20 \text{ \cancel{mg}}}{50 \text{ \cancel{mg}}} \times 1 \text{ mL} = 0.4 \text{ mL}$$

Administer 0.4 mL.

110. **Medication Ordered:** Clindamycin 0.2 g IV
Medication Available: Clindamycin 150 mg/mL

You would administer _____ mL. Calculate the correct dosage using the formula method.

$$\frac{200 \text{ mg}}{150 \text{ mg}} \times 1 \text{ mL}$$

$$\frac{200 \text{ \cancel{mg}}}{150 \text{ \cancel{mg}}} = 1 \text{ mL} = 1.33 \text{ mL} \qquad \text{(Round to 1.3 mL)}$$

Administer 1.3 mL.

Dimensional Analysis

In addition to the two methods discussed in Chapter 6 (formula method and ratio-proportion method), another method of solving dosage calculations can be used. This method is dimensional analysis. The following information is reproduced with permission from Gloria P. Craig's *Clinical Calculations Made Easy* (3rd ed., 2005). The following excerpt provides a simple explanation of how the problems are set up.

TERMS USED IN DIMENSIONAL ANALYSIS

Dimensional analysis is a problem-solving method that can be used whenever two quantities are directly proportional to each other and one quantity must be converted to the other by using a common equivalent, conversion factor, or conversion relation. All medication dosage calculation problems can be solved by dimensional analysis.

It is important to understand the following four terms that provide the basis for dimensional analysis.

- **Given quantity:** the beginning point of the problem
- **Wanted quantity:** the answer to the problem
- **Unit path:** the series of conversions necessary to achieve the answer to the problem
- **Conversion factors:** equivalents necessary to convert between systems of measurement and to allow unwanted units to be canceled from the problem

Each conversion factor is a ratio of units that equals 1.
Dimensional analysis also uses the same terms as fractions: numerators and denominators.

- *The numerator* = the top portion of the problem
- *The denominator* = the bottom portion of the problem

Some problems will have a given quantity and a wanted quantity that contain only numerators. Other problems will have a given quantity and a wanted quantity that contain both a numerator and a denominator. This chapter contains only problems with numerators as the given quantity and the wanted quantity.

Once the beginning point in the problem is identified, then a series of conversions necessary to achieve the answer is established that leads to the problem's solution.

Below is an example of the problem-solving method, showing the placement of basic terms used in dimensional analysis.

	Unit Path			
Given Quantity	Conversion Factor for Given Quantity	Conversion Factor for Wanted Quantity	Conversion Computation	Wanted Quantity
1 liter (L)	1000 mL	1 oz	1 × 1000 × 1 / 1000	= 33.3 oz
	1 liter (L)	30 mL	1 × 30 / 30	

THE FIVE STEPS OF DIMENSIONAL ANALYSIS

Once the given quantity is identified, the unit path leading to the wanted quantity is established. The problem-solving method of dimensional analysis uses the following five steps.

1. Identify the *given quantity* in the problem.
2. Identify the *wanted quantity* in the problem.
3. Establish the *unit path* from the given quantity to the wanted quantity using equivalents as *conversion factors.*
4. Set up the conversion factors to permit cancellation of unwanted units. Carefully choose each conversion factor and ensure that each factor is correctly placed in the numerator or denominator portion of the problem to allow the unwanted units to be canceled from the problem.
5. Multiply the numerators, multiply the denominators, and divide the product of the numerators by the product of the denominators to provide the numerical value of the wanted quantity.

The following examples use the five steps of dimensional analysis to solve problems.

Example

1 liter (L) equals how many ounces (oz)?

STEP 1 Identify the *given quantity* in the problem.

The given quantity is *1 L.*

Unit Path

Given Quantity	Conversion Factor for Given Quantity	Conversion Factor for Wanted Quantity	Conversion Computation	Wanted Quantity
1 liter (L)				=

STEP 2 Identify the *wanted quantity* in the problem.

The wanted quantity is the number of *ounces* (oz) in 1 L.

Unit Path

Given Quantity	Conversion Factor for Given Quantity	Conversion Factor for Wanted Quantity	Conversion Computation	Wanted Quantity
1 liter (L)				= oz

STEP 3 Establish the *unit path* from the given quantity to the wanted quantity. You must determine what conversion factors are needed to convert the given quantity to the wanted quantity.

Given quantity: 1 L = 1000 mL

Wanted quantity: 1 oz = 30 mL

STEP 4 Write the unit path for the problem so that each unit cancels out the preceding unit until all unwanted units are canceled from the problem except the wanted quantity.

The wanted quantity must be within the numerator portion of the problem to identify that the problem is set up correctly.

Unit Path

Given Quantity	Conversion Factor for Given Quantity	Conversion Factor for Wanted Quantity	Conversion Computation	Wanted Quantity
1 liter (L)	1000 mL	1 oz		= oz
	1 liter (L)	30 mL		

Unit Path

Given Quantity	Conversion Factor for Given Quantity	Conversion Factor for Wanted Quantity	Conversion Computation	Wanted Quantity
1 ~~liter (L)~~	1000 ~~mL~~	1 ⓞⓩ		= oz
	1 ~~liter (L)~~	30 ~~mL~~		

STEP 5   After the unwanted units are canceled from the problem, only the numerical values remain. Multiply the numerators, multiply the denominators, and divide the product of the numerators by the product of the denominators to provide the numerical value for the wanted quantity.

One (1) times ($\times$) any number equals that number, therefore 1s may be automatically canceled from the problem. Other factors that can be canceled from the problem include like numerical values in the numerator and denominator portion of the problem and the same number of zeroes in the numerator and denominator portion of the problem.

Unit Path

Given Quantity	Conversion Factor for Given Quantity	Conversion Factor for Wanted Quantity	Conversion Computation		Wanted Quantity
1 ~~liter (L)~~	1000 ~~mL~~	1 ⓞⓩ	1000 × 1	1000	= 33.3 oz
	1 ~~liter (L)~~	30 ~~mL~~	1 × 30	30	

33.3 oz is the wanted quantity and the answer to the problem.

Example

Consider the example given in Chapter 6, page 104. The physician prescribes 100 mg of a medication. The medication is available in 50 mg tablets. The problem would be solved like this using dimensional analysis:

Given Quantity	Conversion Factor for Wanted Quantity	Conversion Computation	Wanted Quantity
100 ~~mg~~	1 tablet	100	= 2 tablets
	50 ~~mg~~	50	

More complex calculations can also be solved using this method by adding more columns to the unit path as more conversions are needed. Again, this method is more fully explained and can be studied in the Craig text.

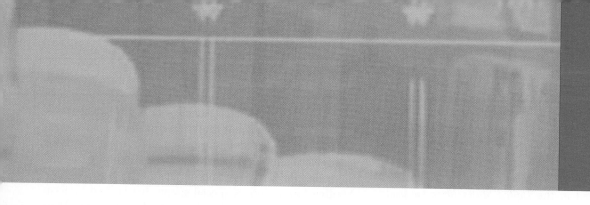

Glossary

Apothecary system. A system for ordering medication dosages that is not generally used. The two basic units are weight and volume. The basic unit of weight is expressed in grains. Volume is expressed in minim, dram, or ounce.

Arabic numbers. Numbers that you use daily, such as 0 to 9.

Brand name. The name given to a medication by the manufacturer. The brand name has the symbol ® or ™ after it, indicating a registered trademark. It starts with an uppercase letter or is in all uppercase letters on the label and is also called a trade name or proprietary name.

Body Surface Area (BSA) method. A reliable method used to calculate therapeutic dosages that requires use of a chart called a nomogram, which converts the weight to square meters of BSA.

Calibrated medication dropper. A device that is used to measure and administer small dosages of medications. The dropper has markings specific to the medication with which it is provided so that accurate measurement of the medication occurs.

Capsule. A method of delivering medication wherein the medication is enclosed in a dissolvable shell of hard or soft gelatin.

Complex fraction. A type of fraction wherein the numerator, denominator, or both can be a whole number, proper fraction, or mixed number. The value of the fraction can be less than, greater than, or equal to 1. Example:

$$\frac{\frac{3}{4}}{\frac{3}{8}} \quad \text{is greater than 1}$$

Compute. The second step in safely calculating medication dosages. This step requires you to determine the data needed to solve the dose problem, to set up the problem correctly, and to calculate an answer.

Convert. The first step in safely calculating medication dosages. This step requires you to make sure that the medication dose ordered is in the same system and unit of measurement as the medication available.

Critically Think. The third step in safely calculating medication dosages. This step requires asking yourself if the answer obtained after converting and computing seems correct, logical, and plausible.

Decimal. A fraction with a denominator that is a multiple of ten. The value of the decimal is determined by the position of the numbers in relation to the decimal point. In a decimal, the value of the numbers to the right of the decimal point is less than one and the value of the numbers to the left of the decimal point is greater than one.

Denominator. The bottom number of a fraction. In the fraction $\frac{2}{4}$, 4 is the denominator.

Drop factor. Number of drops per milliliter that is delivered by intravenous tubing.

Drug order. An order for a medication written by an authorized prescriber on an appropriate medication order form.

Elixir. A liquid medication that is generally a combination of the medication, water, and ethanol.

Emulsion. A combination of two drugs that does not mix well. When shaken, one drug evenly distributes itself through the other drug.

Enteric coating. A wax-like hard coating on the outside of a tablet. This coating prevents the acid environment in the stomach from dissolving the tablet, thereby allowing the tablet to dissolve in a neutral or alkaline environment.

Expiration date. The date after which a medication cannot be used. It typically appears as month/year. The medication is no longer usable after the last day of the month stated.

Formula method. A method for calculating medication doses. It uses a standard formula equation to set up the calculation of the medication dose, and is also called rule method. The formula method is:

$$\frac{D}{H} \times V = A$$

where:

D = desired or prescribed dosage of the medication

H = dosage of medication available or on hand

V = volume that the medication is available in, such as one tablet or milliliters

A = amount of medication to administer

Fraction. A part or piece of the whole that has been divided into equal parts. Fractions are written as $\frac{1}{3}$.

Generic name. Nonproprietary name of a medication; the official name listed in the *United States Pharmacopeia* (USP). Each medication has only one generic name. The generic name is written in lowercase letters.

Household measurement system. A measurement system for medication dosages that uses such items as a teaspoon, tablespoon, cup, pint, quart, and even a medicine dropper.

Improper fraction. A type of fraction wherein the numerator is larger than the denominator. The result of dividing the numerator by the denominator is greater than or equal to 1. Example:

$$\frac{4}{2}$$

Insulin syringe. A type of syringe, marked in units rather than in milliliters or minims, used for the accurate measurement and administration of insulin. The standard insulin syringe is the U-100 syringe that holds 100 units of U-100 insulin, which is equal to 1 mL. Syringe labeling is in 5 unit increments.

International System of Units. The standard system of abbreviations for the metric units of measurement, from the French Système International d'Unités. It is abbreviated as SI units.

Intradermal route. A route of medication administration in which the medication is injected into the dermis or the layer of tissue directly beneath the outer layer of skin.

Intramuscular route. A route of medication administration in which the medication is injected into the muscle below the subcutaneous tissue, with the needle inserted at a 90 degree angle.

Intravenous. Administration of fluids, medications, or electrolyte solutions directly into a vein.

Loading dose. The initial dosage of a medication given over a specified time period to increase serum blood levels to a therapeutic level or achieve the desired effect rapidly.

Lot number. Required by federal law, a label component in the form of a number identifying the batch of medication from which a medication came. It is used to identify medication in the event of a recall by the manufacturer.

Lowest common terms. A mathematical process to simplify or reduce fractions so that both the numerator and denominator are the lowest numbers possible to still correctly represent the fraction.

Macro-drip tubing. Intravenous tubing that delivers 10, 15, or 20 drops per milliliter.

mcg/kg/min. A prescribed dosage of a medication based on a specific number of micrograms per kilograms of body weight per minute.

Medication administration record. The form the nurse uses to document administration of medications. The form may be computer-generated or handwritten.

Medication label. Found on the external packaging of medication, this provides information about the medications for calculating the correct dosage and administering the medication safely and appropriately.

Medication spoon. A special spoon that is used to accurately measure and administer liquid medications. Used most often with children, the typical medicine spoon holds 5 mL of medicine.

Medication syringe. A type of syringe that is marked in mL and is used to measure and administer dosages of medicine.

Medicine cup. A small cup used for measuring and administering liquid medications. The medicine cup typically holds 30 mL of liquid medicine.

Meniscus. The natural curve that liquid makes when poured into a container.

Metric system. An international system of weights and measures that uses meter, liter, and gram as the measurement units and is based on multiples of 10. The metric system is used exclusively in the *United States Pharmacopeia* and is a common system used worldwide.

Micro-drip tubing. Intravenous tubing that delivers 60 drops per mL.

Milligram. A weight unit in the metric system. One thousand milligrams is equivalent to one gram.

Mixed number. A type of fraction wherein a whole number is combined with a proper fraction. The value of this number is always greater than 1. Example:

$$2\frac{2}{3}$$

Multi-dose packaging. The packaging of medications in containers in which there is more than one dosage of the medication.

NDC number. Stands for National Drug Code. Required by federal law, a unique number that is assigned to each prescription medication and must appear on the manufacturer's label. The NDC number consists of the letters NDC followed by three groups of numbers.

Numerator. The top number in a fraction. In the fraction $\frac{2}{4}$, 2 is the numerator.

Osmolarity. The number of particles, or amount of substance, that is in a liter of solution. Osmolarity is reported as milliosmoles per liter (mOsm/L).

Parenteral route. A route for medication administration whereby the medication is injected into body tissues.

Precautions. Printed warnings or alerts from the manufacturer of a medication. They contain information related to medication safety, effectiveness, or administration.

Primary tubing. A type of macro-drip intravenous tubing used for intravenous solution administration or when larger amounts of fluid are delivered.

Proper fraction. A fraction wherein the numerator is smaller than the denominator. The result of dividing the numerator by the denominator is less than 1. Example:

$$\frac{2}{3}$$

Proportion. A statement that two ratios are equal. Proportions can be written in an equivalent fraction form or in a form that uses colons to express the equality. A proportion using the fraction form would be written as: $\frac{2}{3} = \frac{6}{9}$. The equal sign is read as "as." The proportion would be read as "2 is to 3 as 6 is to 9." You can verify that the fractions or ratios are equal by multiplying the numerator of each fraction by the opposite denominator, or the extremes (outer numbers) and the means (inner numbers).

Proprietary name. The name given to a medication by the manufacturer. The proprietary name has the symbol ® or ™ after it, which indicates a registered trademark. It starts with an uppercase letter or is in all uppercase letters on the label, and is also called a trade name or brand name.

Ratio. The expression of the relationship between two units or quantities. To write ratios, use the symbols of a slash (/) or colon (:) between the numbers. The slash or colon is read as "is to" or "per." The ratio 4/5 is read as "4 is to 5." The symbols indicate that division of the two numbers should be done. Fractions are ratios.

Ratio-proportion method. A method that can be used to calculate medication doses. It is useful when the medication dosage prescribed is different from the dosage of the medication available and it is only necessary to find one unknown quantity. The equation for the ratio-proportion method is:

$$\frac{\text{Dosage on hand (D)}}{\text{Amount on hand (H)}} = \frac{\text{Dosage prescribed (Q)}}{(x) \text{ Amount desired}}$$

Roman numerals. Letters of the alphabet that are used to express numbers. The most commonly used letters are: I or i (1), V or v (5), and X or x (10).

Safe Dose Range (SDR). The amount of a drug that is verified in an approved drug reference. Each medication for a child must have the SDR calculated by the nurse prior to administration.

Secondary tubing. A type of macro-drip intravenous tubing used to administer intravenous medications. Secondary tubing is attached to an injection port on the primary tubing.

Six Rights of Medication Administration. A standard of practice that nurses are required to use each time a medication is administered to ensure accuracy in medication administration. The Six Rights are: Right patient, Right medication, Right dosage, Right route, Right time, and Right documentation.

Storage. A section of the medication label that provides information related to how the medication should be stored to prevent the drug from losing its potency or effectiveness.

Subcutaneous route. A route for medication administration whereby the medication is injected into the tissue below the skin and above the muscle with the needle inserted at 45–90° angle.

Suspension. A liquid form of medication that contains a finely divided solid medication mixed into a liquid.

Sustained release. A form of medication whereby a set amount of a medication is released over an extended period of time. It is also called time release.

Syrup. A liquid form of medication within a concentrated solution of sugar.

Tablet. A type of oral medication that is compressed into a solid form.

Titration. A process wherein medication dosages are increased or decreased to achieve a specified desired effect.

Trade name. The name given to a medication by the manufacturer. The trade name has the symbol ® after it, which indicates a registered trademark. It starts with an uppercase letter or is in all uppercase letters on the label, and is also called a brand name or proprietary name.

Tuberculin syringe. A 1 mL syringe that has lines marked in hundredths (0.01) of a milliliter, with each tenth (0.1) printed on the syringe. Useful in measuring and administering small dosages of medications, it generally comes with an attached 25-gauge, $\frac{1}{2}$-inch needle.

Unit-dose packaging. The packaging and labeling of each individual dosage of medication. A single capsule, tablet, or liquid dosage of medication is sealed in an individual package.

Z-track method. A route of medication administration used to prevent the medication from leaking out after the injection. The skin is pulled to the side, the needle is inserted at a 90-degree angle, and the medication is injected. After the needle is removed, the skin is released and forms a seal so that the medication does not leak out.

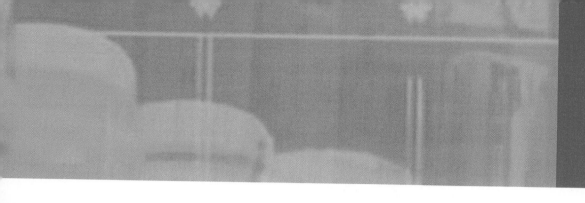

Index

Note: Page numbers followed by *f* indicate figures; those followed by *b* indicate boxed material.

A

Abbreviations
  apothecary system, 39
  for cups, 42
  for drops, 42
  in household measurement system, 42
  for length, 37
  for medication orders, 77, 78*b*, 79, 79*b*
    drug preparation, 78*b*
    route, 78*b*
    time, 78*b*
  metric, 36–37
  for ounces, 42
  for pint, 42
  on prescriptions
    apothecary system, 39
    in household measurement system, 42
    metric, 36–37
    SI, 36
  for quart, 42
  Système Internationale d'Unités, 36
  for tablespoon, 42
  for teaspoon, 42
  unaccepted, 79*b*
  for volume, 37, 39
  for weight, 37, 39
Administration, of drugs, rights of, 110–111
  documentation, 111
  dose, 110
  medication, 110
  patient, 111
  route, 110
  time, 111
Administration routes
  on drug labels, 97–98
  oral, 125
    multi-dose packaging for, 98
    unit-dose packaging for, 97
  parenteral, 125
    multi-dose packaging for, 98
    unit-dose packaging for, 97

  topical
    multi-dose packaging for, 98
    unit-dose packaging for, 97
  transdermal, unit-dose packaging for, 97
Adults, body surface area, nomograms for, 255, 256*f*
Apothecary system, 38–41
  abbreviations in, 39
  conversion in
    of liquid, 40
    to metric, 41
    of weight, 39
Arabic numbers, conversion to Roman numerals, 2–3
Arithmetic, for calculation of drug dosage, 1–20

B

Body surface area (BSA)
  m², 263, 265
  nomograms for, 255, 256*f*
  pediatric dosage calculation with, 255, 256*f*, 263–267
Brand name, on drug labels, 91, 92*f*
BSA. *See* Body surface area

C

Calculation
  of combined drugs in, syringes, 170–173
    formula method, 170–172
    ratio-proportion method, 172–173
  with different units of measurement, 168–170
  of dosage, arithmetic for, 1–20
  dosage, dimensional analysis in, 311–313
  dosage, with different units of measurement, 163–170
  of drugs
    in combination, 269–271
    for pediatric administration, 271–272

  formula method, 104–105
    of combined drugs in syringes, 170–172
    with different units of measurement, 163–168
    with same system of measurement, 157–160
  pediatric dosage
    with body surface area, 255, 256*f*, 263–267
    flow rate, 271–272
    intravenous flow rates, 271–272
    with milligrams/kilograms, 255
      for weight stated in kilograms, 256–259
      for weight stated in ounces, 259–261
      for weight stated in pounds, 259–261
    weight stated in ounces, 259–260
  ratio-proportion method
    in combination, 270–271
    of combined drugs in syringes, 172–173
    with different units of measurement, 168–170
    with same system of measurement, 160–163
    for weight stated in kilograms, 258–259
    for weight stated in ounces, 261
    for weight stated in pounds, 261
    with same system of measurement, 157–163
  solute, per intravenous solutions, 195–196
Calibrated medication dropper, equipment for liquid oral medications, 53, 53*f*
Capsules, 125
  formula method for, 125–129
  ratio-proportion method for, 129–133
Central intravenous insertion sites, 190*f*
Colloid intravenous solutions, 190, 191*f*
Complex fractions, 5–6
Computing, in 3-Step Approach, 104
Concentration, of intravenous solutions, 191
Controller-type electronic infusion devices, 194

Conversion factors, in dimensional analysis, 311, 313
Conversions
  in 3-Step Approach, 103–104
  in apothecary system
    of liquid, 40
    to metric, 41
    of weight, 39
  of fractions, 6–8
    to decimals, 7–8
    to improper, 6–7
    to mixed numbers, 7
  liters to milliliters, 37
  milliliters to liters, 37
Critical thinking, in 3-Step Approach, 104
Crystalloid intravenous solutions, 190, 191f
Cups
  abbreviation for, 42
  equivalent of
    household, 42
    metric, 42
  medicine
    measurements on, 51f, 52f
    use of, 50–52

D

Decimals
  addition of, 13–15
  conversion of fractions to, 7–8
  division of, 17–18
  multiplication of, 15–17
  subtraction of, 13–15
Denominator, 4
Dimensional analysis, in dosage calculation, 311–313
Dobutamine hydrochloride, in micrograms/kilograms/minute, 222
Documentation, in drug administration, 111
Dopamine, dosage of, in micrograms/kilograms/minute, 222
Dosage
  calculation of,
    arithmetic for, 1–20
    with different units of measurement, 163–170
      formula method, 163–168
      ratio-proportion method, 168–170
    with same system of measurement, 157–163
      formula method, 157–160
      ratio-proportion method, 160–163
    dimensional analysis, 311–313
    of Dopamine, in micrograms/kilograms/minute, 222
    on drug labels, 92f, 94, 94f
    formula method
      with different units of measurement, 163–168
      drops/minute, of intravenous drugs in, 200–201

grams/hour, dosage of intravenous drugs in, 229–230
  heparin, in units/hour, dosage of, 223
  insulin, in units/hour, dosage of, 224–225
  milligrams/hour, dosage of intravenous drugs in, 229–230
  milliliters/hour, dosage of intravenous drugs in, 197–198
  pediatric dosage calculation
    for weight stated in kilograms, 256–258
    for weight stated in ounces, 259–260
    for weight stated in pounds, 259–260
  with same system of measurement, 157–160
  of intravenous drugs in
    drops/minute, 200–203
      quick method, 202–203
    grams/hour, 229–231
      formula method, 229–230
      ratio-proportion method, 230–231
    units/hour, 222–226
      heparin, 223, 224
      insulin, 224–225, 225–226
  measurement system for
    apothecary, 38–41
    household, 41–43
    metric, 36–38
  ordered as flow rate, 227–228, 236–237
    heparin, 227–228
    insulin, 228
  pediatric
    with body surface area, 255, 256f, 263–267
    flow rate, 271–272
    intravenous flow rates, 271–272
    with milligrams/kilograms, 255
      for weight stated in kilograms, 256–259
      for weight stated in ounces, 259–261
      for weight stated in pounds, 259–261
    weight stated in ounces, 259–260
  proportions in, 18–19
  ratio-proportion method, 168–170
    grams/hour, dosage of intravenous drugs in, 230–231
    heparin
      flow rate, dosage ordered as, 227–228
      in units/hour, dosage of, 224
    insulin
      flow rate, dosage ordered as, 228
      in units/hour, dosage of, 225–226
    milliliters/hour, dosage of intravenous drugs in, 198–199
    pediatric dosage calculation
      for weight stated in kilograms, 258–259
      for weight stated in ounces, 261
      for weight stated in pounds, 261
  ratios in, 18–19

Dram, equivalent of, 40
Drop factor, 192
Drops
  abbreviation for, 42
  equivalent of, 40
    household, 42
    metric, 42
Drops/minute, dosage of intravenous drugs in, 200–203
  quick method, 202–203
Drug labels, 91–96, 92f
  dosage on, 92f, 94, 94f
  drug form on, 92f, 93, 94f
  drug quantity on, 92f, 93, 93f
  drug strength on, 92f, 93, 93f
  expiration date on, 92f, 95, 95f
  generic name on, 92, 92f, 93f
  lot number on, 92f, 95, 95f
  manufacturer on, 92f, 95, 95f
  NDC number on, 92f, 96, 96f
  precautions on, 92f, 94–95
  storage method on, 92f, 94, 94f
  trade name on, 91, 92f
Drug packaging, 97–98
  multi-dose, 98
  unit-dose, 97
Drug preparation, abbreviations, for medication orders, 78b
Drugs
  administration of, titration, 222
  administration, rights of, 110–111
    documentation, 111
    dose, 110
    medication, 110
    patient, 111
    route, 110
    time, 111
  calculation of
    in combination, 269–271
    for pediatric administration, 271–272
  form of, on labels, 92f, 93, 94f
  orders for, 74, 75f, 76
  quantity of, on labels, 92f, 93, 93f
  strength of, on labels, 92f, 93, 93f

E

Electronic infusion devices, 193–195, 194f
  controller-type, 194
  patient-controlled analgesia, 194–195
  positive-pressure, 194
  syringe pumps, 194
Elixirs, 125
Emulsions, 125
Enteric-coated tablets, 125
Equipment
  administration, intravenous fluids, 190–195
    electronic infusion devices, 193–195, 194f
    solutions, 190–191

added components to, 191
concentration of, 191
osmolarity, 190
packaging of, 191
strength of, 191
tubing, 192–193, 192*f*, 193*f*
injection
parenteral administration routes,
155–156, 156*f*
for liquid oral medications, 50–54
calibrated medication dropper, 53, 53*f*
measuring spoons, 52
medication syringes, 52
medicine cup, 50–52, 51*f*, 52*f*
meniscus, 50, 51*f*
pediatric, 52, 52*f*
Expiration date, on drug labels, 92*f*, 95, 95*f*
Extremes, 18

F
Flow rate
dosage ordered as, 227–228, 236–237
heparin, 227–228
insulin, 228
pediatric, dosage calculation in, 271–272
Formula method
calculation of combined drugs in syringes,
170–172
calculation of dosages
with different units of measurement,
163–168
with same system of measurement,
157–160
for capsules, 125–129
drops/minute, dosage of intravenous drugs
in, 200–201
drugs, calculation of, in combination,
269–270
grams/hour, dosage of intravenous drugs
in, 229–230
heparin, in units/hour, dosage of, 223
insulin, in units/hour, dosage of, 224–225
for liquid medications, 133–135
milligrams/hour, dosage of intravenous
drugs in, 229–230
milliliters/hour, dosage of intravenous
drugs in, 197–198
parenteral medication preparation, from
powders, 174–175
pediatric dosage calculation
for weight stated in kilograms,
256–258
for weight stated in ounces, 259–260
for weight stated in pounds, 259–260
for tablets, 125–129
Fractions, 4–13
addition of, 8–10
complex, 5–6
conversion of, 6–8
to decimals, 7–8

to improper, 6–7
to mixed numbers, 7
denominator of, 4
division of, 12–13
improper, 5
lowest common terms of, 6
mixed number, 5
multiplication of, 10–11
numerator of, 4
proper, 5
reduction of, 6
subtraction of, 8–10
types of, 5–6

G
Gallon, equivalent of, 40
Generic name, on drug labels, 92, 92*f*, 93*f*
Given quantity, in dimensional analysis, 311,
312
Grains, 39
conversion to grams, 39
conversion to micrograms, 39
conversion to milligrams, 39
Grams
conversion to microgram, 39
milligrams conversion to, 39
Grams/hour, dosage of intravenous drugs in,
229–231
formula method, 229–230
ratio-proportion method, 230–231

H
Heparin
flow rate, dosage ordered as, 227–228
in units/hour, dosage of, 223–224
formula method, 223
ratio-proportion method, 224
Household measurement system, 41–43
abbreviations in, 42
metric system to, 42
Hypertonic solutions, 191
Hypotonic solutions, 191

I
ID. *See* Intradermal parenteral administration
routes
IM. *See* Intramuscular parenteral
administration routes
Improper fractions, 5
Infant. *See* Pediatric
Insulin
flow rate, dosage ordered as, 228
in units/hour, dosage of, 224–226
formula method, 224–225
ratio-proportion method, 225–226
Insulin injections, syringes for, 50, 59,
59*f*
International System of Units (SI), 36

Intradermal (ID) parenteral administration
routes, 157
Intramuscular (IM) parenteral administration
routes, 157
Intravenous (IV) administration, 189
insertion sites for, 190*f*
Intravenous drugs
in drops/minute, 200–203
formula method, 200–201
quick method, 202–203
in grams/hour, 229–231
formula method, 229–230
ratio-proportion method, 230–231
in micrograms/kilograms/minute, 231,
234–236
in micrograms/minute, 231, 233–234
in milligrams/hour, 229–231
formula method, 229–230
ratio-proportion method, 230–231
in milligrams/minute, 231, 232–233
in milliliters/hour, 197–199
formula method, 197–198
ratio-proportion method, 198–199
in units/hour, 222–226
heparin, 223, 224
formula method, 223
ratio-proportion method, 224
insulin, 224–225, 225–226
formula method, 224–225
ratio-proportion method, 225–226
Intravenous fluids, administration equipment,
190–195
electronic infusion devices, 193–195, 194*f*
solutions, 190–191
added components to, 191
concentration of, 191
osmolarity, 190
packaging of, 191
strength of, 191
tubing, 192–193, 192*f*
Intravenous solutions
added components to, 191
colloid, 190, 191*f*
concentration of, 191
crystalloid, 190, 191*f*
Intravenous solutions (*continued*)
packaging of, 191
solute calculation per, 195–196
strength of, 191
Isotonic solutions, 191
IV. *See* Intravenous administration

L
Labels, drug
See Drug labels
Large-volume intravenous syringes, 50
Length
abbreviations for, 37
equivalent of, 37
units of, 37

Liquid, apothecary system, conversion in, 40
Liquid medications
    formula method for, 133–135
    ratio-proportion method for, 135–139
Liquid oral medications, equipment for, 50–54
    calibrated medication dropper, 53, 53f
    measuring spoons, 52
    medication syringes, 52
    medicine cup, 50–52, 51f, 52f
    meniscus, 50, 51f
    pediatric, 52, 52f
Liters, conversion to milliliters, 37
Lot number, on drug labels, 92f, 95, 95f
Lowest common terms, 6

M

m², body surface area in, 263, 265
Macro-drip tubing, 192–193, 193f
Manufacturer, on drug labels, 92f, 95, 95f
MAR. See Medication Administration Record
Means, 18
Measurement system. See also specific
    apothecary, 38–41
    household, 41–43
    metric, 36–38
Measuring spoons, equipment for liquid oral medications, 52
Medication Administration Record (MAR), 80–83, 81f
Medication orders, abbreviations for, 77, 78b, 79, 79b
    drug preparation, 78b
    route, 78b
    time, 78b
Medications. See also Drugs; specific names
    abbreviations for
        drug preparation, 78b
        time, 78b
    administration of, rights of, 110
    correct measurement of, 61
    of drug administration, 110
    equipment for liquid oral
        calibrated medication dropper, 53, 53f
        meniscus, 50, 51f
    error prevention in, administration of, 61
    liquid oral
        formula method for, 133–135
        measuring spoons, 52
        pediatric, 52, 52f
        ratio-proportion method for, 135–139
    liquid oral equipment for, 50–54
        calibrated medication dropper, 53, 53f
        measuring spoons, 52
        medication syringes, 52
        medicine cup, 50–52, 51f, 52f
        meniscus, 50, 51f
        pediatric, 52, 52f

parenteral
    preparation of, from powders, 174–176
        formula method, 174–175
        ratio-proportion method, 175–176
    in syringes, 50
    syringes for, 56
    powders, parenteral medication preparation from, 174–176
        formula method, 174–175
        ratio-proportion method, 175–176
    syringes
        equipment for liquid oral medications, 52
        parenteral, 56
Medicine cups
    measurements on, 51f, 52f
    use of, 50–52
Meniscus, equipment for liquid oral medications, 50, 51f
Metric system, 36–38
    abbreviations for, 36–37
    apothecary equivalents in, 41
    apothecary system, conversion in, 41
    conversion to household, 42
Micro-drip tubing, 192–193, 193f
Micrograms/kilograms/minute, dosage of intravenous drugs in, 231, 234–236
Micrograms/minute, dosage of intravenous drugs in, 231, 233–234
Milligrams
    conversion to grams, 39
    conversion to micrograms, 39
Milligrams/hour, dosage of intravenous drugs in, 229–231
    formula method, 229–230
    ratio-proportion method, 230–231
Milligrams/kilograms, pediatric dosage calculation with, 255
    for weight stated in kilograms, 256–259
    for weight stated in ounces, 259–261
    for weight stated in pounds, 259–261
Milligrams/minute, dosage of intravenous drugs in, 231, 232–233
Milliliters/hour, dosage of intravenous drugs in, 197–199
    formula method, 197–198
    ratio-proportion method, 198–199
Milliliters, conversion to liters, 37
Minims, equivalent of, 40
Mixed number fractions, 5
Mixed numbers, 5
Multi-dose drug packaging, 98

N

National Drug Code (NDC) number, on drug labels, 92f, 96, 96f
NDC. See National Drug Code number
Nomograms, for body surface area, 255, 256f
Numbers, mixed, 5
Numerator, 4

O

Oral administration routes, 125
    multi-dose packaging for, 98
    unit-dose packaging for, 97
Order form, physician, 75f
Orders
    abbreviations for, 77, 78b, 79, 79b
        drug preparation, 78b
        route, 78b
        time, 78b
    for drugs, 74, 75f, 76
Osmolarity, 190
Ounces
    abbreviation for, 42
    equivalent of, 40
        household, 42
        metric, 42
    weight stated in
        formula method, pediatric dosage calculation, 259–260
        milligrams/kilograms, pediatric dosage calculation with, 259–261
        pediatric dosage calculation, ratio-proportion method, 261

P

Packaging, of intravenous solutions, 191
Parenteral administration routes, 125
    injection equipment, 155–156, 156f
    intradermal, 157
    intramuscular, 157
    multi-dose packaging for, 98
    packaging for, 155, 155f
    subcutaneous, 157
    unit-dose packaging for, 97
Parenteral medications
    preparation of, from powders, 174–176
        formula method, 174–175
        ratio-proportion method, 175–176
    in syringes, 50
    syringes for, 56
Patient-controlled analgesia (PCA) pumps, electronic infusion devices, 194–195
Patients, of drug administration, 111
PCA. See Patient-controlled analgesia pumps
Pediatric
    body surface area, nomograms for, 255, 256f
    dosage calculation in
        body surface area (BSA), 255, 256f
        intravenous flow rates, 271–272
        milligrams/kilograms, 255
    equipment for liquid oral medications, 52, 52f
Peripheral intravenous insertion sites, 190f
Physician order form, 75f
Pint
    abbreviation for, 42
    equivalent of, 40
        household, 42
        metric, 42

Positive-pressure pumps, electronic infusion devices, 194
Powders, parenteral medication preparation from, 174–176
    formula method, 174–175
    ratio-proportion method, 175–176
Precautions, on drug labels, 92f, 94–95
Prescriptions, abbreviations on
    apothecary system, 39
    in household measurement system, 42
    metric, 36–37
    SI, 36
Primary tubing, 193
Proper fractions, 5
Proportions, 18–19
    solving for x, 19
Proprietary name, on drug labels, 91, 92f

Q
Quart
    abbreviation for, 42
    equivalent of, 40
        household, 42
        metric, 42
Quick method, drops/minute, dosage of intravenous drugs in, 202–203

R
Ratio-proportion method, 107–108
    calculation of combined drugs in syringes, 172–173
    calculation of dosages
        with different units of measurement, 168–170
        with same system of measurement, 160–163
    for capsules, 129–133
    drugs, calculation of, in combination, 270–271
    grams/hour, dosage of intravenous drugs in, 230–231
    heparin
        flow rate, dosage ordered as, 227–228
        in units/hour, dosage of, 224
    insulin
        flow rate, dosage ordered as, 228
        in units/hour, dosage of, 225–226
    for liquid medications, 135–139
    milliliter/hour, dosage of intravenous drugs in, 198–199
    parenteral medication preparation, from powders, 175–176
    pediatric dosage calculation
        for weight stated in kilograms, 258–259
        for weight stated in ounces, 261
        for weight stated in pounds, 261
    for tablets, 129–133

Ratios, 18–19
    solving for x, 19
Roman numerals, conversion to Arabic numbers, 2–3
Routes
    abbreviations of, for medication orders, 78b
    administration
        on drug labels, 97–98
        oral, 125
            multi-dose packaging for, 98
            unit-dose packaging for, 97
        parenteral, 125
            multi-dose packaging for, 98
            unit-dose packaging for, 97
        topical
            multi-dose packaging for, 98
            unit-dose packaging for, 97
        transdermal, unit-dose packaging for, 97
    of drug administration, 110
    intradermal parenteral administration, 157
    intramuscular parenteral administration, 157
    parenteral administration, 125
        injection equipment, 155–156, 156f
        intradermal, 157
        intramuscular, 157
        multi-dose packaging for, 98
        packaging for, 155, 155f
        subcutaneous, 157
        unit-dose packaging for, 97
    subcutaneous parenteral administration, 157
    topical administration
        multi-dose packaging for, 98
        unit-dose packaging for, 97
    transdermal administration, unit-dose packaging for, 97

S
Safe dose range (SDR), 255
Safety syringes, 50
SDR. See Safe dose range
Secondary tubing, 193
SI. See International System of Units
Storage, of drugs, instructions on labels, 92f, 94, 94f
Strength, of intravenous solutions, 191
Subcutaneous (SubQ) parenteral administration routes, 157
SubQ. See Subcutaneous parenteral administration routes
Suspensions, 125
Sustained release, 125
Syringe pumps, electronic infusion device, 194

Syringes, 56–60, 56f
    calculation of combined drugs in, 170–173
        formula method, 170–172
        ratio-proportion method, 172–173
    insulin, 50, 59, 59f
    large-volume intravenous, 50
    medication, equipment for liquid oral medications, 52
    1-mL, 57–58, 58f
    for parenteral medications, 56
    parenteral medications in, 50
    parts of, 156f
    safety, 50
    3-mL, 56–57, 56f
    tuberculin, 50, 57–58, 58f
    U-100, 59, 59f
Syrups, 125
Système Internationale (SI) d'Unités abbreviations, 36

T
Tablespoons, 42–43
    abbreviations for, 42
    household equivalent of, 42
    metric equivalent of, 42
Tablets
    administration of, sublingual, 125
    formula method for, 125–129
    ratio-proportion method for, 129–133
    types of, 125
Teaspoons, 42–43
    abbreviations for, 42
    household equivalent of, 42
    metric equivalent of, 42
3-Step Approach, 103–104
    compute in, 104
    convert in, 103–104
    critically think in, 104
Time
    abbreviations of, for medication orders, 78b
    of drug administration, 111
Timed release, 125
Topical administration routes
    multi-dose packaging for, 98
    unit-dose packaging for, 97
Trade name, on drug labels, 91, 92f
Transdermal administration routes, unit-dose packaging for, 97
Tuberculin syringes, 50, 57–58, 58f
Tubing, intravenous, 192–193, 192f
    macro-drip, 192–193, 193f
    micro-drip, 192–193, 193f
    primary, 193
    secondary, 193

U

U-100 syringe, 59, 59*f*
Unit-dose packaging, 97
United States Pharmacopeia (USP), 92
Unit path, in dimensional analysis, 311,
    312–313
Units/hour, dosage of intravenous drugs in,
    222–226
  heparin
    formula method, 223
    ratio-proportion method, 224
  insulin
    formula method, 224–225
    ratio-proportion method, 225–226
USP. *See* United States Pharmacopeia

V

Volume
  abbreviations for, 37, 39
  apothecary system, 39, 40–41
  equivalent of, 37
  units of, 37

W

Warranted quantity, in dimensional analysis,
    311, 312
Weight
  abbreviations for, 37, 39
  apothecary system, 39–40
  equivalent of, 37
  stated in ounces
    formula method, pediatric dosage
      calculation, 259–260
    milligrams/kilograms, pediatric dosage
      calculation with, 259–261
    pediatric dosage calculation, ratio-
      proportion method, 261
  units of, 37

Z

Z-track technique, of intramuscular injection,
    157, 158*f*